Progress
in Neurotherapeutics and
Neuropsychopharmacology
2008

Published annually, volumes in this series provide readers with updates of recent clinical trial results, impacts of trials on guidelines and evidence-based practice, advances in trial methodologies, and the evolution of biomarkers in trials. The series focuses on trials in neurotherapeutics, including disease-modifying and symptomatic agents for neurological diseases, psychopharmacological management of neurological and psychiatric illnesses, and non-drug treatments. Each article is authored by a leader in the area of neurotherapeutics and clinical trials, and the series is guided by an Editor-in-Chief and Editorial Board with broad experience in drug development and neuropsychopharmacology. *Progress in Neurotherapeutics and Neuropsychopharmacology* is an essential update of recent trials in all aspects of the management of neurological and neuropsychiatric disorders, and will be an invaluable resource for practising neurologists as well as clinical and translational neuroscientists. Articles also available at http://www.cambridge.org/jid_PNN

Progress in Neurotherapeutics and Neuropsychopharmacology 2008

VOL. 3(1)   2008

Editor-in-Chief

Jeffrey L. Cummings, MD

The Augustus S. Rose Professor of Neurology
Professor of Psychiatry and Biobehavioral Sciences
Director, Mary S. Easton Center for Alzheimer's Disease Research
Director, Deane F. Johnson Center for Neurotherapeutics
David Geffen School of Medicine at UCLA

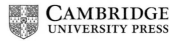

CAMBRIDGE
UNIVERSITY PRESS

PUBLISHED BY THE PRESS SYNDICATE OF THE UNIVERSITY OF CAMBRIDGE
The Pitt Building, Trumpington Street, Cambridge, United Kingdom

CAMBRIDGE UNIVERSITY PRESS
The Edinburgh Building, Cambridge CB2 8RU, UK
40 West 20th Street, New York, NY 10011-4211, USA
477 Williamstown Road, Port Melbourne, VIC 3207, Australia
Ruiz de Alarcón 13, 28014 Madrid, Spain
Dock House, The Waterfront, Cape Town 8001, South Africa

http://www.cambridge.org

© Cambridge University Press 2008

First published 2006

Printed in the United Kingdom at the University Press, Cambridge

A catalogue record for this book is available from the British Library

ISBN 9780521862554
ISSN 17482321

Dedicated

Kate (Zhong) Cummings

There is only one happiness in life – to love and be loved.
                                            – George Sand

Progress in Neurotherapeutics and Neuropsychopharmacology, 3:1, vii–viii © 2008 Cambridge University Press
Printed in the United Kingdom

Contents

Progress in Neurotherapeutics and Neuropsychopharmacology, 3:1, ix–xii © 2008 Cambridge University Press
Printed in the United Kingdom

Contributors

P.S. Aisen
Department of Neurology
Georgetown University Medical Center
Washington DC, USA

Neil Allen
Consultants in Neurology
Northbrook, IL, USA

Kelly C. Allison
Weight & Eating Disorders Program
Department of Psychiatry
University of Pennsylvania
Philadelphia, PA, USA

Fred Askari
Department of Internal Medicine
University of Michigan
Ann Arbor, MI, USA

Andrew D. Barreto
Department of Neurology
Stroke Division
The University of Houston-Texas
Houston, TX, USA

Javier Borja
Drug Safety Manager
J. Uriach y Compañía, S.A.
Polígon Industrial Riera de Caldes
Avinguda Camí Reial
Palau-solità i Plegamans
Barcelona, Spain

George J. Brewer
Department of Human Genetics
Department of Internal Medicine
University of Michigan
Ann Arbor, MI, USA

R. Briand
Neurochem Inc.
Laval, Quebec, Canada

Martha Carlson
Department of Pediatrics-Neurology
University of Michigan
Ann Arbor, MI, USA

E. Cittadini
Headache Group
Institute of Neurology
The National Hospital for Neurology
   and Neurosurgery
Queen Square, London, UK

Suzanne Craft
Geriatric Research, Education, and
   Clinical Center (GRECC)
Veterans Affairs Puget Sound Health
   Care System
and
Department of Psychiatry and Behavioral
   Sciences
University of Washington School
   of Medicine
Seattle, WA, USA

Antonio Culebras
Department of Neurology
Upstate Medical University
Syracuse, NY, USA

Jefrey L. Cummings
Departments of Neurology and
   Psychology and Behavioral Sciences
David Geffen School of Medicine
   at UCLA
Los Angeles, CA, USA

D. Deforce
Laboratory of Pharmaceutical
  Biotechnology
Ghent University
Ghent, Belgium

D.A.J.P. Denys
AMC
University of Amsterdam
Amsterdam, The Netherlands

Robert B. Dick
Department of Human Genetics
University of Michigan
Ann Arbor, MI, USA

A. Duong
Neurochem Inc.
Laval, Quebec, Canada

Robert H. Dworkin
Departments of Anesthesiology
  and Neurology
University of Rochester School
  of Medicine and Dentistry
Rochester, NY, USA

John K. Fink
Department of Neurology
University of Michigan
Ann Arbor, MI, USA

Paul B. Fitzgerald
Alfred Psychiatry Research Centre
The Alfred and Monash University
  School of Psychiatry, Psychology
  and Psychological Medicine
Melbourne, Victoria, Australia

D. Garceau
Neurochem Inc.
Laval, Quebec, Canada

Julián García-Rafanell
Director of Medical Affairs
J. Uriach y Compañía, S.A.
Polígon Industrial Riera de Caldes
Avinguda Camí Reial
Palau-solità i Plegamans
Barcelona, Spain

Leif Gjerstad
Department of Neurology
Rikshospitalet
University of Oslo
Norway

P.J. Goadsby
Headache Group
Institute of Neurology
The National Hospital for Neurology
  and Neurosurgery
Queen Square, London, UK
and
Department of Neurology
University of California
San Francisco, CA, USA

Teresa Griesing
Pfizer, Inc.
New York, NY, USA

Karen E. Groff
Weight & Eating Disorders Program
Department of Psychiatry
University of Pennsylvania
Philadelphia, PA, USA

James C. Grotta
Department of Neurology
Stroke Division
The University of Houston-Texas
Houston, TX, USA

Peter Hedera
Department of Neurology
Vanderbilt University
Nashville, TN, USA

Esa Heinonen
University of Helsinki
Institute of Biotechnology
Helsinki, Finland

Erik Hessen
Helse Øst Health Services and
  Department of Neurology
Akershus University Hospital
Norway

Kamyar Keramatian
Neuroscience Program
University of British Columbia
Vancouver, Canada

Hossein A. Khalili
Department of Neurosurgery
Amiralmomenin Hospital
Shiraz University of Medical Sciences
Grash, Iran

Karen J. Kluin
Department of Neurology
Department of Speech Pathology
University of Michigan
Ann Arbor, MI, USA

J. Laurin
Neurochem Inc.
Laval, Quebec, Canada

Matthew T. Lorincz
Department of Neurology
University of Michigan
Ann Arbor, MI, USA

Morten I. Lossius
Helse Øst Health Services and
   Department of Neurology
Akershus University Hospital
Norway
and
National Center for Epilepsy
Rikshospitalet
University of Oslo
Norway

Kelly E. Lyons
Department of Neurology
University of Kansas Medical Center
Kansas City, USA

Catherine Meyer
Consultants in Neurology
Northbrook, IL, USA

Paolo Moretti
Departments of Neurology and
   Molecular and Human Genetics
Baylor College of Medicine
Houston, TX, USA

Dennis O'Brien
Billings Clinic
Billings, MT, USA

John P. O'Reardon
Weight & Eating Disorders Program
Department of Psychiatry
University of Pennsylvania
Philadelphia, PA, USA

Rajesh Pahwa
Department of Neurology
University of Kansas Medical Center
Kansas City, USA

Sven E. Pålhagen
Department of Neurology
Karolinska University Hospital
Huddinge, Stockholm, Sweden

John H. Peloian
Department of Psychiatry
VA Greater Los Angeles Healthcare
   System

Joseph M. Pierre
Department of Psychiatry
VA Greater Los Angeles Healthcare
   System
and
Department of Psychiatry and
   Biobehavioral Sciences
Geffen School of Medicine at the
   University of California
Los Angeles, USA

Ivar Reinvang
Department of Psychology
University of Oslo
Norway

D. Saumier
Neurochem Inc.
Laval, Quebec, Canada
Michael Schilsky
Department of Internal Medicine
Cornell University
New York, NY, USA

Uma Sharma
Pfizer, Inc.
Ann Arbor, MI, USA

Julia Sitterly
Department of Human Genetics
University of Michigan
Ann Arbor, MI, USA

Albert J. Stunkard
Weight & Eating Disorders Program
Department of Psychiatry
University of Pennsylvania
Philadelphia, PA, USA

Roberta Tankanow
College of Pharmacy
University of Michigan
Ann Arbor, MI, USA

Rajbala Thakur
Department of Anesthesiology
University of Rochester School
  of Medicine and Dentistry
Rochester, NY, USA

Guochuan Emil Tsai
Department of Psychiatry
Harbor-UCLA Medical Center
Torrance, CA, USA

F. Van Nieuwerburgh
Laboratory of Pharmaceutical
  Biotechnology
Ghent University
Ghent, Belgium

G. Stennis Watson
Geriatric Research, Education, and
  Clinical Center (GRECC)
Veterans Affairs Puget Sound Health
  Care System
and
Department of Psychiatry and
  Behavioral Sciences
University of Washington School
  of Medicine
Seattle, WA, USA

Daniel Wynn
Consultants in Neurology
Northbrook, IL, USA

James P. Young
Pfizer, Inc.
Ann Arbor, MI, USA

Progress in Neurotherapeutics and Neuropsychopharmacology, 3:1, 1–11 © 2008 Cambridge University Press
DOI: 10.1017/S1748232107000183   Printed in the United Kingdom

Progress in Neurotherapeutics and Neuropsychopharmacology 2008

Jeffrey L. Cummings

Departments of Neurology and Psychiatry and Behavioral Sciences, David Geffen School of Medicine at UCLA, Los Angeles, CA, USA; Email:jcummings@mednet.ucla.edu

ABSTRACT

There has been continuous progress in neurotherapeutics and neuropsychopharmacology in the past year. Notable are the reports of successful preliminary disease-modifying trials in Niemann-Pick disease and Friedreich's ataxia. Progress also has been made in treatment of migraine, stroke, epilepsy, multiple sclerosis, traumatic brain injury, and pain. Biomarkers are increasingly used to establish proof of pharmacology including measures of cerebrospinal fluid constituents and brain changes on magnetic resonance imaging. There is an increasing diversity of patient populations participating in clinical trials, including pediatric migraine and traumatic brain injury.

Key words: argatroban, atorvastatin, biomarkers, bipolar depression, clinical trials, deep brain stimulation, depression, disease modification, duloxetine, epilepsy, fingolimod, Friedreich's ataxia, glatiramer acetate, Huntington's disease, Idebenone, methylphenidate, Miglustat, migraine, modafinil, multiple sclerosis, neuropathic pain, nicardipine, Niemann-Pick Type C disease, Parkinson's disease, pharmacogenetics, pregabalin, retigabin, riluzole, ritogitine, rivastigmine, rizatripan, schizophrenia, spinal cord injury pain, testosterone, tramiprosate, transcranial magnetic stimulation, traumatic brain injury, zolmitriptan, zonisamide.

Progress in Neurotherapeutics and Neuropsychopharmacology 2008

Neurologic and psychiatric disorders are among the most common afflictions of human kind and continue to produce enormous disability globally. It is incumbent on the scientific community to search for means to relieve of neurologic and psychiatric disorders, to improve understanding of disease mechanisms, and to enhance neuropsychopharmacology. There continue to be advances in neurotherapeutics based on an improved understanding of disease mechanisms and improved access to tractable therapeutic targets. Progress in neurotherapeutics in neuropsychopharmacology 2008 captures some of the recent advances in the treatment of neurologic and psychiatric illnesses.

Correspondence should be addressed to: Jeffrey L. Cummings, MD, UCLA Alzheimer Disease Center, 10911 Weyburn Ave., Suite 200, Los Angeles, CA 90095, USA; Ph: +1 310 794 3665; Fax: +1 310 794 3148; Email: jcummings@mednet.ucla.edu

Disease-Modifying Therapies

Niemann-Pick Type C disease is an inherited neurodegenerative disorder with an intracellular lipid trafficking defect leading to accumulation of glycosphingolipids. It heretofore has been an untreatable progressive neurodegenerative disorder. Based on understanding of glycosphingolipid synthesis, a new agent capable of ameliorating the synthetic process was tested in a clinical trial. Miglustat was tested in 29 patients randomly assigned to receive active treatment or standard care for 12 months in a phase IIa proof-of-concept (CPOC) trial. The primary outcome measure was horizontal saccadic eye movement velocity, chosen because of its correlation with disease progression. At study termination patients receiving miglustat had improved eye movement velocity as well as improved swallowing, stabilization of auditory function, and slower deterioration in ambulation. Adverse events included diarrhea, flatulence, weight loss, and abdominal pain. This study represents one of the first successful interventions in a neurodegenerative disease with a disease-modifying therapy (Patterson *et al.*, 2007).

Use of Idebenone to treat patients with Friedreich's ataxia also suggested an ability to intervene in a neurodegenerative disease. Forty-eight patients with Friedreich's ataxia were randomized to active treatment or placebo in a 6-month double-blind trial. The primary endpoint was a biological marker indicative of oxidated DNA damage; secondary endpoint included clinical ratings. At trial termination there was no difference in the biological marker. An overall analysis showed no clinical impact. A pre-specified analysis excluding patients who required wheelchair assistance showed a significant clinical improvement with a dose–response relationship (Di Prospero *et al.*, 2007). The results are sufficiently promising to warrant further investigation of debenon and other potent anti-oxidants.

A neuroprotective trial of riluzole in Huntington's disease in a 3-year randomized trial involving 379 patients found no benefit of treatment (Landwehrmeyer *et al.*, 2007).

Cerebrovascular Disease

Recent trials have improved our understanding of optimal treatment of patients with various types of cerebrovascular disease. A comparison of oral anticoagulant therapy with aspirin showed that oral anti-coagulants are not more effective than aspirin for secondary prevention after transient ischemic attacks or minor stroke of arterial origin (ESPRIT Group, 2007).

Greater benefit in stroke prevention was observed in a double-blind placebo-controlled trial of atorvastatin after stroke or transient ischemic attack in secondary stroke prevention. The reduction in stroke risk was 3.5% (statistically significant) (SPARCL, 2006).

Sugg *et al.* (2006) provide preliminary evidence on a small number of patients suggesting that low dose argatroban combined with intravenous rtPA may produce greater recanelization following stroke than use of rtPA alone. This trial is discussed in detail in this volume.

A double-blind trial of nicardipine prolonged release implants in patients with aneurysmal subarachnoid hemorrhage suggests that the incidence of vasospasm and delayed ischemic deficit was reduced with treatment (Barth *et al.*, 2007).

Parkinson's Disease

There has been substantial activity in the development of new symptomatic therapies for Parkinson's disease. There has been particular interest in the testing of a transdermal therapy, rotigotine. Two studies (Giladi *et al.*, 2007; Jankovic *et al.*, 2007) assessed the efficacy of transdermal rotigotine in early Parkinson's disease. In both double-blind placebo-controlled trials, patients on rotigotine had improved motor performance compared to patients receiving placebo. The most common adverse events observed were site reactions, nausea, and somnolence. In a third study, rotigotine was compared with pramipexole to assess the impact on motor fluctuations in patients with advanced Parkinson's disease and wearing-off type motor functions. Rotigotine was shown to be non-inferior to pramipexole (Poewe *et al.*, 2007). These studies demonstrate that transdermal rotigotine offers a viable alternative to oral medications for patients with both early and advanced Parkinson's disease.

A prolonged release form of ropinirole was assessed in a double-blind placebo-controlled trial. Compared to patients receiving placebo, those on prolonged release ropinirole were able to reduce their daily dosage of levodopa and had reductions in daily "off" time. There was improvement of a variety of secondary outcome measures including time "on", dyskinesias, activities of daily living, depression, and sleep quality (Pahwa *et al.*, 2007). A similar study compared "on" time in patients receiving entacapone to those receiving placebo (Mizuno *et al.*, 2007). Both entacapone doses (100 mg or 200 mg administered with levodopa) were equally efficacious and superior to placebo. The most common adverse event observed was an increase in dyskinesias. These two strategies are alternatives for reducing "off" time and improving "on" time for patients with advanced Parkinson's disease.

Murata *et al.* (2007) explored the utility of zonisamide in improving motor function in patients with Parkinson's disease. Improved motor function and diminished "off" time was observed with both zonisamide dosage groups (50 mg and 100 mg) compared to placebo. Dyskinesia was not higher in the zonisamide treated patients. The authors concluded that zonisamide is a useful adjunctive therapy to levodopa in Parkinson's disease patients with suboptimal therapeutic responses.

Deuschl *et al.* (2006) conducted a randomized trial of deep brain stimulation for Parkinson's disease. They showed that compared with medication management alone, those with deep brain stimulation had improvement on measures of mobility, activities of daily living, emotional well being, stigma, and bodily discomfort. There were more serious adverse events in the neurostimulation group including one fatal intracerebral hemorrhage. Deep brain stimulation offers an alternative to medication-resistant patients, but patient selection must be scrupulous and installation of stimulation devices should be confined to highly experienced centers and neurosurgeons.

Another study investigated the utility of deep brain stimulation in patients with early Parkinson's disease (Schupbach et al., 2007). In an unblinded comparison study where matched pairs of patients were randomly assigned to either deep brain stimulation or medication management; improvement in quality of life was shown in those receiving surgical management; and there was as improvement in motor function after 18 months of therapy. This provocative study suggests that consideration of deep brain stimulation earlier in the course of Parkinson's disease is warranted.

Epilepsy

In a study comparing early versus delayed anti-convulsant therapy in patients whose physicians were uncertain as to whether or not to intervene with anti-epileptic drugs, carbamazepine as monotherapy was strongly associated with a delay of seizure recurrence; there was mixed evidence for an effect of valproate (Marson et al., 2007).

Three doses of retigabin were compared to placebo in a multiarm double-blind placebo-controlled trial of patients with partial seizures. Doses compared to placebo were 600, 900, and 1200 mg/day. Median percent change in seizure frequency from baseline was -23%, -29%, and -35%, respectively compared to -13% for placebo. Treatment-emergent adverse events included somnolence, dizziness, confusion, speech disorder, vertigo, tremor, amnesia, abnormal thinking, abnormal gait, paresthesia, and diplopia. The study suggests that retigabin is an effective adjunctive therapy and reduces the frequency of partial onset seizures. Side effects must be carefully monitored (Porter et al., 2007).

Hessen et al. (2007) executed a double-blind placebo-controlled withdrawal study of patients who had been seizure free for at least 2 years and were on monotherapy with an anti-convulsant. Those in the discontinuation group improved on tests that require complex cognitive processing under time pressure. Simple tasks of attention and reaction time revealed no significant differences between the discontinuation group and the non-discontinuation group. The results suggest that patients who had been seizure free for at least 2 years and are on monotherapy may experience cognitive benefits with anti-convulsant withdrawal.

Transcranial magnetic stimulation is gaining in popularity as a treatment for epilepsy. Fregni et al. (2006) treated 21 patients with malformations of cortical development and refractory epilepsy with five consecutive sessions of low frequency repetitive transcranial magnetic stimulation. This was a randomized double-blind sham-controlled trial. Those receiving active transcranial magnetic stimulation experienced a significant decrease in the number of seizures compared to those receiving sham therapy. The effect persisted for 2 months. Adverse events were limited. This preliminary study suggests that repetitive transcranial magnetic stimulation may represent an important alternative to medication management in certain classes of epilepsy patients.

Multiple Sclerosis

Glatiramer acetate was studied in both primary progressive multiple sclerosis and relapsing remitting multiple sclerosis in recent double-blind placebo-controlled trials. Cohen *et al.* (2007) found a trend favoring the 40-mg group over placebo on the primary endpoint of gadolinum-enhancing lesions on magnetic resonance imaging (MRI) at months 7, 8, and 9. There was also a trend favoring the 40-mg group for relapse rate and proportion of relapse-free subjects. Overall tolerability was acceptable with higher injection site reactions and immediate post-injection reactions with 40 mg compared to 20 mg. The results suggest but do not prove that the 40-mg dose will be more beneficial compared to the 20-mg dose for patients with relapsing remitting disease.

The study group led by Wolinsky *et al.* (2007) failed to demonstrate a significant treatment effect of glatiramer acetate on primary progressive multiple sclerosis. The low event rate and premature discontinuation of study medication decreased the power to detect a treatment effect.

A phase II study of intravenous synthetic peptide MBP8298 in a 24-month double-blind placebo-controlled trial showed no drug-placebo difference on the expanded disability status scale in the analysis of all patients. A contingency analysis in an HLA class 2 sub-group showed a statistically significant benefit of therapy compared to placebo in those with HLA haplotypes BR2 or DR4. The apparent benefit was sustained in long term (5 year) follow up. The study suggests that it may be possible to define responsive sub-groups of patients with progressive multiple sclerosis who benefit from treatment with this intravenous synthetic peptide.

Oral fingolimod (FTY720) was tested in a proof-of-concept (POC) study in relapsing remitting multiple sclerosis (Warren *et al.*, 2006). In the 6-month double-blind placebo-controlled portion of the trial there was a benefit to fingolimod in terms of gadolinium-enhancing MRI lesions and annualized relapse rate for both doses of the active agent (0.125 and 5 mg/day). The benefit continued to be evidenced in the open label extension portion of the study. Adverse events included nasopharyngitis, dyspnea headache, diarrhea, and nausea; 10% of patients had asymptomatic elevations of liver enzyme levels. The authors concluded that the results were sufficiently promising that the agent warrants further study.

Sicotte *et al.* (2007) tested the hypothesis that men with multiple sclerosis might benefit from treatment with testosterone supplementation. They showed in a crossover design with a 6-month treatment period that men receiving testosterone gel evidenced improved cognitive performance and slowing of brain atrophy. There was no effect of testosterone treatment on gadolinium-enhancing lesions or lesion volume. Testosterone was well tolerated.

Traumatic Brain Injury

Rivastigmine, a cholinesterase inhibitor commonly used in Alzheimer disease, was assessed in a double-blind placebo-controlled 12-week trial in patients with traumatic brain injury and persistent cognitive deficit (Silver *et al.*, 2006). Rivastigmine did not perform better than placebo in overall analysis, but sub-group assessment suggested improved memory in those with moderate to severe memory impairment at baseline. Further investigation of the use of cholinesterase inhibitors in traumatic brain injury is needed.

Treatment with methylphenidate of patients with severe and moderate traumatic brain injury has showed that patients receiving active treatment on admission had shorter ICU and hospital lengths of stay compared to patients receiving placebo. Patients with severe traumatic brain injury had reductions in both ICU and hospital length of stay, whereas patients with moderate brain injury had reductions in ICU length of stay only (Moein *et al.*, 2006).

Complications of Spinal Cord Injury

Pregabalin was shown to be effective in relieving central neuropathic pain in patients with spinal cord injury (Siddall *et al.*, 2006). Conclusions were based on a randomized double-blind placebo-controlled trial of flexible dose pregabalin (150–600 mg/day). Pain, disturbed sleep, and anxiety were all improved in patients receiving pregabalin therapy.

The international campaign for cures of spinal cord injury paralysis has provided recent guidance on the conduct of clinical trials in patients with spinal cord injury (Steeves *et al.*, 2007; Fawcett *et al.*, 2007).

Migraine and Cluster Headaches

There has been increased attention to treating neurological disorders in children. Rizatriptan was shown in a double-blind placebo-controlled trial to relieve migraine attacks in children ages 6–17 years (Ahonen *et al.*, 2006). Rizatriptan was well tolerated and no serious adverse events were observed in the trial.

A randomized trial of intranasal zolmitriptan was shown to relieve acute cluster headache within 30 minutes of intranasal administration (Cittadini *et al.*, 2006). Ninety-two patients were included in the randomized trial. No serious adverse events were observed; shortness of breath, vomiting, and rheumatic pain occurred in the group receiving intranasal zolmitriptan.

Neuropathic Pain

Duloxatine is a dual reuptake inhibitor of serotonin and norepinephrine. It has been shown to reduce depression. Wernicke *et al.* (2006) performed a randomized placebo-controlled trial of patients with diabetic peripheral neuropathic pain. Duloxatine was shown to be superior to placebo and had a rapid onset of action. Reductions in pain were approximately 15% in the placebo group and approximately 50% in the duloxatine treated group.

Schizophrenia

The Clinical Antipsychotic Trials of Intervention Effectiveness (CATIE) study sponsored by the National Institute of Mental Health continues to provide interesting and provocative observations into the real world management of schizophrenia. Swartz *et al.* (2007) measured quality of life as an outcome for treatment with first- and second-generation anti-psychotics – olanzapine, perphenazine, quetiapine, risperdone, ziprasdone, for up to 18 months. All anti-psychotic treatment groups in all phases of the trial made modest improvements in psychosocial functioning as measured with the quality of life scale analysis. There were no differences among the pharmacologic agents in producing this response.

In another trial addressing possible treatment differences among therapeutic approaches, Lindenmayer *et al.* (2007) found a significant improvement in negative symptoms in patients treated with olanzapine compared to those treated with haloperidol. There were no treatment differences in positive symptoms, general psychopathology, or depressive symptoms.

A randomized double-blind placebo-controlled trial of modafinil for negative symptoms of schizophrenia (Pierre *et al.*, 2007) failed to establish a benefit of modafinil for negative symptoms.

Depression

Two recent double-blind placebo-controlled trials addressed means of reducing relapse in patients with major depressive disorder. In both studies patients were treated for 1 year following a recovery from an acute depressive episode. Amsterdam & Bodkin (2006) showed that transdermal selegiline was significantly better than placebo in preventing depression relapse. Similarly, Kornstein *et al.* (2006) demonstrated that escitralopram maintenance treatment also was significantly better than placebo in reducing recurrent depression.

Corya *et al.* (2006) compared an olanzapine/fluoxetine combination, olanzapine, fluoxetine, and venlafaxine in patients with treatment-resistant depression. All interventions were similarly effective at study endpoint. The olanzapine/fluoxetine combination showed a more rapid onset of anti-depressant action.

Bipolar depression was also the subject of investigation. Sachs *et al.* (2007) showed that the use of anti-depressant medication as compared to the use of mood stabilizers was not associated with increased efficacy or with increased risk of treatment-emergent affective switching. Patients receiving a mood stabilizer plus adjunctive anti-depressant therapy had similar outcomes to patients receiving a mood stabilizer only.

The anti-depressant venlafaxine also was shown to be effective in reducing symptoms of post-traumatic stress disorder in a 24-week double-blind placebo-controlled trial (Miller *et al.*, 2007).

Incorporation of Biomarkers into Clinical Trials

MRI was used in a 2-year placebo-controlled trial of natalizumab. Nine hundred and forty-two patients with relapsing remitting multiple sclerosis were included in the trial. Relapse rates were reduced by 68% and progression of disability by 42%. MRI showed a 92% decrease in enhancing lesions, an 83% decrease in new or enlarging hyperintense lesions, and a 76% decrease in new hypointense lesions over 2 years (Miller *et al.*, 2007). This study shows a utility of including MRI monitoring in multiple sclerosis trials.

Cerebrospinal fluid amyloid beta protein was used as the primary outcome in a phase II tramiprosate trial (Aisen *et al.*, 2006). Tramiprosate reduced cerebrospinal fluid a beta 42 level in a dose-dependent level over 3 months of treatment. No clinical treatment differences were seen among the treatment groups.

Pharmacogenetics

Genetic profiles may come to play an increasingly important role in prediction of treatment response and adverse event occurrence. In a preliminary study of this type Denys *et al.* (2007) analyzed responders in a trial of paroxetine and venlafaxine for obsessive–compulsive disorder. They found genotype specificity for the responder group for each medication. Larger samples and replication studies would be required to confirm such an effect, but the study is a forward-looking application of pharmacogenetics.

Summary

Patients with neurologic and psychiatric illness require new disease-modifying and symptom relieving medications to improve target indications and quality of life.

Advances in neuroscience are providing consistent improvements in understanding of the basic mechanisms in neurologic and psychiatric illnesses. Mechanistic understanding provides the opportunity for identification of critically vulnerable and exploitable steps in the pathogenic cascade that may surrender to therapeutic intervention. In addition to an urgent need to improve therapeutics, biomarkers that support POC studies are also required to advance clinical trials and to enhance the opportunity for success for developing new therapeutics. As shown in this and the following chapters, success is evolving in the development of new treatments for disabling neurologic and psychiatric disorders.

Disclosures

Dr. Cummings has provided consultation to the following pharmaceutical companies: Avanir, Eisai, EnVivo, Forest, Janssen, Lilly, Lundbeck, Medivation, Merck, Novartis, Ono Pharma, Pfizer, Sanofi-Aventis, and Takeda Pharmaceuticals.

Acknowledgements

Dr. Cummings is supported by an NIA Alzheimer Disease Research Center Grant (P50 AG16570), an Alzheimer Disease Research Center Grant of California, and the Sidell-Kagan Foundation.

References

Ahonen, K., Hämäläinen, M., Eerola, M., & Hoppu, K. (2006). A randomized trial of rizatriptan in migraine attacks in children. *Neurology*, 67, 1135–1140.

Aisen, P.S., Saumier, D., Briand, R., *et al.* (2006). A phase II study targeting amyloid-beta with 3APS in mild-to-moderate Alzheimer disease. *Neurology*, 67, 1757–1763.

Amsterdam, J.D., & Bodkin, J.A. (2006). Selegiline transdermal system in the prevention of relapse of major depressive disorder: a 52-week, double-blind, placebo-substitution, parallel-group clinical trial. *Journal of Clinical Psychopharmacology*, 26, 579–586.

Barth, M., Capelle, H.H., Weidauer, S., Weiss, C., Münch, E., Thomé, C., Luecke, T., Schmiedek, P., Kasuya, H., & Vajkoczy, P. (2007). Effect of nicardipine prolonged-release implants on cerebral vasospasm and clinical outcome after severe aneurysmal subarachnoid hemorrhage: a prospective, randomized, double-blind phase IIa study. *Stroke*, 38, 330–336.

Cittadini, E., May, A., Straube, A., Evers, S., Bussone, G., & Goadsby, P.J. (2006). Effectiveness of Intranasal Zolmitriptan in acute cluster headache. *Archives of Neurology*, 63, 1537–1542.

Cohen, J.A., Rovaris, M., Goodman, A.D., Ladkani, D., Wynn, D., & Filippi, M. (9006 Study Group) (2007). Randomized, double-blind, dose-comparison study of glatiramer acetate in relapsing-remitting MS. *Neurology*, 68, 939–944.

Corya, S., Williamson, D., Sanger, T., Briggs, S., Case, M., & Tollefson, G. (2006). A randomized, double-blind comparison of olanzapine/fluoxetine combination, olanzapine, fluoxetine, and venlafaxine in treatment-resistant depression. *Depression and Anxiety*, 23, 364–372.

Denys, D., Van Nieuwerburgh, F., Deforce, D., & Westenberg, H. (2007). Prediction of response to paroxetine and venlafaxine by serotonin-related genes in obsessive–compulsive disorder in a randomized, double-blind trial. *Journal of Clinical Psychiatry*, 68, 747–753.

Deuschl, G., Schade-Brittinger, C., Krack, O., et al. (2006). A randomized trial of deep-brain stimulation for Parkinson's disease. *New England Journal of Medicine*, 355, 896–908.

Di Prospero, N., Baker, A., Jeffries, N., & Fischbeck, K. (2007). Neurological effects of high-dose idebenone in patients with Friedreich's ataxia: a randomised, placebo-controlled trial. *Lancet Neurology*, 6, 878–886.

ESPRIT Group (2007). Medium intensity oral anticoagulants versus aspirin after cerebral ischaemia of arterial origin (ESPRIT): a randomised controlled trial. *Lancet Neurology*, 6, 115–124.

Fawcett, J., Curt, A., Steeves, J., et al. (2007). Guidelines for the conduct of clinical trials for spinal cord injury as developed by the ICCP panel: spontaneous recovery after spinal cord injury and statistical power needed for therapeutic clinical trials. *Spinal Cord*, 45, 190–205.

Fregni, F., Boggio, P., Lima, M.C., et al. (2006). A sham-controlled, phase II trial of transcranial direct current stimulation for the treatment of central pain in traumatic spinal cord injury. *Pain*, 122, 197–209.

Giladi, N., Boroojerdi, B., Korczyn, A.D., Burn, D.J., Clarke, C.E., & Schapira, A.H. (SP513 Investigators) (2007). Rotigotine transdermal patch in early Parkinson's disease: A randomized, double-blind, controlled study versus placebo and ropinirole. *Movement Disorders*, 22, 2398–2404.

Hessen, E., Lossius, M.I., Reinvang, I., & Gjerstad, L. (2007). Influence of major antiepileptic drugs on neuropsychological function: results from a randomized, double-blind, placebo-controlled withdrawal study of seizure-free epilepsy patients on monotherapy. *Journal of the International Neuropsychological Society*, 13, 393–400.

Jankovic, J., Watts, R., Martin, W., & Boroojerdi, B. (2007). Transdermal rotigotine: double-blind, placebo-controlled trial in Parkinson disease. *Archives of Neurology*, 64, 676–682.

Kornstein, S., Bose, A., Li, D., Saikali, K., & Gandhi, C. (2006). Escitalopram maintenance treatment for prevention of recurrent depression: a randomized, placebo-controlled trial. *Journal of Clinical Psychiatry*, 67, 1767–1775.

Landwehrmeyer, G., Dubois, B., de Yébenes, J., et al. (2007). Riluzole in Huntington's disease: a 3-year, randomized controlled study. *Annals of Neurology*, 62, 262–272.

Lindenmayer, J., Khan, A., Iskander, A., Abad, M., & Parker, B. (2007). A randomized controlled trial of olanzapine versus haloperidol in the treatment of primary negative symptoms and neurocognitive deficits in schizophrenia. *Journal of Clinical Psychiatry*, 68, 368–379.

Marson, A.G., Al-Kharusi, A.M., Alwaidh, M., et al. (2007). The SANAD study of effectiveness of valproate, lamotrigine, or topiramate for generalised and unclassifiable epilepsy: an unblinded randomised controlled trial. *Lancet*, 369, 1016–1026.

Miller, D.H., Soon, D., Fernando, K.T., MacManus, D.G., Barker, G.J., Yousry, T.A., Fisher, E., O'Connor, P.W., Phillips, J.T., Polman, C.H., Kappos, L., Hutchinson, M., Havrdova, E., Lublin, F.D., Giovannoni, G., Wajgt, A., Rudick, R., Lynn, F., Panzara, M.A., & Sandrock, A.W. (AFFIRM Investigators) (2007). MRI outcomes in a placebo-controlled trial of natalizumab in relapsing MS. *Neurology*, 68, 1390–1401.

Mizuno, Y., Kanazawa, I., Kuno, S., Yanagisawa, N., Yamamoto, M., & Kindo, T. (2007). Placebo-controlled, double-blind close-finding study of entacapone in fluctuating Parkinsonian patient. *Movement Disorders*, 22, 75–80.

Moein, H., Khalili, H.A., & Keramatian, K. (2006). Effect of methylphenidate on ICU and hospital length of stay in patients with severe and moderate traumatic brain injury. *Clinical Neurology and Neurosurgery*, 108, 539–542.

Murata, M., Hasegawa, K., Kanazawa, I., & Group TJZoPS (2007). Zonisamide improves motor function in Parkinson disease. *Neurology*, 68, 45–50.

Pahwa, R., Stacy, M., Factor, S., et al. (2007). Ropinirole 24-hour prolonged release. *Neurology*, 68, 1108–1115.

Patterson, M.C., Vecchio, D., Prady, H., Abel, L., & Wraith, J.E. (2007). Miglustat for treatment of Niemann-Pick C disease: a randomised controlled study. *Lancet Neurology*, 6, 765–772.

Pierre, J.M., Peloian, J.H., Wirshing, D.A., Wirshing, W.C., & Marder, S.R. (2007). A randomized, double-blind, placebo-controlled trial of modafinil for negative symptoms in schizophrenia. *Journal of Clinical Psychiatry*, 68, 705–710.

Poewe, W.H., Rascol, O., Quinn, N., et al. (2007). Efficacy of pramipexole and transdermal rotigotine in advanced Parkinson's disease: a double-blind, double-dummy, randomised controlled trial. *Lancet Neurology*, 6, 513–520.

Porter, R.J., Partiot, A., Sachdeo, R., Nohria, V., & Alves, W.M. (2007). Randomized, multicenter, dose-ranging trial of retigabine for partial-onset seizures. *Neurology*, 68, 1197–1204.

Sachs, G., Nierenberg, A., Calabrese, J.R., et al. (2007). Effectiveness of adjunctive antidepressant treatment for bipolar depression. *New England Journal of Medicine*, 357, 1711–1722.

Schupbach, W.M., Maltete, D., Houeto, J.L., et al. (2007). Neurosurgery at an earlier stage of Parkinson disease: a randomized, controlled trial. *Neurology*, 686, 267–271.

Sicotte, N.L., Giesser, B., Tandon, V., et al. (2007). Testosterone treatment in multiple sclerosis. *Archives of Neurology*, 64, 683–688.

Siddall, P., Cousins, M., Otte, A., Griesing, T., Chambers, R., & Murphy, T. (2006). Pregabalin in central neuropathic pain associated with spinal cord injury. *Neurology*, 67, 1792–1800.

Silver, J., Koumaras, B., Chen, M., et al. (2006). Effects of rivastigmine on cognitive function in patients with traumatic brain injury. *Neurology*, 67, 748–758.

SPARCL (2006). High-dose atorvastatin after stroke or transient ischemic attack. *New England Journal of Medicine*, 355, 549–559.

Steeves, J., Lammertse, D., Curt, A., et al. (2007). Guidelines for the conduct of clinical trials for spinal cord injury (SCI) as developed by the ICCP panel: clinical trial outcome measures. *Spinal Cord*, 45, 206–221.

Sugg, R., Pary, J., Uchino, K., et al. (2006). Argatroban tPA stroke study. *Archives of Neurology*, 63, 1057–1062.

Swartz, M.S., Perkins, D.O., Stroup, T.S., et al. (2007). Effects of antipsychotic medications on psychosocial functioning in patients with chronic schizophrenia: findings from the NIMH CATIE study. *American Journal of Psychiatry*, 164, 428–436.

Warren, K.G., Catz, I., Ferenczi, L.Z., & Krantz, J. (2006). Intravenous synthetic peptide MBP8298 delayed disease progression in an HLA class II-defined cohort of patients with progressive multiple sclerosis: results of a 24-month double-blind placebo-controlled clinical trial and 5 years of follow-up treatment. *European Journal of Neurology*, 13, 887–895.

Watts, R.L., Jankovic, J., Waters, C., Rajput, A., Boroojerdi, B., & Rao, J. (2007). Randomized, blind, controlled trial of transdermal rotigotine in early Parkinson disease. *Neurology*, 68, 272–276.

Wernicke, J., Pritchett, Y., D'Souza, D., et al. (2006). A randomized controlled trial of duloxetine in diabetic peripheral neuropathic pain. *Neurology*, 67, 1411–1420.

Wolinsky, J., Narayana, P., O'Connor, P., et al. (2007). Glatiramer acetate in primary progressive multiple sclerosis: results of a multinational, multicenter, double-blind, placebo-controlled trial. *Annals of Neurology*, 61, 14–24.

Progress in Neurotherapeutics and Neuropsychopharmacology, 3:1, 13–33 © 2008 Cambridge University Press
DOI: 10.1017/S1748232107000092   Printed in the United Kingdom

Triflusal versus Aspirin for the Prevention of Stroke

Antonio Culebras
Department of Neurology, Upstate Medical University, 750 E. Adams Street, Syracuse, NY 13210, USA;
Email: aculebras@aol.com

Javier Borja
Drug Safety Manager, J. Uriach y Compañía, S.A., Polígon Industrial Riera de Caldes, Avinguda Camí Reial,
51–57, 08184 Palau-solità i Plegamans, Barcelona, Spain; Email: fv-borja@uriach.com

Julián García-Rafanell
Director of Medical Affairs, J. Uriach y Compañía, S.A., Polígon Industrial Riera de Caldes, Avinguda Camí Reial,
51–57, 08184 Palau-solità i Plegamans, Barcelona, Spain; Email: garcia-rafanell@uriach.com

ABSTRACT

Antiplatelet agents represent an important part of the therapeutic armamentarium in the prevention of stroke. Triflusal is an antiplatelet agent structurally related to salicylates but not derived from acetylsalicylic acid. Like aspirin, triflusal irreversibly acetylates cyclo-oxygenase isoform 1 (COX-1) and therefore inhibits thromboxane biosynthesis. Triflusal is rapidly absorbed after oral administration, with an absorption half life of 0.44 hours. Evidence of the efficacy and safety of triflusal is derived from clinical trials performed in patients with unstable angina, acute myocardial infarction, stroke, aortocoronary bypass, atrial fibrillation, valve replacement, and asthmatic patients intolerant to aspirin and/or non-steroidal antiinflamatory drugs (NSAID). The Triflusal versus Aspirin for the Prevention of Infarction: A Randomized Stroke Study (TAPIRSS) study was performed to explore the efficacy and safety of triflusal versus aspirin in the prevention of vascular complications in patients with a previous TIA or ischemic stroke in a Latin American population. In this pilot study differences between triflusal and aspirin in the prevention of vascular complications after TIA or ischemic stroke were not observed. Hemorrhagic risk was lower with triflusal than with aspirin. The TAPIRSS study contributed evidence on the efficacy and safety of triflusal as a valid alternative to aspirin in the prevention of vascular events in patients with ischemic stroke or TIA.

Key words: antiplatelet agent, aspirin, stroke, transient ischemic attack, triflusal.

Correspondence should be addressed to: Antonio Culebras, Department of Neurology, Upstate Medical University, 750 E. Adams Street, Syracuse, NY 13210, USA; Fax: +1 315 637 6226; Email: aculebras@aol.com

Introduction and Overview

Antiplatelet agents represent an important part of the therapeutic armamentarium in the prevention of stroke. In this regard, the meta-analysis of the Antithrombotic Trialists' Collaboration (2002), formerly the Antiplatelet Trialist's Collaboration (1994), evidenced that in patients with previous stroke/transient ischemic attack (TIA), treatment with antiplatelet agents leads to an absolute reduction in the risk of having a serious vascular event (myocardial infarction, stroke or vascular death) of 3.6%. Aspirin is the most widely studied antiplatelet drug with a recurrent stroke risk reduction of 20% (Weisman & Graham, 2002). Other drugs such as ticlopidine, clopidogrel and triflusal are also considered effective for secondary prevention of stroke and other vascular events in patients with cerebrovascular disease (Albers *et al.*, 2004). In one study, the combination of low-dose aspirin and extended-release dipyridamole was more effective than either agent prescribed separately (Diener *et al.*, 1996).

Aspirin has well known adverse effects such as bleeding, drug-resistance, intolerance or allergy. The blood toxicity associated with ticlopidine, mainly neutropenia and thrombotic thrombocytopenic purpura (White *et al.*, 2001), have made the current role of this drug uncertain. For clopidogrel, efficacy data come from the Clopidogrel versus Aspirin in Patients at risk of Ischemic Events (CAPRIE) study (CAPRIE Steering Committee, 1996), that studied three different clinical entities: myocardial infarction, ischemic stroke and symptomatic peripheral arterial disease. Although overall results were favorable for clopidogrel, no differences compared with aspirin were found when subgroups of ischemic stroke and myocardial infarction were analyzed. Patrono *et al.* (2001) reported that the formal test of heterogeneity of the three treatment effects in the CAPRIE study (CAPRIE Steering Committee, 1996) was statistically significant, suggesting that the true benefit of clopidogrel may not be identical for each type of disease.

Recurrent stroke risk reduction with accepted antiplatelet agents is only partial with adverse effects and in consequence new studies are desirable proposition. Such is the case of the recently published Triflusal versus Aspirin for the Prevention of Infarction: A Randomized Stroke Study (TAPIRSS) study (Culebras *et al.*, 2004), which compared triflusal with aspirin for the secondary prevention of stroke and will be described with more detail in this review.

Agent

Triflusal is an antiplatelet agent structurally related to salicylates but not derived from acetylsalicylic acid (ASA).

Pharmacodynamic Profile

Like aspirin, triflusal irreversibly acetylates cyclo-oxygenase isoform 1 (COX-1) and therefore inhibits thromboxane biosynthesis (Cruz-Fernández, 2001; Mc Neely & Goa, 1998). The main metabolite of triflusal, 2-hydroxy-4-(trifluoro-methyl) benzoic acid (HTB) also has reversible inhibitory effects on the COX pathway. Aspirin, triflusal and HTB are able to stimulate nitric oxide (NO) synthase, increasing NO synthesis in several cell lines including monocytes (Cruz-Fernández 2001). NO can be transferred to platelets, where it exerts an antiaggregant effect by potentiating cGMP synthesis (Sánchez de Miguel *et al.*, 2000). Triflusal, in addition, inhibits platelet phosphodiesterase, the enzyme responsible for degrading cAMP and cGMP, both of which have antiaggregant effects (García-Rafanell *et al.*, 1986). Triflusal blocks the activation of nuclear transcription factor (NF-κB) and therefore is able to inhibit the expression of both vascular and neuronal inflammatory markers and adhesion molecules (Acarin *et al.*, 2002; Bayón *et al.*, 1999). Unlike to aspirin, the endothelial synthesis of prostacyclin is unaffected with triflusal (Cruz-Fernández, 2001).

In vitro and *ex vivo* studies in healthy volunteers (Albors *et al.*, 1987), patients with type 1 diabetes (De La Cruz *et al.*, 1998) and patients with prosthetic heart valves (Domínguez *et al.*, 1985) have revealed that thromboxane B_2 (TxB_2) production was significantly reduced by both triflusal and aspirin. In patients with type 1 diabetes (De La Cruz *et al.*, 1998), serum levels of TxB_2 were greatly reduced with both triflusal and aspirin after 15 days (85% and 99%, respectively; $p < 0.05$). However, reductions in serum 6-keto-prostaglandin-$F_{1\alpha}$ (6-keto-PG $F_{1\alpha}$) levels were negligible with triflusal compared with aspirin (8.8% versus 97.8%; $p < 0.001$). These data suggest that triflusal has selective activity on platelet arachidonic acid metabolism, whereas aspirin inhibits both platelet and endothelial arachidonic acid metabolism (Mc Neely & Goa, 1998). One *ex vivo* study in human platelet rich plasma (PRP) evidenced that 65% inhibition of arachidonic acid-induced platelet aggregation was apparent 24 hours after a single 600 mg dose of triflusal ($p < 0.05$) (Albors *et al.*, 1987). Repeated administration of triflusal (600 mg daily for 7 days) resulted in 50–75% inhibition of platelet aggregation induced by arachidonic acid, adenosine diphosphate, epinephrine and collagen. Ten days after discontinuation of treatment, inhibition was still significant when using arachidonic acid as the inducer of platelet aggregation. Otherwise platelet response was fully recovered. In one *ex vivo* study in whole blood of healthy volunteers triflusal reduced ADP-induced platelet aggregation more than aspirin (De La Cruz *et al.*, 1995a). Triflusal reduced also thrombus formation on rabbit vascular subendothelium (De La Cruz *et al.*, 1995b) as well as the formation of microthrombi subsequent to experimentally induced brain ischemia in rats (Heye *et al.*, 1991).

A recent study demonstrated that triflusal reduced pathological and inflammatory markers and functional deficits in rats receiving β-amyloid or endotelin injections, suggesting a neuroprotective effect for Alzheimer disease (AD) and cerebral ischemia (Whitehead *et al.*, 2005).

Pharmacokinetic Profile

Triflusal is rapidly absorbed after oral administration, with an absorption half life ($t_{1/2} k_a$) of 0.44 hours (Mc Neely & Goa, 1998). In 8 healthy volunteers (mean age 27 years) who received a single 900 mg oral dose of triflusal, mean maximum plasma concentrations (C_{max}) of triflusal and HTB were 11.6 mg/l and 92.7 mg/l, respectively (Ramis *et al.*, 1991). The time to C_{max} was much shorter for the parent compound than the metabolite (0.88 versus 4.96 hours). However, both compounds were detectable in the plasma at similar time intervals after triflusal administration (t_{lag}: 0.23 and 0.31 hours for triflusal and HTB, respectively) which suggests a rapid biotransformation of the parent compound (Ramis *et al.*, 1991). The area under the concentration-time curve (AUC) was 20.26 mg/l/hour for triflusal 900 mg and 4227 mg/l/hour for HTB. Volume of distribution was 34 l for triflusal and 8.96 l for HTB, respectively. Clearance was 45.4 l/hour for triflusal and 0.18 l/hour for HTB and terminal elimination half life ($t_{1/2β}$) values were 0.53 hour and 34.29 hours for triflusal and HTB, respectively (Ramis *et al.*, 1991). Pharmacokinetic parameters of triflusal 900 mg single dose are shown in Table 1.

There was no plasma accumulation of the parent compound in elderly volunteers (mean age 80 years) after 13 days' administration of twice-daily triflusal 300 mg (Ferrari *et al.*, 1996). However, C_{max} values of the active metabolites increased significantly from day 1 to day 13 (39.88 versus 120.42 mg/l) with an accumulation factor of 6.64 (Ferrari *et al.*, 1996). Similar results were seen in young volunteers (mean age 23 years) who received triflusal 300 mg every 8 hours for 13 days: C_{max} values for HTB were 36.4 mg/l on day 1 and 177.8 mg/l on day 13 with an accumulation factor of 6.35 (Ramis *et al.*, 1990). C_{max} values for HTB also increased (to

Table 1. **Pharmacokinetic Parameters of Triflusal After a 900 mg Single Dose**

Absorption	Fast, not affected by food
Metabolism	Plasma hydrolysis, giving rise to active metabolite HTB
Maximum concentration	Triflusal: 1 hour
	HTB: 5 hours
Biological half life ($t_{1/2}$)	Triflusal: 30 minutes
	HTB: 35 hours
Elimination	Renal
Initial activity	2 hours after intake

152.9 mg/l) after 13 days' triflusal 600 mg every 24 hours in the young volunteers, however, the accumulation factor was reduced (2.77) (Ramis *et al.*, 1990).

In elderly volunteers, steady-state plasma HTB concentrations (mean 102.21 mg/l) were attained after 4–5 days' administration of twice-daily triflusal 300 mg therapy (Ferrari *et al.*, 1996). In younger volunteers, mean steady-state plasma HTB concentrations were 168 mg/l with triflusal 300 mg every 8 hours and 123 mg/l with triflusal 600 mg every 24 hours (Ramis *et al.*, 1990).

Mean HTB AUC values after a single 300 mg dose of triflusal were 1624 mg/l/hour in young (Ramis *et al.*, 1990) and 2156 mg/l/hour in elderly volunteers (Ferrari *et al.*, 1996). After 13 days' therapy in young volunteers, the mean steady-state AUC values for HTB were 1301 mg/l/hour with once daily triflusal 600 mg (Ramis *et al.*, 1990). In the elderly, the mean HTB AUC value was 1226 mg/l/hour with twice-daily triflusal 300 mg (Ferrari *et al.*, 1996). The $t_{1/2\beta}$ values for HTB were similar in the elderly (Ferrari *et al.*, 1996) and in the young (Ramis *et al.*, 1990) and after single (300 mg) or repeated (600–900 mg/day for 13 days) administration of triflusal (Ferrari *et al.*, 1996; Ramis *et al.*, 1990). Reported values ranged from 44.5 to 54.6 hours (Ferrari *et al.*, 1996; Ramis *et al.*, 1990).

In a recent study in healthy volunteers, HTB penetrated into the cerebrospinal fluid in a range of concentrations experimentally proven to have protective effects in AD (Valle *et al.*, 2005).

Clinical Efficacy and Safety

Evidence of the efficacy and safety of triflusal is derived from clinical trials performed in patients with unstable angina (Plaza *et al.*, 1993), acute myocardial infarction (AMI) (Cruz-Fernández *et al.*, 2000), stroke (Culebras *et al.*, 2004; Matías-Guíu *et al.*, 2003; 1997; Smirne *et al.*, 1994), aortocoronary bypass (Guiteras *et al.*, 1989), atrial fibrillation (Pérez-Gómez *et al.*, 2004), valve replacement (Aramendi *et al.*, 2005) and asthmatic patients intolerant to aspirin and/or non-steroidal antiinflamatory drugs (NSAID) (Dela Cruz *et al.*, 2002). The evidence is reinforced by a recently published systematic review comparing efficacy and safety of triflusal with aspirin in patients with stroke or TIA or AMI (Costa *et al.*, 2005). Two pharmaco-epidemiological studies (Ibáñez *et al.*, 2006; Lanas *et al.*, 2003) assessed the risk of upper gastrointestinal bleeding associated with triflusal and other drugs.

UNSTABLE ANGINA

In a randomized, double-blind, parallel, placebo-controlled, multicenter clinical trial, performed in 281 patients aged 70 or less admitted to the coronary care unit with unstable angina, triflusal at a dose of 300 mg t.i.d. during 6 months led to a marked risk reduction of non-fatal myocardial infarction (risk reduction: 65.8%; 95% confidence interval (CI): 58.8–71.2%; $p = 0.013$) (Plaza *et al.*, 1993); 18.1% of placebo recipients and 27.9% of those treated with triflusal reported at

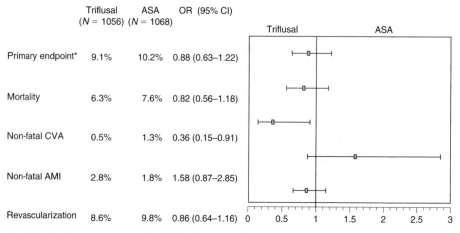

Fig. 1.
Cardiovascular events in patients with AMI treated with triflusal or aspirin (ASA) in the TIM study.
Cruz-Fernández *et al.* (2000). *European Heart Journal*, 21, 457–465.

least one adverse event ($p = 0.05$). Six patients in the placebo group and 7 in the triflusal group withdrew due to adverse events (placebo group: severe epigastric burning 5, and skin reaction 1; triflusal group: gastrointestinal complaints 5, and minor bleeding 2).

AMI

The Triflusal in Myocardial Infarction (TIM) study (Cruz-Fernández *et al.*, 2000) was a randomized, double-blind, sequential, multicenter clinical trial to compare the efficacy and tolerability of triflusal with aspirin in the prevention of cardiovascular events following myocardial infarction. 2275 patients with AMI were randomized to triflusal 600 mg or aspirin 300 mg, once daily for 35 days. Treatment was started within 24 hours of symptom onset.

2270 patients were evaluated for safety and 2224 patients were validated for sequential monitoring. The primary composite endpoint of death, non-fatal myocardial infarction or non-fatal cerebrovascular events within the first 35 days occurred in 99 (9.06%) of 1056 patients receiving triflusal and 105 (10.15%) of 1068 patients receiving aspirin (odds ratio (OR): 0.882; 95% CI: 0.634 to 1.227; $p = 0.582$). The risk of non-fatal cerebrovascular events was significantly lower with triflusal than with aspirin: 5 (0.48%) versus 14 (1.31%) patients, respectively (OR: 0.364; 95% CI: 0.146 to 0.908; $p = 0.030$) (Figure 1).

Differences between groups in incidence of adverse events possibly related to treatment were not evidenced. However, the incidence of bleeding events in the brain was lower in patients receiving triflusal in comparison with patients receiving aspirin (0.27% versus 0.97%, $p = 0.03$) (Figure 2).

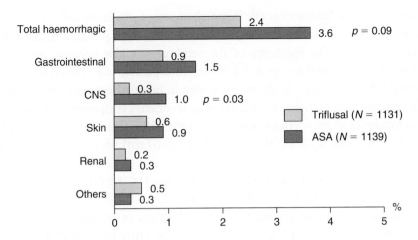

Fig. 2.
Hemorrhagic events in patients with AMI treated with triflusal or aspirin (ASA) in the TIM study.
Cruz-Fernández et al. (2000). *European Heart Journal*, 21, 457–465.

STROKE

Promising results obtained in two preliminary studies (Matías-Guíu *et al.*, 1997; Smirne *et al.*, 1994) of triflusal compared with aspirin in stroke prevention prompted to perform larger studies.

Two main studies (Culebras *et al.*, 2004; Matías-Guíu *et al.*, 2003) have been performed with triflusal in stroke patients. The Triflusal versus Aspirin in Cerebral Infarction Prevention (TACIP) study (Matías-Guíu *et al.*, 2003) was a randomized, double-blind, parallel, multicenter clinical trial to assess the potential benefit of triflusal for secondary prevention of stroke compared with aspirin in patients with stroke or TIA. 2113 patients aged 40 years or older who had suffered a transient ischemic attack or non-disabling stroke within the previous 6 months were randomized to receive triflusal 600 mg/day or aspirin 325 mg/day, over 1–3 years.

2107 patients were evaluated for safety and for intention-to-treat (ITT) efficacy analysis. The primary composite endpoint of vascular death, non-fatal ischemic stroke or non-fatal myocardial infarction occurred in 138 (13.1%) of 1055 triflusal treated patients and in 130 (12.4%) of 1052 aspirin treated patients (hazard ratio (HR): 1.09; 95% CI: 0.85 to 1.38).

Safety evaluation showed that 54.3% of patients in the triflusal group and 52.8% in aspirin group presented at least one adverse event ($p = 0.485$). Dyspepsia was lower in the aspirin group than in the triflusal group (21.7% versus 27.4%; $p = 0.002$) whereas gastric/peptic ulcer was lower in the triflusal group than in aspirin group (0.1% versus 0.8%; $p = 0.021$).

The incidence of major systemic hemorrhage was 1.2% in the triflusal group and 2.9% in the aspirin group (HR: 0.42; 95% CI: 0.22 to 0.81; $p = 0.006$), a finding of particular interest. The incidence of any cerebral or major systemic hemorrhage was 1.9% in the triflusal group and 4.0% in the aspirin group (HR: 0.48; 95% CI: 0.28 to 0.82; $p = 0.004$). Both, major systemic hemorrhage and any cerebral or major systemic hemorrhage, were defined as secondary endpoints of the trial. The overall incidence of hemorrhage was lower in the triflusal group than in the aspirin group: 16.7% versus 25.2% (OR: 0.76; 95% CI: 0.67 to 0.86; $p < 0.001$) (Table 2).

THE COCHRANE COLLABORATION SYSTEMATIC REVIEW
OF TRIFLUSAL VERSUS ASPIRIN IN STROKE AND AMI

A systematic review comparing efficacy and safety of triflusal with aspirin in patients with stroke or TIA or AMI has been recently published (Costa *et al.*, 2005). Five studies (four in stroke or TIA (2994 patients) and one in AMI (2275 patients)) comparing triflusal with aspirin were included.

The comparative efficacy of triflusal versus aspirin (OR > 1 favours triflusal), showed no significant differences between triflusal and aspirin neither for the primary outcome, defined as non-fatal myocardial infarction, non-fatal ischemic or hemorrhagic stroke, or vascular death (OR: 1.04; 95% CI: 0.87 to 1.23) nor for each of the individual outcomes that contributed to the primary outcome: vascular death (OR: 1.11; 95% CI: 0.86 to 1.45), non-fatal stroke (OR: 1.1; 95% CI: 0.86 to 1.40), and non-fatal AMI (OR: 0.90; 95% CI: 0.61 to 1.31). In general, differences for the secondary outcomes were not found. The exceptions, all favouring triflusal, were non-fatal hemorrhagic stroke (OR: 2.83; 95% CI: 1.2 to 6.68), fatal and non-fatal hemorrhagic stroke (OR: 2.15; 95% CI: 1.15 to 4.04) and fatal ischemic stroke (OR: 2.71; 95% CI: 1.12 to 6.55).

Table 2. **Hemorrhagic Adverse Events in Patients with TIA or Stroke Treated with Triflusal or Aspirin in the TACIP Study**

	TREATMENT				*p*-VALUE
	ASPIRIN ($N = 1052$)		TRIFLUSAL ($N = 1055$)		
Any minor	233	22.10%	160	15.20%	<0.001
Any major*	42	4.00%	20	1.90%	0.004
Any major or minor	265	25.20%	176	16.70%	<0.001
Gastrointestinal	89	8.50%	59	5.60%	0.01
Skin hematoma	82	7.80%	47	4.50%	0.001
Respiratory	74	7.00%	56	5.3%	n.s.
Urinary	24	2.30%	20	1.9%	n.s.
Cerebral	11	1.00%	7	0.70%	n.s.
Ocular	11	1.00%	6	0.60%	n.s.

*Include: systemic and cerebral hemorrhage, fatal and non-fatal.
Matías-Guíu *et al.* (2003). *Stroke*, 34, 840–848.

The comparative safety of triflusal versus aspirin (OR > 1 favours triflusal) was also studied. No differences were detected in the number of patients with at least one adverse event, although the number of patients with serious adverse events related to medication was higher with aspirin than with triflusal (OR: 1.36; 95% CI: 1.04 to 1.78). Triflusal was safer than aspirin concerning the following variables: overall hemorrhagic adverse events (OR: 1.73; 95% CI: 1.44 to 2.08), number of patients with any intracranial hemorrhage or other major systemic hemorrhage (OR: 2.34; 95% CI: 1.58 to 3.46), number of patients with any major systemic hemorrhage (OR: 2.34; 95% CI: 1.41 to 3.86), number of patients with any minor hemorrhage (OR: 1.60; 95% CI: 1.31 to 1.95) and number of patients with gastrointestinal hemorrhage (OR: 1.83; 95% CI: 1.35 to 2.48). The number of patients with non-hemorrhagic gastrointestinal adverse events was lower in the aspirin treated patients (OR: 0.84; 95% CI: 0.75 to 0.95).

PREVENTION OF AORTOCORONARY VEIN-GRAFT OCCLUSION

In a randomized, double-blind study, performed in 209 patients, comparing the efficacy of triflusal 300 mg plus dipyridamole 75 mg three times daily with aspirin 50 mg plus dipyridamole 75 mg three times daily and with placebo, on saphenous vein aortocoronary bypass graft patency, triflusal plus dipyridamole was superior to low-dose aspirin plus dipyridamole in the prevention of vein-graft occlusion after 6 months of surgery (Smirne *et al.*, 1994).

ATRIAL FIBRILLATION

The recently published National Study for Prevention of Embolism in Atrial Fibrillation (NASPEAF) study (Pérez-Gómez *et al.*, 2004) studied the efficacy and tolerability of triflusal plus moderate intensity anticoagulation in patients with atrial fibrillation. This was a prospective, multicenter, randomized clinical trial, performed in 1209 patients with atrial fibrillation. Patients were divided into two groups based on risk for thromboembolism: the high-risk group included patients with nonvalvular disease plus prior embolism and patients with mitral stenosis with and without prior embolism. All others were included in the intermediate-risk group. Patients in the intermediate-risk group were randomized to one of the three arms: oral anticoagulation with acenocoumarol (a vitamin K antagonist commonly used in Europe) to a target international normalized ratio (INR) of 2–3, triflusal 600 mg daily, or a combination of both with a target INR of 1.25–2. In the high-risk group, the triflusal-only arm was omitted and subjects were assigned to anticoagulation with a target INR of 2–3 or the combination therapy with a target INR of 1.4–2.4. Primary outcome was a composite of vascular death, TIA and non-fatal stroke or systemic embolism, whichever came first. After a median follow-up of 2.76 years, primary outcome was lower in the combined therapy than in the anticoagulant arm in both the intermediate (hazard ratio (HR): 0.33; 95% CI: 0.12 to 0.91; $p = 0.02$) (Figure 3) and the high-risk

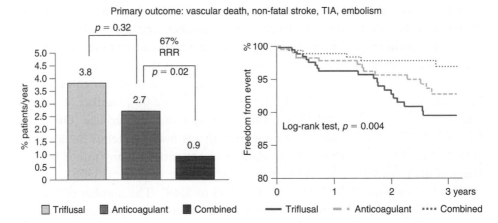

Fig. 3.
Efficacy results in the intermediate-risk group of patients with atrial fibirllation in the NASPEAF study.
Pérez-Gómez *et al.* (2004). *Journal of the American College of Cardiology,* 44, 1557–1566.

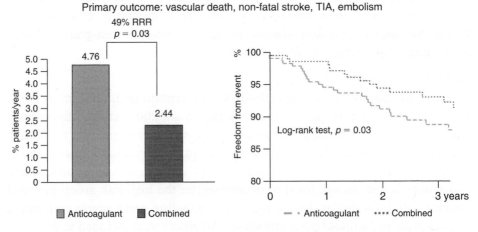

Fig. 4.
Efficacy results in the high-risk group of patients with atrial fibirllation in the NASPEAF study.
Pérez-Gómez *et al.* (2004). *Journal of the American College of Cardiology,* 44, 1557–1566.

group (HR: 0.51; 95% CI: 0.27 to 0.96; $p = 0.03$) (Figure 4). Primary outcome plus severe bleeding was lower with combined therapy in the intermediate-risk group.

The NASPEAF study (Pérez-Gómez *et al.*, 2004) was of interest because it included patients with mitral stenosis but more importantly because it demonstrated for the first time that the addition of antiplatelet therapy (triflusal) to reduced intensity anticoagulation in atrial fibrillation stratified for risk of thrombo-embolism, significantly decreases subsequent vascular events compared with patients receiving standard anticoagulation, without increasing bleeding risk. Similar results were not demonstrated in previous trials combining low-dose warfarin and aspirin (Stroke Prevention in Atrial Fibrillation III Investigators, 1996; Gullov *et al.*, 1998; Edvarson *et al.*, 2003).

PREVENTION OF THROMBOEMBOLISM AFTER VALVE REPLACEMENT
A randomized, multicenter clinical trial comparing the efficacy and safety of triflusal versus acenocoumarol for primary prevention of thromboembolism in the early postoperative period after implantation of a bioprosthesis was recently published (Aramendi *et al.*, 2005). Patients were assigned to treatment with triflusal (600 mg daily) or acenocoumarol (target INR 2.0–3.0). Study medication was started 24–48 hours after valve replacement with a bioprosthesis, and continued for 3 months. The primary endpoint was a composite of the rate of thromboembolism, severe hemorrhage and valve-related mortality. A total of 193 patients were included, with a mean age of 72.5 years. Aortic valve replacement was performed in 181 patients (93.8%), mitral valve replacement in 10 patients (5.2%) and double valve replacement in 2 (1.0%). Primary outcome was recorded in 9 patients with triflusal (9.4%) and in 10 patients with acenocumarol (11%) ($p = 0.79$). A total of 10 (10%) patients assigned to the acenocoumarol group reported at least one hemorrhagic adverse event as compared with three (3.1%) in the triflusal group ($p = 0.048$). Six episodes in the acenocoumarol group and three in the triflusal group were recorded.

TRIFLUSAL IN PATIENTS INTOLERANT TO ASPIRIN AND/OR NSAIDS
A single-blind placebo-controlled study to evaluate the tolerance to triflusal was performed in 26 asthmatic patients intolerant to aspirin and/or NSAIDs (Dela Cruz *et al.*, 2002). In visit 1 one placebo capsule was administered followed by two placebo capsules after 2 hours. Total doses of triflusal were 225 mg in visit 2 (one 75 mg capsule and two 75 mg capsules after 2 hours), 450 mg in visit 3 (one 150 mg capsule and two 150 mg capsules after 2 hours) and 900 mg in visit 3 (one 300 mg capsule and two 300 mg capsules after 2 hours). No patient presented intolerance to triflusal, defined as the appearance of respiratory, nasal, ocular or cutaneous symptoms and/or a decrease of 20% or more of forced expiratory volume in 1 second (FEV_1) or peak expiratory flow (PEF) with respect to the basal value.

PHARMACOEPIDEMIOLOGICAL STUDIES ASSESSING THE RISK
OF UPPER GASTROINTESTINAL BLEEDING
Two case-control studies evaluated the risk of upper gastrointestinal bleeding associated with non-aspirin cardiovascular drugs, analgesics and NSAID (Lanas *et al.*, 2003) and with antiplatelet drugs (Ibáñez *et al.*, 2006), respectively. In the first study (Lanas *et al.*, 2003), including 1122 cases and 2231 controls, triflusal was not associated with increased risk of upper gastrointestinal bleeding. In the

second study (Ibáñez *et al.*, 2006), including 2813 cases and 7193 controls, the individual risks of upper gastrointestinal bleeding for the studied antiplatelet agents were (OR; 95% CI) aspirin: 4.0 (3.2–4.9), clopidogrel: 2.3 (0.9–6.0), dipyridamole: 0.9 (0.4–2), ticlopidine: 3.1 (1.8–5.1) and triflusal: 1.6 (0.9–2.7). These results are compatible with those found in triflusal clinical trials.

Clinical Trial

The TAPIRSS study (Culebras *et al.*, 2004) was performed to explore the efficacy and safety of triflusal versus aspirin in the prevention of vascular complications in patients with a previous TIA or ischemic stroke in a Latin American population.

Subjects

Subjects older than 40 years with a diagnosis of TIA or established cerebral infarction within the previous 6 months were selected for the study. TIA was defined as an episode of reversible neurological deficit of ischemic origin lasting at least 15 minutes and resolving completely within a period of 24 hours or as three or more episodes of ischemic neurological deficit lasting <15 minutes within a period of 24 hours. Cerebral infarction was defined as a neurological deficit of rapid onset lasting >24 hours, attributable to a vascular event. Baseline confirmation of the qualifying event was required by either brain CT or MRI within 1 month after onset of symptoms. Qualifying cerebral infarctions were classified according to neuroimaging findings into lacunar (small-vessel), non-lacunar (large-vessel), and brainstem infarcts. Written informed consent was obtained prior to inclusion to the study.

Patients were excluded if they had disabling stroke (Oxford Scale score above 2 at the time of inclusion), brain hemorrhage, stroke of non-atherothrombotic cause, cardioembolic source of stroke (valvular prosthesis, atrial fibrillation, myocardial infarction within the last 4 months, or other embolic heart disease), a previous carotid endarterectomy or were awaiting one.

Other reasons for exclusion were cognitive impairment (Mini-Mental State Examination score of <22 at inclusion); renal or liver failure; moderate or severe heart failure; HIV infection; alcohol or drug abuse; active peptic ulcer; receiving unavoidable treatment with NSAID, anticoagulant or antiplatelet agents; malignancy with high bleeding risk; pregnancy; breast-feeding or childbearing potential; hypersensitivity to study drugs; inclusion in other clinical studies; inability to comply with study visits or unable to give informed consent; and life expectancy of <2 years.

Trial Methods

This was a multicenter, double-blind, randomized, parallel groups, pilot clinical trial. Patients were recruited at 19 hospital centers in Buenos Aires, Argentina.

To avoid interference with acute-phase treatments, patients were enrolled after 15 days from onset of the qualifying event. Patients were randomized to receive treatment with a daily single dose of either triflusal 600 mg or aspirin 325 mg. Both treatment forms were indistinguishable in color, shape, form and packaging. Study drugs were packed in blisters grouped in white boxes with 60 capsules each. Boxes were identified by a unique number according to randomization in blocks of 10. Both treatment products were manufactured by J. Uriach & Cía, S.A. (Barcelona, Spain).

The randomization schedule was computer generated and was kept unknown to all study-related personnel until closure of the database. The randomization system allowed centers to unblind treatment allocation in case of emergency. Medication was supplied to patients at each follow-up visit, and compliance was then assessed by asking patients at each follow-up visit whether they were taking the medication as indicated in the protocol. At each visit, non-compliance was defined as the use by the patient of <70% of the prescribed medication, unless early withdrawal occurred. Non-compliance with treatment protocol was determined in the event of failure to adhere to treatment in two consecutive follow-up visits.

Concurrent treatment for >10 days with anticoagulants, other antiplatelet agents or NSAID was not allowed during the study period. Concurrent medication consumption was investigated and recorded at each visit.

Patient treatment and follow-up extended from a minimum of 1 year to a maximum of 2 years from inclusion. Endpoint (see below) and safety assessments were done at each follow-up visit (1, 2, 3, 6, 9, 12, 15, 18, 21 and 24 months) following randomization. Baseline clinical assessments included neurological examination and recent neuroimaging brain study, NIH Stroke Scale (NIHSS), Oxford Handicap Scale, Mini-Mental State Examination, blood tests, ECG and chest radiographs. General and neurological examinations, including the NIHSS, were done at each visit. Blood tests and ECG were obtained 12 and 24 months after inclusion.

Withdrawal from the study was mandated for the following reasons: insufficient eligibility criteria identified after randomization, occurrence of serious adverse events possibly due to study drugs, concurrent treatment with drugs not allowed during the study for ⩾10 days, pregnancy, or if voluntarily requested. All patients withdrawn from the study were followed until the end of the 2-year period.

General coordination and centralized data management were carried out by the Clinical Stroke Research Center of Syracuse, NY. Computer data transmission via direct telephone link was performed twice weekly over the duration of the study, and monitors from Syracuse audited all Buenos Aires centers every 6 months. The study received favorable review from local research ethics committees and was authorized by the Argentinian Ministry of Health.

Primary and Secondary Outcomes

Primary endpoint was the first occurrence of the composite of either vascular death, non-fatal ischemic stroke, non-fatal AMI, or major bleeding, defined as follows: (1) vascular death attributable to stroke, myocardial infarction, congestive heart failure, systemic bleeding causing hemodynamic failure, or sudden unexpected cardiac death occurring within the first hour following appearance of symptoms or within the first 24 hours after a convincing vascular event; (2) non-fatal ischemic stroke manifested by a neurological deficit of rapid onset, with a duration of >24 hours, attributable to an ischemic cerebrovascular event; (3) non-fatal myocardial infarction defined as concurrence of at least two of the three items: (a) chest pain, (b) cardiac enzyme increases in blood twice above the upper limit of normal, (c) Q wave in a standard 12-lead ECG; (4) major bleeding defined as fatal bleeding, documented by convincing clinical manifestations or autopsy, gastrointestinal bleeding, cerebral bleeding, subdural hematoma, rupture of an aortic aneurysm, retinal bleeding, or any non-fatal bleeding requiring a hospital visit and treatment.

Secondary endpoints were the occurrence of each of the above events separately as well as the following: (1) episodes of minor bleeding not requiring hospitalization; (2) non-vascular death defined as death of any cause not included in the vascular death definition; (3) systemic thromboembolism characterized by spontaneous episodes of sudden vascular failure associated with clinical or radiological evidence of arterial occlusion.

Adjudication of a stroke diagnosis was based on neurological assessment and verified with CT or MRI. The initial determination was done by local investigators in Buenos Aires. A subsequent determination was made by the principal study medical coordinator in the Data Management Center of Syracuse, NY. In case of conflict, an Adjudication Committee was available made up of the safety monitor, the principal study medical coordinator, and two local investigators.

Analysis

The efficacy analysis was based on the ITT sample, defined as those patients with a confirmed qualifying event who took at least one dose of the study drug. If no follow-up visit was available, the patient was declared free of events with only 1 day of follow-up. Safety analysis included all patients who took at least one dose of study drug.

Survival curves were estimated with the Kaplan–Meier method, and differences were determined with the log-rank test. Incidences were described for each single event and compared between treatments by χ^2 or Fischer tests, OR were calculated for primary and secondary variables and 95% CI according to the Miettinen method when required.

Adverse events were coded according to the World Health Organization Adverse Reaction Terminology dictionary and analyzed by preferred term and system organ. The number of patients with at least one adverse event pertaining to each system organ was tabulated. Repeated adverse events pertaining to the same system and involving the same patient were recorded only once. Bleeding complications were studied separately and grouped by location of the hemorrhage. Incidences were compared by χ^2 or Fischer tests, as required.

Data listings, descriptive tables and statistical analysis were generated by the SPSS version 10.0 (Chicago, IL). All statistical tests were two tailed, with a significance level of 0.05.

Results

Patients were recruited between October 1996 and December 1997. Follow-up of the last patient was completed in November 1999 and the analysis was completed in July 2000.

A total of 431 patients were enrolled to receive either aspirin (216 patients) or triflusal (215 patients). The safety sample consisted of 430 patients who took at least one dose of study medication. In one patient the qualifying event was not confirmed and, thus, the efficacy sample was 429 patients (216 in the aspirin group and 213 in the triflusal group).

The eligible patients were predominantly men (68.3%) and had a mean age of 64.7 years. There were no significant differences in demographic characteristics, personal risk factors, or previous antiplatelet therapy between the two treatment groups. Recent ischemic stroke was the qualifying event for most cases (81.5% aspirin, 80.3% triflusal).

The duration of the follow-up period was similar for patients in the aspirin and triflusal groups (mean (SD) 580.3 (239.6) and 595.4 (229.1) days). The duration of the study treatment was also similar between groups (mean (SD) 579.5 (239.7) and 592.2 (232.3) days).

EFFICACY

There were 57 primary endpoints. No significant differences were observed between groups (30/216 (13.9%) in the aspirin group versus 27/213 (12.7%) in the triflusal group; OR: 1.11, 95% CI: 0.64 to 1.94, $p = 0.711$).

The analysis of secondary endpoints did not show significant differences between groups. However, the triflusal-treated group showed a favorable trend in hemorrhagic events, with an incidence of major hemorrhages of 7 patients (3.2%) in the aspirin group versus 1 patient (0.5%) in the triflusal group (OR: 7.1, 95% CI: 1.15 to 43.52, $p = 0.068$) and an incidence of minor hemorrhages of 13 patients (6%) in the aspirin group versus 5 (2.3%) in the triflusal group (OR: 2.66, 95% CI: 0.93 to 7.61, $p = 0.058$). Endpoints by treatment group are shown in Table 3.

In a post hoc analysis, all bleeding episodes, including first major and minor hemorrhages, were significantly more frequent in the aspirin group (OR: 3.13, 95% CI: 1.22 to 8.06, $p = 0.013$) (Figure 5). The gastrointestinal tract was the most frequently reported bleeding site, with a favorable trend toward fewer

Table 3. **Endpoints by Treatment Groups in Patients with Stroke or TIA in the TAPIRSS Study**

	TREATMENT				*p*-VALUE
	ASPIRIN (*N* = 216)		TRIFLUSAL (*N* = 213)		
Primary endpoint					
Combined primary endpoint	30	13.9%	27	12.7%	n.s.
Secondary endpoints					
Non-fatal cerebral infarction	16	7.40%	17	8.00%	n.s.
Non-fatal AMI	5	2.30%	4	1.90%	n.s.
Vascular death	8	3.70%	5	2.30%	n.s.
Major hemorrhage	7	3.20%	1	0.50%	0.068
Non-vascular death	5	2.30%	1	0.50%	n.s.
Overall mortality	13	6.00%	6	2.80%	n.s.
Minor systemic hemorrhage	13	6.00%	5	2.30%	0.058
Overall hemorrhage	18	8.30%	6	2.80%	0.013
Non-fatal systemic thrombo-embolism	2	0.90%	3	1.40%	n.s.

Culebras *et al.* (2004). *Neurology*, 62, 1073–1080.

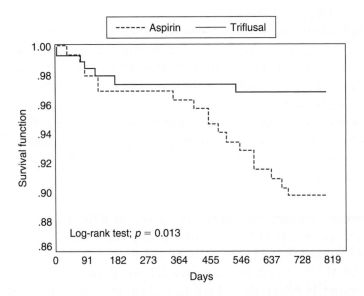

Fig. 5.
Overall hemorrhagic events in patients with stroke or TIA in the TAPIRSS study.
Culebras *et al.* (2004). *Neurology*, 62, 1073–1080.

episodes in triflusal treated patients (p = 0.062). Differences were particularly evident after the first year of follow-up.

SAFETY AND TOLERABILITY

Six hundred and ninety-two adverse events (358 aspirin, 334 triflusal) were reported by 248 patients, 127 (58.8%) had been assigned to aspirin and 121 (56.5%) to triflusal. Less than one half of adverse events were considered treatment related (35.7% in aspirin and 43.1% in triflusal). A total of 69 serious adverse events were reported (43 aspirin, 26 triflusal); 17 (14 aspirin, 3 triflusal) were considered treatment related. The most frequently reported were dyspepsia (three aspirin, none triflusal), angina pectoris (three aspirin, none triflusal), and cerebrovascular disorder (one aspirin two triflusal).

The most frequently affected body system was the gastrointestinal tract with an incidence of 30.1% (65 patients) in the aspirin group (related: 21.3%, 46 patients) and 34.6% (74 patients) in the triflusal group (related: 25.2%, 54 patients). However, only 13 (6%) patients in the aspirin group and 11 (5.1%) in the triflusal group interrupted their treatment because of gastrointestinal adverse events. This difference was not significant.

Unique Aspects of the Trial

The TAPIRSS study (Culebras *et al.*, 2004) was a pilot intercontinental study with the data management center located in Syracuse, NY, the study centers located in Buenos Aires and the data analysis center located in Barcelona. Results obtained were similar to those of the TACIP study (Matías-Guíu *et al.*, 2003), performed in an European population. This data allows to assume that results of future clinical trials in stroke performed in Buenos Aires can be valid for both American and European populations. Feasibilities for these studies are derived of the possibility to concentrate a big number of hospitals in a relatively small geographic area. The feasibility of clinical trials in Buenos Aires is enhanced by the concentration of a large number of hospitals and population in a relatively small geographical area.

Conclusions

In this pilot study differences between triflusal and aspirin in the prevention of vascular complications after TIA or ischemic stroke were not observed. Hemorrhagic risk is lower with triflusal than with aspirin.

Influence on the Field

How the Results Fit into the Secondary Prevention of Stroke

The TAPIRSS study (Culebras *et al.*, 2004) provided additional evidence of the efficacy and safety of triflusal for the secondary prevention of stroke and suggested that triflusal is a valid alternative to aspirin in the prevention of cardiovascular events in patients with ischemic stroke or TIA. It may add efficacy without increasing hemorrhagic risk when combined with other antithrombotic agents.

Translation to Clinical Practice

Influence on Clinical Guidelines

Triflusal should be included in the clinical guidelines of stroke treatment, as a valid alternative to aspirin, either alone or in combination with other antithrombotic agents, specially in patients with bleeding risk or aspirin intolerance.

Treatment Algorithm

ETIOLOGICAL EVALUATION
Appropriate blood tests.
Cardiac monitor and 12-lead ECG.
Carotid duplex and transcranial Doppler.
Transthoracic echocardiography.
Magnetic resonance imaging.
Magnetic resonance angiography (intracranial).
Hypercoagulable evaluation (if patients ≤55 years old).
Transesophageal echocardiography, if indicated.
Catheter angiography, if indicated.

TREATMENT
In all cases: control of risk factors

Non-cardioembolic Stroke or TIA (atherothrombotic, lacunar or cryptogenic)
Aspirin or triflusal or aspirin and extended-release dipyridamole.
Patients with moderate to high risk of bleeding: triflusal or clopidogrel.
Patients with allergy to aspirin: clopidogrel or triflusal.
Patients undergoing carotid endarterectomy: aspirin.
Patients with well documented prothrombotic disorders: oral anticoagulation may be considered.

Cardioembolic Stroke
Patients with atrial fibrillation: reduced intensity oral anticoagulation plus triflusal or oral anticoagulation.
Patients with stroke associated with aortic atherosclerotic lesions: antiplatelet therapy.
Patients with cryptogenic ischemic stroke associated with mobile aortic arch thrombi: oral anticoagulation or antiplatelet agents.
Patients with cryptogenic ischemic stroke and a patent foramen ovale: antiplatelet therapy.
Patients with mitral valve strands and prolapse: antiplatelet therapy.

Cerebral Venous Sinus Thrombosis

Heparin or low molecular weight heparin during the acute phase; then oral anticoagulation.

Summary

Therapeutic strategies for secondary stroke prevention are based on risk factor modification, surgical interventions and antithrombotic agents. The American College of Chest Physicians (Albers *et al.*, 2004) and the American Heart Association (Goldstein *et al.*, 2001) have published guidelines for the secondary stroke prevention. Aspirin has been considered the gold standard against which other antiplatelet agents have been measured. However, 21% of subjects will abandon treatment or develop adverse effects. The hemorrhagic complication is generally considered one of the most serious adverse effects with any adminis-tered dose of aspirin. Triflusal offers a therapeutic alternative for the secondary prevention of vascular events and may be considered appropriate for combined therapy with other antithrombotic agents. Factors related to tolerability, efficacy, toxicity and cost modulate the clinical use of all available antiplatelet agents and suggest that the quest to find a more efficacious agent should continue.

References

Acarin, L., González, B., & Castellano, B. (2002). Decrease of proinflammatory molecules correlates with neuroprotective effect of the fluorinated salicylate triflusal after postnatal excitotoxic damage. *Stroke*, 33, 2499–2505.

Albers, G.W., Amarenco, P., Easton, J.D., & Sacco, R.L. (2004). Antithrombotic and thrombolytic therapy for ischemic stroke. The seventh ACCP Conference on antithrombotic and thrombolytic therapy. *Chest*, 126, 483S–512S.

Albors, M., de Castellarnau, C., Vila, L., *et al.* (1987). Inhibition of thromboxane production and platelet function by triflusal in healthy volunteers. *Revista de Farmacología Clínica y Experimental* 4, 11–16.

Antiplatelet Trialist's Collaboration (1994). Collaborative overview of randomised trials of antiplatelet therapy. I. Prevention of death, myocardial infarction, and stroke by prolonged antiplatelet therapy in various categories of patients. *British Medical Journal*, 308, 81–106.

Antithrombotic Trialists' Collaboration (2002). Collaborative meta-analysis of randomised trials of antiplatelet therapy for prevention of death, myocardial infarction, and stroke in high risk patients. *British Medical Journal*, 324, 71–86.

Aramendi, J.I., Mestres, C.A., Martínez-León, J., *et al.* (2005). Triflusal versus oral anticoagulation for primary prevention of thromboembolism after bioprosthetic valve replacement (trac): prospective, randomized, co-operative trial. *European Journal of Cardio-Thoracic Surgery*, 27, 854–860.

Bayón, Y., Alonso, A., & Sánchez Crespo, M. (1999). 4-Trifluoromethyl derivatives of salicylate, triflusal and its main metabolite 2-hydroxy-4-trifluoromethylbenzoic acid, are potent inhibitors of nuclear factor κ B activation. *British Journal of Pharmacology*, 126, 1359–1366.

CAPRIE Steering Committee (1996). A randomised, blinded, trial of clopidogrel versus aspirin in patients at risk of ischaemic events (CAPRIE). *Lancet*, 1996, 348, 1329–1339.

Costa, J., Ferro, J.M., Matías-Guíu, J., Alvarez-Sabín, J., & Torres, F. (2005). Triflusal for preventing serious vascular events in people at high risk. *The Cochrane Database of Systematic Reviews 2005*, 3, Art. N.: CD004296.pub2. DOI: 10.1002/14651858.CD004296.pub.2.

Cruz-Fernández, J.M. (2001). Antiplatelet drugs in the treatment of acute coronary syndromes: focus on cyclooxigenase inhibitors. *European Heart Journal*, 3(Suppl. I), 123–130.

Cruz-Fernández, J.M., López-Bescós, L., García-Dorado, D., et al. (2000). Randomized comparative trial of triflusal and aspirin following acute myocardial infarction. *European Heart Journal*, 21, 457–465.

Culebras, A., Rotta-Escalante R., Domínguez, R., et al. (2004). Triflusal vs aspirin for prevention of cerebral infarction. *Neurology*, 62, 1073–1080.

Dela Cruz, G., Sorio, F., Pérez, I., et al. (2002). Estudio de seguridad del triflusal, en pacientes asmáticos con intolerancia a aspirina y/o AINES. *Revista de medicina de la Universidad de Navarra*, 14, 5–46.

De La Cruz, J.P., Pavía, J., García-Arnes, J., et al. (1998). Effects of triflusal and acetylsalicylic acid on platelet aggregation in whole blood of diabetic patients. *European Journal of Haematology*, 40, 232–236.

De La Cruz, J.P., Pavía, J., Bellido, I., et al. (1995a). Effects of triflusal and its main metabolite HTB on platelet interaction with subendothelium in healthy volunteers. *European Journal of Clinical Pharmacology*, 47, 497–502.

De La Cruz, J.P., Villalobos, M.A., García, P.J., et al. (1995b). Effects of triflusal and its main metabolite HTB on platelet interaction with subendothelium in healthy volunteers. *European Journal of Clinical Pharmacology*, 47, 497–502.

Diener, H.C., Cunha, L., Forbes, C., Sivenius, J., Smets, P., & Lowenthal, A. (1996). European stroke prevention study. 2. Dipyridamole and acetylsalicylic acid in the secondary prevention of stroke. *Journal of the Neurological Sciences*, 143, 1–13.

Domínguez, M.J., Vacas, M., Sáez, Y., et al. (1985). Effects of triflusal in patients with prosthetic valves. *Clinical Therapeutics*, 7, 357–360.

Edvarson, N., Juul-Moller, S., Omblus, R., & Pehersson, K. (2003). Effect of low dose warfarin and aspirin on stroke versus no treatment on stroke in a medium-risk patient population with atrial fibrillation. *Journal of Internal Medicine*, 254, 95–101.

Ferrari, E., Reboldi, G., Marenco, P., et al. (1996). Pharmacokinetic study of triflusal in elderly subjects after single and repeated oral administration. *American Journal of Therapeutics*, 3, 630–636.

García-Rafanell, J., Ramis, J., Gómez, L., et al. (1986). Effect of triflusal and other salicylic acid derivatives on cyclic AMP levels in rat platelets. *Archives Internationales de Pharmacodynamie et de Therapie*, 284, 155–165.

Goldstein, L.B., Adams, R., Becker, K., et al. (2001). Primary prevention of ischemic stroke: a statement for healthcare professionals from the Stroke Council of the American Heart Association. *Stroke*, 32, 280–299.

Guiteras, P., Altimiras, J., Arís, A., et al. (1989). Prevention of aortocoronary vein-graft attrition with low-dose aspirin and triflusal, both associated with dipyridamole: a randomized, double-blind, placebo-controlled trial. *European Heart Journal*, 10, 159–167.

Gullov, A.L., Koefoed, B.G., Petersen, P., et al. (1998). Fixed minidose warfarin and aspirin alone and in combination vs adjusted-dose warfarin for stroke prevention in atrial fibrillation: second copenhagen atrial fibrillation, aspirin and anticoagulation study. *Archives of Internal Medicine*, 158, 1513–1521.

Heye, N., Campos, A., Kannuki, S., et al. (1991). Effects of triflusal and acetylsalicylic acid on microthrombi formation in experimental brain ischemia. *Experimental Pathology*, 41, 31–36.

Ibáñez, L., Vidal, X., Vendrell, L., Moretti, U., & Laporte, J.R. (2006). Upper gastrointestinal bleeding associated with antiplatelet drugs. *Alimentary Pharmacology & Therapeutics*, 23, 235–242.

Lanas, A., Serrano, P., Bajador, E., Fuentes, J., & Sainz, R. (2003). Risk of upper gastrointestinal bleeding associated with non-aspirin cardiovascular drugs, analgesics and nonsteroidal anti-inflammatory drugs. *European Journal of Gastroenterology and Hepatology*, 15, 173–178.

Matías-Guíu, J., Ferro, J.M., Alvarez-Sabín, J., et al. (2003). Comparison of triflusal and aspirin for prevention of vascular events in patients after cerebral infarction. The TACIP study: a randomized, double-blind, multicenter trial. *Stroke*, 34, 840–848.

Matías-Guíu, J., Alvarez-Sabín, J., & Codina, A. (1997). Estudio comparativo del efecto del ácido acetilsalicílico en dosis bajas y el triflusal en la prevención de eventos cardiovasculares en adultos jóvenes con enfermedad cerebrovascular isquémica. *Revista de Neurologia*, 25, 1669–1672.

Mc Neely, W., & Goa, K.L. (1998). Triflusal. *Drugs*, 55, 823–833.

Patrono, C., Coller, B., Dalen, J.E., et al. (2001). Platelet-active drugs: the relationship among dose, effectiveness, and side effects. *Chest*, 119, 39S–63S.

Pérez-Gómez, F., Alegría, E., Berjón, J., et al. for the NASPEAF Investigators (2004). Comparative effects of antiplatelet, anticoagulant, or combined therapy in patients with valvular and nonvalvular atrial fibrillation. *Journal of the American College of Cardiology*, 44, 1557–1566.

Plaza, L., López-Bescós, L., Martín-Jadraque, L., et al. (1993). Protective effect of triflusal against acute myocardial infarction in patients with instable angina: results of a Spanish multicenter trial. *Cardiology*, 82, 388–398.

Ramis, J., Mis, R., Forn, J., et al. (1991). Pharmacokinetics of triflusal and its main metabolite HTB in healthy subjects following a single oral dose. *European Journal of Drug Metabolism and Pharmacokinetics*, 16, 269–273.

Ramis, J., Torrent, J., Mis, R., et al. (1990). Pharmacokinetics of triflusal after single and repeated doses in man. *International Journal of Clinical Pharmacology, Therapy, & Toxicology*, 28, 344–349.

Sánchez de Miguel, L., Montón, M., Arriero, M.M., et al. (2000). Effect of triflusal on human platelet aggregation and secretion: role of nitric oxide. *Revista Espanola DeCardiologia*, 53, 205–211.

Smirne, S., Ferini-Strambi, L., Cucinotta, D. (1994). Triflusal and prevention of cerebrovascular attacks: a double-blind clinical study versus ASA. *Journal of Neurology*, 241(Suppl. 1), S130.

Stroke Prevention in Atrial Fibrillation III Investigators (1996). Adjusted-dose warfarin versus low-intensity, fixed dose warfarin plus aspirin for high-risk patients with atrial fibrillation: Stroke Prevention in Atrial Fibrillation III randomised clinical trial. *Lancet* 1996, 348, 633–638.

Valle, M., Barbanoj, M.J., Donner, A., et al. (2005). Access of HTB, main metabolite of triflusal, to cerebrospinal fluid in healthy volunteers. *European Journal of Clinical Pharmacology*, 61, 103–111.

White, H.D., Gersh, B.J., & Opie, L.H. (2001). Antithrombotic agents: platelet inhibitors, anticoagulants and fibrinolytics. In: Opie, L.H., & Gersh, B.J. (eds.), *Drugs for the Heart* (5th ed.). Philadelphia: W.B. Saunders Company, pp. 273–322.

Whitehead, S., Cheng, G., Hachinski, V., & Cechetto, D.F. (2005). Interaction between a rat model of cerebral ischemia and β-amiloid toxicity. II. Effects of triflusal. *Stroke*, 36, 1782–1789.

Weisman, S.M., & Graham, D.Y. (2002). Evaluation of the benefits and risks of low-dose aspirin in the secondary prevention of cardiovascular and cerebrovascular events. *Archives of Internal Medicine*, 162, 2197–2202.

Progress in Neurotherapeutics and Neuropsychopharmacology, 3:1, 35–47 © 2008 Cambridge University Press
DOI: 10.1017/S1748232107000158   Printed in the United Kingdom

The Argatroban and tPA Stroke Study

Andrew D. Barreto

Department of Neurology, Stroke Division, The University of Houston-Texas, Houston, TX, USA;
Email: andrew.d.barreto@uth.tmc.edu

James C. Grotta

Department of Neurology, Stroke Division, The University of Houston-Texas, Houston, TX, USA;
Email: james.c.grotta@uth.tmc.edu

ABSTRACT

Background: The benefit of intravenous recombinant tissue plasminogen activator (rtPA) in acute ischemic stroke is related to clot lysis and arterial recanalization. Argatroban is a direct thrombin inhibitor that safely augments the benefit of rtPA in animal stroke models. However, human data on this combination are limited. *Design*: We report an update of the Argatroban tPA Stroke Study, an ongoing prospective, open-label, dose escalation, safety, and activity study of argatroban and rtPA in patients with ischemic stroke. The primary outcome was incidence of intracerebral hemorrhage; secondary outcome, complete recanalization at 2 h. After standard dose intravenous rtPA administration, a 100-µg/kg bolus of argatroban followed by infusion of 1 µg/kg per min for 48 h was adjusted to a target partial thromboplastin time of 1.75 times baseline. *Results*: Twenty patients with middle cerebral artery occlusions (including 13 men) have been enrolled, with a mean ± SD age of 61 ± 13 years. Baseline median National Institute of Health Stroke Scale score was 12.5 (range, 3–25). The mean ± SD time from symptom onset to argatroban bolus administration was 177 ± 56 min. Symptomatic intracerebral hemorrhage occurred in 2 patients, including 1 with parenchymal hemorrhage type 2. Asymptomatic bleeding occurred in 2 patients and there was 1 death. Recanalization was complete in 7 patients and partial in another 7, and reocclusion occurred in 4 within 2 h of rtPA bolus administration. *Conclusion*: The combination of low-dose argatroban and intravenous rtPA may be safe, and produce faster and more complete recanalization, but a larger cohort of patients is required to confirm this pilot study.

Key words: acute stroke, anticoagulation, argatroban, thrombin inhibitor, thrombolysis.

Correspondence should be addressed to: Andrew D. Barreto, MD, Department of Neurology, Stroke Division, The University of Houston-Texas, 6431 Fannin – MSB 7.128, Houston, TX 77030, USA; Ph: +1 713 500 7002; Fax: +1 713 500 0660; Email: andrew.d.barreto@uth.tmc.edu

Introduction

The thrombin inhibitor Argatroban (GLAXOSmithKline, Philadelphia, PA), directly and selectively inhibits the action of free and clot-associated thrombin (Tanaka *et al.*, 2004; Walenga, 2002; Investigator's Brochure for Argatroban, 2001) Argatroban is approved for treatment of heparin-induced thrombocytopenia. Safety has been demonstrated with and without thrombolytics or aspirin in patients with acute myocardial infarction (Wykrzykowska *et al.*, 2003; Moledina *et al.*, 2001; Arg-231 Clinical Study Report, 1999; Jang *et al.*, 1999). In animal stroke models, argatroban safely augments the benefit of recombinant tissue plasminogen activator (rtPA) by improving flow in the microcirculation, increasing the speed and completeness of recanalization, and preventing reocclusion (Morris *et al.*, 2001; Tamao *et al.*, 1997; Kawai *et al.*, 1995; Jang *et al.*, 1990; Tanaka *et al.*, 1987). Kobayashi & Tazaki (1997) gave argatroban to 60 stroke patients within 48 h of onset and found a significant improvement in neurological outcome compared with placebo. The Argatroban Anticoagulation in Patients with Acute Ischemic Stroke (ARGIS-1) study showed that argatroban (mean doses of 1.2 and 2.7 µg/kg per min) given within 12 h of ischemic stroke provides safe anticoagulation without an increase in intracerebral hemorrhage (ICH). No clinical benefit was observed but it should be noted that rtPA treatment was excluded (LaMonte *et al.*, 2004).

Intravenous (IV) rtPA is the only proven effective treatment for acute stroke patients, but it has limitations in efficacy and application. Fifty-seven percent of the patients in the National Institute of Neurological Disorders and Stroke (NINDS) rt-PA Stroke Study and 58% in the Second European-Australian Cooperative Acute Stroke Study (ECASS-II) failed to show a favorable clinical response (Hacke *et al.*, 1999; 1998; NINDS, 1995). The benefit of rtPA in acute stroke is linked to the speed and degree of clot lysis and artery recanalization (Labiche *et al.*, 2003; Alexandrov *et al.*, 2001; Demchuk *et al.*, 2001). However, only 20–30% of patients will have complete recanalization on transcranial Doppler imaging (TCD) within 2 h of IV rtPA therapy, as many as 60% will have only partial recanalization, and 34% of those with any recanalization will experience reocclusion (Alexandrov *et al.*, 2004a; Alexandrov & Grotta, 2002). Because of its short half-life, allowing careful titration of the anticoagulant effect, we hypothesized that argatroban might be safely added to full-dose IV rtPA. Further, we also hypothesized that the addition of argatroban to rtPA would increase recanalization rates and therefore increase clinical benefit.

Purpose

The primary purpose of this study was to assess the safety of combined argatroban and rtPA treatment in an ischemic stroke population as measured by the incidence of ICH. Symptomatic hemorrhage was defined as ICH present on cerebral computed tomography (CT) temporally related to a decline in neurological status and consistent with new or worsening symptoms in the judgment of the clinical investigator. We defined parenchymal hemorrhage type 2 (PH-2) as confluent bleeding occupying more than 30% of the infarct volume and causing significant mass effect (Fiorelli *et al.*, 1999). The secondary objectives of this study were to evaluate drug activity by determining the speed and completeness of arterial recanalization and reocclusion on TCD. We prospectively planned to compare our results with those of a control cohort from the previously reported Combined Lysis of Thrombus in Brain Ischemia Using Transcranial Ultrasound and Systemic tPA (CLOTBUST) trial (Alexandrov *et al.*, 2004b). This cohort received rtPA alone and underwent the same selection criteria and TCD monitoring of activity and safety as the patients in this trial (Alexandrov *et al.*, 2004c).

Methods

Design

The Argatroban tPA Stroke Study is a prospective single-arm, dose-escalation, safety, and activity study evaluating the rate of bleeding and successful recanalization with combined rtPA and argatroban administration in acute ischemic stroke. This was an open-label, noncontrolled study. Because this was designed to be the first ever exposure of patients with acute stroke to the combination of rtPA and argatroban, a prespecified group size of 15 patients was to be treated in phase 1 to obtain a preliminary assessment of safety. If the drug combination demonstrated adequate safety (described below), then continued enrollment would occur.

Subjects

Study subjects met the following inclusion criteria (1) age 18–85 years; (2) ischemic stroke symptoms with onset within 3 h; (3) demonstration of a clot causing complete or partial occlusion (Thrombolysis in Brain Ischemia (TIBI) flow grades of 0, 1, 2, or 3) identified by TCD before argatroban infusion in the middle cerebral artery (MCA) M1 (45- to 65-mm depth) or M2 (<45-mm depth of worst TIBI signals on TCD findings) segment; and (4) being eligible by NINDS criteria for IV rtPA treatment.

Exclusion criteria were (1) National Institutes of Health Stroke Scale (NIHSS) level-of-consciousness score of 2 or more; (2) baseline NIHSS total score less than 5; (3) baseline NIHSS total score of greater than 17 (modified to >15) for right hemisphere strokes and greater than 22 (modified to >20) for left hemisphere strokes; (4) preexisting disability with modified Rankin Scale score of 2 or more; (5) ICH or significant bleeding episode within the past 3 months; (6) stroke, myocardial infarction, pericarditis, intracranial surgery, or significant head trauma within 3 months; (7) alcohol or other substance abuse; (8) life expectancy of less than 3 months; (9) need for concomitant use of anticoagulants other than argatroban; and (10) participation in any investigational drug or device study within the past 30 days.

After informed consent was obtained from the patient or their legal representative and before starting argatroban treatment, all patients had blood drawn for complete blood cell and platelet counts and underwent measurement of activated partial thromboplastin time (aPTT), prothrombin time, and international normalized ratio. Other tests included electrolyte and liver function panels, urinalysis, measurement of serum β human chorionic gonadotropin level (in premenopausal women), electrocardiography, noncontrast brain CT, TCD, and evaluation of NIHSS and modified Rankin Scale score. All patients received standard rtPA dosing of 0.9 mg/kg (10% of the total dose given in 1 min and the remainder infused in 59 min). Next, argatroban was administered intravenously within 1 h of starting rtPA treatment initiated as an initial 100-μg/kg bolus over 3–5 min, followed by a continuous infusion of 1.0 μg/kg per min for 48 h adjusted to a mean ± SD target aPTT of 1.75 times baseline (±10%). A dosing algorithm was utilized so that standardized increments or decrements of argatroban infusion rate took place in response to the aPTT. The aPTT was monitored at baseline and 2, 6, 12, and 24 h after initiation of argatroban infusion; at the end of argatroban infusion; within 2–4 h of any adjustment in the argatroban infusion; and in the event of a major bleed. If major bleeding or symptomatic ICH was suspected, the infusion was terminated immediately. Major bleeding was defined as any overt bleeding associated with a fall in the hemoglobin level of 2 g/dl or more, requiring a blood transfusion. There was no delay in the start of IV rtPA treatment in any patient enrolled in this trial. Concomitant administration of other defibrinogenating agents, heparinoids, platelet glycoprotein IIb/IIIa inhibitors, other direct thrombin inhibitors, other thrombolytic agents, dextran, other anticoagulants, and antiplatelet agents was not permitted. Cerebral CT was performed at baseline, 48 h after the rtPA bolus administration, and at any neurological deterioration associated with an increase in the NIHSS score of 2 points more than baseline. Follow-up CT scans were interpreted by a treatment-blinded neuroradiologist. NIHSS scores were measured at 2, 24, and 48 h after rtPA bolus administration and any time of neurological deterioration. A modified Rankin Scale score, Barthel index, and Glasgow Outcome Score were obtained at 48 h and 7 days after rtPA bolus administration. A diagnostic TCD was initiated before administration of the rtPA bolus in order to confirm vessel occlusion. Brief vessel assessments (<1 min of ultrasound exposure) were performed at the start of argatroban infusion, and at 30, 60, 90, and 120 min and 24 and 48 h after rtPA bolus administration. Signals from the proximal, middle, and distal portions of the MCA were recorded. Proximal and middle portions were considered to represent the M1 segment of the MCA, and the distal portion the M2 segment. Arterial recanalization was determined with the use of the previously validated TIBI grading system (Alexandrov *et al.*, 2001; Demchuk *et al.*, 2001). Recanalization and reocclusion were determined from data using the most proximal portion of the MCA with the lowest qualifying TIBI score. Exceptions were that if flow was absent in a segment, the segment immediately proximal to it was used. If the flow grade was 3 in all segments, the most distal segment was used. Recanalization was defined as an increase in TIBI flow by 1 grade or more compared with baseline and an overall TIBI grade of 2 or more. Partial recanalization was defined as improvement of flow to grade 2 or 3. Complete recanalization was defined as improvement of flow to grade 4 or 5. Reocclusion was defined as a worsening of TIBI flow signals by 1 grade or more in sequential measurements (whether or not recanalization had occurred), with the following exceptions: TIBI grade 2 or 3 had to result in the disappearance of diastolic flow where it was previously present, that is, nonpulsatile flow (TIBI grade 0 or 1), and TIBI grade 4 or 5 had to decrease to a TIBI grade of 3 or less. A blinded central reader from the University of Texas–Houston Stroke Team interpreted all TCD waveforms.

This study was approved by the University of Texas–Houston Committee for the Protection of Human Subjects and an independent data and safety monitoring committee provided safety oversight. Two neurologists unaffiliated with the study reviewed the clinical record, case report forms, and CT findings of each patient. A prospective stopping rule mandated enrollment cessation if more than 2 symptomatic hemorrhages or PH-2 events occurred at any time during the enrollment of the first 15 patients. After the first 15 patients were enrolled, the results were compiled, analyzed, published (Sugg *et al.*, 2006), and sent to the FDA for their review. At their request, the current dose level sample size was repowered based on the data from the first 15 patients. It was determined that a total of 65 patients will enable us to be 90% certain that the true PH-2 rate was no higher than 10%.

When designing this study, we prospectively intended to compare our results with those of the control cohort from our previously reported CLOTBUST trial as a historical comparison group (Alexandrov *et al.*, 2004b). We used χ^2, Fisher exact, unpaired t tests and analysis of confidence (Stata statistical software; StataCorporation, College Station, Texas) to compare data within and between cohorts. A p value of <0.05 was considered statistically significant. All values are presented as mean $\pm$ SD or median.

Outcomes

From May 1, 2003, through July 16, 2007, 20 patients (including 13 men) have been enrolled, with a mean age of 61 ± 13 (median age, 59; range, 43–82) years.

All patients had MCA occlusions, including 50% in the M1 and 50% in the M2 segments, 60% in the left hemisphere, and 40% in the right hemisphere. The median baseline NIHSS score was 12.5 (range, 3–25) points, with 70% having a score of 10 points or more (Table 1). Time from symptom onset to rtPA bolus administration averaged 117 ± 48 min. Nineteen patients received the intended argatroban dose. Eleven of 19 patients (58%) received the argatroban before the end of the tPA infusion, while 8 (42%) experienced a minimal delay of 15 ± 15 min. One patient received only the argatroban bolus without the infusion, due to suspected hemorrhagic transformation, which was later not confirmed. The average time to argatroban bolus was 177 ± 56 (median, 156; range, 100–276 min). The average time to target aPTT was 528 ± 297 (median, 422; range, 139–1150 min); however, 9 (47%) of 19 patients had reached or exceeded the target range within 2 h. One patient never reached the target aPTT range. Symptomatic hemorrhage occurred in 2 (10%) of 20 patients (95% confidence interval, 2–33%). Treatment in 1 of these patients involved a protocol violation owing to a high baseline NIHSS score of 21 with right hemisphere MCA stroke. Despite the hemorrhage, his NIHSS score decreased to 16 at 7 days. In response to this patient's hemorrhage, on the recommendation of the data and safety monitoring board, the upper limit of the NIHSS score was reduced to 15 (right hemisphere) and 20 (left hemisphere) after the 10th patient was enrolled. The other patient with symptomatic hemorrhage also had PH-2 and a 7-day NIHSS score (15) that was unchanged from initial presentation (PH-2 incidence, 5%; 95% CI, 1–27%). Asymptomatic hemorrhage occurred in two patients and one death resulted from malignant cerebral edema. No patients experienced major bleeding requiring transfusion. At 7 days, the median NIHSS score was 4 (range, 0–19) points; median modified Rankin Scale score was 1.5 (range, 0–6); median Barthel index was 83 (range, 0–100); and median Glasgow Outcome Score was 4 (range, 3–5). There was a mean decrease (improvement) in NIHSS scores at day 7 by 5.7 ± 6.4 points ($p = 0.001$). Monitoring of recanalization with TCD was performed for the 19 patients who received the continuous argatroban infusion (Table 2). Of these, 7, 10, 13, 14, 18, and 18 patients achieved any recanalization at 30, 60, 90, and 120 min and 24 and 48 h, respectively. Complete recanalization occurred in 2, 4, 6, 7, 15, and 15 patients at the same time intervals, respectively. Two patients (15 and 17) experienced two separate partial recanalizations within the first 2 h (e.g. TIBI 0–2, then 2–3). Reocclusion occurred in 4 of 19 patients; 1 patient with early reocclusion had subsequent recanalization (patient 2).

Our results were compared with those from the CLOTBUST control group ($n = 63$) which received IV rtPA alone (Figure 1). Patient demographic characteristics were similar, but not identical, with 10 (50%) of 20 patients with M1- and 10 (50%) with M2-segment occlusion versus CLOTBUST findings of 44 (70%) of 63 patients with M1- and 19 (30%) with M2-segment occlusion

Table 1. Clinical Data for All 20 Patients

PATIENT NO./ SEX/AGE	RACE/ ETHNICITY	HEMISPHERE	NIHSS PRE-rtPA	NIHSS PRE-ARGATROBAN	NIHSS 7-DAY	mRS*	SYMPT ICH	PH-2	ASYMPT ICH
1/M/78	W	L	18	11	1	1	N	N	N
2/F/75	W	L	3	10	2	1	N	N	N
3/F/51†	AA	L	25	22	Died	Died	Y	Y	Y
4/M/77	AA	L	17	15	15	4	N	N	N
5/M/62	AA	L	13	16	15	4	N	N	N
6/F/55	H	R	9	9	2	0	N	N	N
7/M/52	W	R	18	18	5	3	N	N	N
8/F/58	A	R	21	21	16	4	Y	N	N
9/M/60	H	L	12	9	9	2	N	N	N
10/M/78	W	R	5	5	0	0	N	N	N
11/M/44	W	L	14	13	5	3	N	N	N
12/M/62	W	R	4	5	7	3	N	N	N
13/M/48	W	R	14	7	0	0	N	N	N
14/M/51	AA	R	14	13	4	0	N	N	N
15/F/81	W	L	7	6	1	1	N	N	N
16/F/82	W	L	12	3	0	1	N	N	N
17/F/64	H	L	12	11	19	5	N	N	N
18/M/43	H	L	16	8	18	5	N	N	N
19/M/46	AA	L	9	8	1	1	N	N	N
20/M/56	A	R	10	10	0	1	N	N	Y

Abbreviations: Asympt, asymptomatic; ICH, intracerebral hemorrhage; L, left; mRS, modified Rankin Scale score; N, no; NIHSS, National Institutes of Health Stroke Scale; PH-2, parenchymal hemorrhage type 2; R, right; Sympt, symptomatic; Y, yes.

*At 7 days.

†Patient 3 had cerebral edema.

Table 2. **TCD Data for All 20 Patients**

PATIENT NO./ SEX/AGE	MCA SEGMENT	RECANALIZATION		REOCCLUSION
		PARTIAL	COMPLETE	
1/M/78	Prox	NA	1 h	N
2/F/75	Mid	NA	1 h	1.5 h, then complete recanalization at 24 h
3/F/51[†]	Mid	24 h	N	N
4/M/77	Prox	1 h	1.5 h	N
5/M/62	Distal	NA	1.5 h	2 h
6/F/55	Distal	NA	24 h	N
7/M/52	Distal	NA	24 h	N
8/F/58	Prox	1.5 h	N	N
9/M/60	Mid	NA	30 min	2 h
10/M/78	Distal	2 h	24 h	N
11/M/44	Distal	NA	24 h	N
12/M/62	NA	NA	NA	N
13/M/48	Mid	30 min	24 h	N
14/M/51	Distal	30 min	2 h	N
15/F/81	Distal	1.5 h & 2 h	24 h	1 h
16/F/82	Mid	30 min	24 h	N
17/F/64	Mid	30 min & 2 h	N	48 h
18/M/43	Mid	N	N	N
19/M/46	Mid	NA	30 min	N
20/M/56	Prox	30 min	24 h	N

Abbreviations: MCA, middle cerebral artery; N, no; NA, not applicable; R, right; TCD, transcranial Doppler; Y, yes.
[†] Patient 3 had cerebral edema.

($p = 0.388$). The baseline NIHSS median score was 12.5 (range, 3–25; $\geqslant$10 in 14 [70%] of 20 patients) compared with the CLOTBUST control median score of 17 (range, 5–29; $\geqslant$10 in 52 [83%] of 63) ($p = 0.019$). The time from symptom onset to rtPA bolus administration averaged 117 ± 48 min in the present study versus 137 ± 32 min in the CLOTBUST controls ($p = 0.09$). Parenchymal hemorrhage type 2 occurred in 1 (5%) of 20 patients in the present study versus 3 (5%) of the 63 CLOTBUST controls, and symptomatic ICH occurred in 2 (10%) of 20 patients in the present study versus 3 (5%) of the 63 CLOTBUST controls. Recanalization rates by 2 h after treatment occurred more often in our study compared to CLOTBUST controls (14 [74%] of 19 patients versus 24 [38%] of 63, $p = 0.02$). However, the rate of complete recanalization was not significantly different between groups (7 [37%] of 19 argatroban patients versus 11 [17%] of 63 CLOTBUST controls, $p = 0.39$). Two-hour reocclusion rates were 21% (4 of 19 patients in our study) versus 22% (14 of 63 CLOTBUST controls).

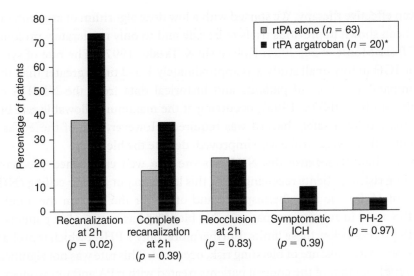

Fig. 1.
Outcome data in patients treated with argatroban combined with recombinant tissue plasminogen activator (rtPA) compared with rtPA alone. ICH indicates intracerebral hemorrhage; PH-2, parenchymal hemorrhage type 2. *For symptomatic ICH and PH-2, $n = 19$ for rtPA and argatroban.

Influence on the Field

This preliminary study highlights the potential hazards and possible benefits of argatroban therapy used in combination with rtPA in patients with acute stroke. The drug was chosen because of its multiple possible actions of increasing the speed and completeness of recanalization while improving flow in the microcirculation (Tanaka *et al.*, 2004; Walenga, 2002). In addition, safety has been demonstrated in combination with rtPA in both experimental models (Morris *et al.*, 2001; Jang *et al.*, 1990) and clinical cardiac trials (Wykrzykowska *et al.*, 2003; Arg-231 Clinical Study Report, 1999; Jang *et al.*, 1999). An advantage of argatroban compared with some other thrombin inhibitors is its short halflife, which allows rapid offset of action in case of bleeding, and the ease of monitoring its antithrombotic effect by means of the aPTT. Although, platelet glycoprotein IIb/IIIa antagonists or other antithrombotic agents such as heparin might also be used advantageously in combination with rtPA, none of these agents, including argatroban, have been shown to be useful when given as monotherapy in patients with acute stroke (Ciccone *et al.*, 2007; LaMonte *et al.*, 2004; TOAST Investigators, 1998). We chose the argatroban dose based on 2 considerations. We wanted to give standard dose rtPA so that patients would not be deprived of proven effective therapy. We started with a low dose algorithm of argatroban that had been shown in previous trials to be safe and to only moderately prolong the aPTT (LaMonte et al., 2004; Kobayashi & Tazaki, 1997). The rate of symptomatic ICH in this small study was approximately 1.5–2 times greater than that of a comparable cohort of patients and historical data from the NINDS rt-PA Stroke Study (NINDS, 1995), occurring at the maximum allowable rate before termination for a safety hazard was required. However, one of these was in a patient with a severe stroke who improved, despite the bleeding.

Nevertheless, because the NIHSS score is a well established predictor of bleeding risk in patients receiving rtPA, this led us to put a lower ceiling (NIHSS score of 15 for the right hemisphere and of 20 for the left) on the admission NIHSS score in subsequent patients. No bleeding has occurred in patients with NIHSS scores below these limits. Furthermore, only 1 PH-2, which is probably a more objective measure of bleeding risk, occurred. This rate was not significantly different from that of the control patients treated with rtPA and ultrasonography in the CLOTBUST group (Alexandrov et al., 2004b). Because of the small sample size, the 95% confidence interval for symptomatic ICH was 2–33%; for PH-2, 1–27%. To be 90% certain that the true PH-2 rate is less than 10%, we will need to enroll a total of 65 patients. This second phase is ongoing (www.clinicaltrials.gov).

Our safety and recanalization results can be compared with those of the control cohort of the CLOTBUST trial (Alexandrov et al., 2004b). The two studies share the same patient selection criteria and protocols for monitoring recanalization and safety (Alexandrov et al., 2004c), thereby providing us with a cohort of patients treated with rtPA only as a comparison group. As expected, we had similar patient populations; however, the argatroban cohort had a non-significant higher percentage of M2-segment occlusions. This difference in occlusion site could contribute to recanalization outcome because larger vessel occlusions are known to be more resistant to thrombolytic treatment. Furthermore, the strokes in the argatroban-treated patients were slightly less severe and were treated with rtPA earlier than in the CLOTBUST study, introducing additional bias in favor of argatroban. Our results showed a significant improvement in recanalization rates of 74% compared with 38% with rtPA alone. Furthermore, although not significant, we found higher complete recanalization rates at 2 h in 37% versus 17% of patients with rtPA alone. These findings will require a larger patient cohort to confirm.

We found no difference in reocclusion rates between the 2 groups. If argatroban increased the rate of recanalization, one would expect it would also prevent reocclusion. It is possible that failure to detect even a trend in this direction may be owing to the small number of patients experiencing reocclusion. Another explanation could be the prolonged time to achieve target levels of anticoagulation in

10 (53%) of the 19 patients. Future studies should evaluate a dosing algorithm that would result in a more consistent and rapid time to target aPTT. Other study limitations include possible selection bias, investigators nonblinded to treatment, historical controls, and a lack of long-term outcome data. However, these design characteristics are typical of small, pilot safety analyses and are offset by the potential patient benefits of new appropriately controlled and monitored therapies.

Relevant FDA Issues

Despite being approved as monotherapy for acute ischemic stroke within 48 h of symptom onset in Japan, argatroban only holds approval for anticoagulation in heparin-induced thrombocytopenia in the United States. As part of safety concerns in combination with rtPA, the FDA has required the additional enrollment of 50 patients at the current 1 μg/kg per min dose in order to be 90% certain that the true PH-2 rate is less than 10%. If the rates of hemorrhage are acceptable, we plan to request permission from the FDA to enroll another cohort of patients who will receive high dose argatroban (3.0 μg/kg/min) infusion for 48 h with a target aPTT of 2.25 times baseline.

Influence on Clinical Guidelines

Current stroke guidelines do not allow antiplatelets, antithrombotics, or anticoagulants until after 24 h from thrombolysis. Despite small numbers, our study provides preliminary evidence that anticoagulation with argatroban during this time frame may be safe. Whether this will lead to changes in the ischemic stroke guidelines will depend on larger cohorts of treated patients as well as double-blinded, randomized phase III trials.

Summary

In conclusion, argatroban in combination with IV rtPA may be safe and may produce faster and more complete recanalization than rtPA alone. Historical comparison described herein reveals the potential for clinical benefit, as well as the possibility of increased risk associated with the use of both drugs. Careful patient selection with moderately severe strokes may offset this risk. The next phase of the study, enrollment of a total of 65 patients in the open-label trial to ensure that hemorrhage rates are below 10%, is currently under way. Balancing the risk–benefit ratio of this combined therapy can ultimately be established only in an adequately powered, blinded clinical trial with appropriate interim monitoring for early benefit and harm.

Conflict of Interest

Dr. Grotta received grant support from Texas Biotechnology Corporation. Other officials of The University of Texas Health Science Center at Houston, not connected with this study, had equity interest in Texas Biotechnology Corporation.

References

Alexandrov, A.V., & Grotta, J.C. (2002). Arterial reocclusion in stroke patients treated with intravenous tissue plasminogen activator. *Neurology*, 59, 862–867.

Alexandrov, A.V., Burgin, W.S., Demchuk, A.M., El-Mitwalli, A., & Grotta, J.C. (2001). Speed of intracranial clot lysis with intravenous tissue plasminogen activator therapy: sonographic classification and short-term improvement. *Circulation*, 103, 2897–2902.

Alexandrov, A.V., Demchuk, A.M., Burgin, W.S., Robinson, D.J., & Grotta, J.C. (2004a). Ultrasound-enhanced thrombolysis for acute ischemic stroke, phase I: findings of the CLOTBUST trial. *Journal of Neuroimaging*, 14, 113–117.

Alexandrov, A.V., Molina, C.A., Grotta, J.C., *et al.* (2004b). Ultrasound enhanced systemic thrombolysis for acute ischemic stroke. *New England Journal of Medicine*, 351, 2170–2178.

Alexandrov, A.V., Wojner, A.W., & Grotta, J.C. (2004c). CLOTBUST: design of a randomized trial of ultrasound-enhanced thrombolysis for acute ischemic stroke. *Journal of Neuroimaging*, 14, 108–112.

Arg-231 Clinical Study Report (1999). *A Randomized, Single-Blind Study of Two Doses of Novastan Versus Heparin as Adjunctive Therapy to Recombinant Tissue Plasminogen Activator in Acute Myocardial Infarction: MINT Study.* Houston, TX: Texas Biotechnology Corporation.

Ciccone, A., Abraha, I., & Santilli, I. (2007). Glycoprotein IIb-IIIa inhibitors for acute ischemic stroke. *Stroke*, 38, 1113–1114.

Demchuk, A.M., Burgin, W.S., Christou, I., *et al.* (2001). Thrombolysis in brain ischemia (TIBI) transcranial Doppler flow grades predict clinical severity, early recovery, and mortality in patients treated with intravenous tissue plasminogen activator. *Stroke*, 32, 89–93.

Fiorelli, M., Bastianello, S., von Kummer, R., *et al.* (1999). Hemorrhagic transformation within 36 hours of a cerebral infarct: relationships with early clinical deterioration and 3-month outcome in the European Cooperative Acute Stroke Study I (ECASS I) cohort. *Stroke*, 30, 2280–2284.

Hacke, W., Kaste, M., Fieschi, C., *et al.* (1998). Second European-Australian Acute Stroke Study Investigators. Randomised double-blind placebo-controlled trial of thrombolytic therapy with intravenous alteplase in acute ischaemic stroke (ECASS II). *Lancet*, 352, 1245–1251.

Hacke, W., Brott, T., Caplan, L., *et al.* (1999). Thrombolysis in acute ischemic stroke: controlled trials and clinical experience. *Neurology*, 53, S3–S14.

Investigator's Brochure for Argatroban (2001). Houston, TX: Texas Biotechnology Corporation.

Jang, I.K., Gold, H.K., Leinbach, R.C., Fallon, J.T., & Collen, D. (1990). *In vivo* thrombin inhibition enhances and sustains arterial recanalization with recombinant tissue-type plasminogen activator. *Circulation Research*, 67, 1552–1561.

Jang, I.K., Brown, D.F., Giugliano, R.P., *et al.* (1999). A multicenter, randomized study of argatroban versus heparin as adjunct to tissue plasminogen activator (Tpa) in acute myocardial infarction: Myocardial Infarction with Novastan and TPA (MINT) study. *Journal of the American College of Cardiology*, 33, 1879–1885.

Kawai, H., Umemura, K., & Nakashima, M. (1995). Effect of argatroban on microthrombi formation and brain damage in the rat middle cerebral artery thrombosis model. *Japanese Journal of Pharmacology*, 69, 143–148.

Kobayashi, S., & Tazaki, Y. (1997). Effect of the thrombin inhibitor argatroban in acute cerebral thrombosis. *Seminars in Thrombosis and Hemostasis*, 23, 531–534.

Labiche, L.A., Al-Senani, F., Wojner, A.W., Grotta, J.C., Malkoff, M.A., & Alexandrov, V. (2003). Is the benefit of early recanalization sustained at 3 months? a prospective cohort study. *Stroke*, 34, 695–698.

LaMonte, M.P., Nash, M.L., Wang, D.Z., et al. (2004). Argatroban anticoagulation in patients with acute ischemic stroke (ARGIS-1): a randomized, placebo-controlled safety study. *Stroke*, 35, 1677–1682.

Moledina, M., Chakir, M., & Gandhi, J.P. (2001). A synopsis of the clinical uses of argatroban. *Journal of Thrombsis and Thrombolysis*, 12, 141–149.

Morris, D.C., Zhang, L., Zhang, Z.G., et al. (2001). Extension of the therapeutic window for recombinant tissue plasminogen activator with argatroban in a rat model of embolic stroke. *Stroke*, 32, 2635–2640.

National Institute of Neurological Disorders and Stroke rt-PA Stroke Study Group (1995). Tissue plasminogen activator for acute ischemic stroke. *New England Journal of Medicine*, 333, 1581–1587.

Sugg, R.M., Pary, J.K., Uchino, K., et al. (2006). Argatroban tPA stroke study: study design and results in the first treated cohort. *Archievs of Neurology*, 63, 1057–1062.

Tamao, Y., & Kikumoto, R. (1997). Effect of argatroban, a selective thrombin inhibitor, on animal models of cerebral thrombosis. *Seminars in Thrombosis and Hemostasis*, 23, 523–530.

Tanaka, K.A., Szlam, F., Katori, N., Sato, N., Vega, J.D., & Levy, J.H. (2004). The effects of argatroban on thrombin generation and hemostatic activation *in vitro*. *Anesthesia and Analgesia*, 99, 1283–1289.

Tanaka, Y., Kawabata, S., Sin, R., et al. (1987). Therapeutic effect of argatroban (MD-805), antithrombotic agent, in the acute stage of cerebral thrombosis. *Journal of Clinical and Therapeutic Medicine*, 3, 133–142.

The Publications Committee for the Trial of ORG 10172 in Acute Stroke Treatment (TOAST) Investigators (1998). Low molecular weight heparinoid, ORG 10172 (danaparoid), and outcome after acute ischemic stroke: a randomized controlled trial. *JAMA*, 279, 1265–1272.

Walenga, J.M. (2002). An overview of the direct thrombin inhibitor argatroban. *Pathophysiology of Haemostasis and Thrombosis*, 32(Suppl. 3), 9–14.

www.clinicaltrials.gov Identifier: NCT00268762. Accessed September 28, 2007.

Wykrzykowska, J.J., Kathiresan, S., & Jang, I.K. (2003). Clinician update: direct thrombin inhibitors in acute coronary syndromes. *Journal of Thrombsis and Thrombolysis*, 15, 47–57.

Progress in Neurotherapeutics and Neuropsychopharmacology, 3:1, 49–71 © 2008 Cambridge University Press
DOI: 10.1017/S174823210700002X   Printed in the United Kingdom

Use of Selegiline as Monotherapy and in Combination with Levodopa in the Management of Parkinson's Disease: Perspectives from the MONOCOMB Study[*]

Sven E. Pålhagen

Department of Neurology, Karolinska University Hospital, Huddinge, Stockholm, Sweden;
Email: sven.palhagen@karolinska.se

Esa Heinonen

University of Helsinki, Institute of Biotechnology, Helsinki, Finland; Email: esa.heinonen@helsinki.fi

ABSTRACT

The MONOCOMB study was a double-blind, randomized, controlled trial initiated to examine the impact of selegiline monotherapy on time to the start of levodopa therapy and, subsequently, to compare the progression of PD in patients treated with individualized levodopa plus selegiline or placebo.

Previously untreated patients with idiopathic PD (N 5 157) were randomized to receive selegiline 10 mg/day or placebo until levodopa was required; experimental medication was then withdrawn for 8 weeks. Patients were then randomized to levodopa (50 mg/day, titrated in 50 mg/day increments to 150 mg/day) plus either selegiline or placebo. Treatment was continued until patients required additional antiparkinsonian therapy or up to 7 years after initial randomization. The primary efficacy outcome for the monotherapy phase of the study was time to introduction of levodopa. Primary efficacy endpoints for the combined therapy phase were: time to development of fluctuations in disability; and time to the addition of supplementary antiparkinsonian treatment.

Selegiline significantly delayed the time when levodopa therapy became necessary during the monotherapy phase, although mean total UPDRS scores at time of initiation of levodopa were similar in both groups. Selegiline was also associated with improvements in PD symptom status and disability as reflected in a broad range of well-established indices. After the 8 week wash out period the disability of the clinical condition of the patients in the selegiline group was still significantly better in the selegiline group than in the placebo group.

*The MONOCOMB study was sponsored by Orion Corporation, Orion Pharma, Espoo, Finland.

Correspondence should be addressed to: Sven E. Pålhagen, Department of Neurology, Karolinska University Hospital, Huddinge, SE-141 86 Stockholm, Sweden; Ph: +46 8 585 800 00; Fax: +46 8 585 820 90; Email: sven.palhagen@karolinska.se

49

During the combination phase of the study, the use of selegiline as an adjunct to levodopa enabled a given degree of therapeutic effect to be achieved with a demonstrably lower total consumption of levodopa. Patients treated with selegiline plus levodopa also exhibited a distinct ($p = 0.005$) slowing in the anticipated increase in the UPDRS scores over time, as for example in a mean UPDRS total score after 5 years 10 points lower than in patients on levodopa and placebo. The emergence of motor (wearing-off) fluctuations was delayed by selegiline, and the proportion of patients experiencing these events was lower than with placebo (20% versus 34%; $p = 0.053$).

Mild gastrointestinal events were significantly more common with selegiline monotherapy than with placebo (12 versus 3; $p = 0.028$). The overall rates of AEs during the combination therapy phase were 69% in the selegiline group and 54% in the placebo group ($p = 0.053$). Significantly more patients in the selegiline group reported nausea. Of the five deaths that occurred during the combination therapy phase of the study (selegiline $N = 4$, placebo $N = 1$) none was expressly attributed to study medication.

The results of MONOCOMB, among the largest and longest-duration placebo-controlled studies to report experience with selegiline monotherapy in early-phase PD, confirm that selegiline is effective in retarding the progression of early PD, that it has levodopa-sparing qualities in more advanced disease, and that it is reasonably well-tolerated in long-term use.

Key words: controlled trial, levodopa, monoamine oxidase-B inhibitor, Parkinson's disease, selegiline.

Introduction and Overview

The selective monoamine oxidase (MAO)-B inhibitor selegiline has been used as monotherapy in the early phase of Parkinson's disease (PD) (The Parkinson Study Group, 1993; Tetrud and Langston, 1989; Myllylä et al., 1997; 1995; 1992), and in combination therapy with levodopa both in the early phase (Przuntek et al., 1999; Olanow et al., 1995; Presthus et al., 1987) and in fluctuating patients (Shoulson et al., 2002; Shan & Yeh, 1996; Golbe et al., 1988; Golbe & Duvoisin, 1987; Presthus & Hajba, 1983; Schachter et al., 1980; Rinne et al., 1978; Stern et al., 1978). Selegiline monotherapy in early PD has been reported to slow the progression of symptoms and delay the need for levodopa (Larsen et al., 1999) whereas its inclusion in early-phase combination therapy enables levodopa to be used at lower dose while maintaining or enhancing its clinical benefits (Przuntek et al., 1999; Olanow et al., 1995; Presthus et al., 1987). There are indications from clinical studies that selegiline may delay the time to the start of wearing-off fluctuations in patients receiving levodopa (Larsen et al., 1999; Lees, 1995; Myllylä et al., 1995) or ameliorate such effects (Shoulson et al., 2002; Shan & Yeh, 1996; Golbe & Duvoisin, 1987; Schachter et al., 1980; Rinne et al., 1978).

Methodological differences between earlier trials mean, however, that it is still uncertain whether the effects of selegiline can be explained by symptomatic relief or by a slowing of the progression of PD (or some combination of both). The MONOCOMB study was a double-blind, randomized, controlled trial initiated to examine this issue by investigating, first, the impact of selegiline monotherapy on time to the start of levodopa therapy and, subsequently, to compare the progression of PD in patients treated with individualized levodopa plus selegiline or placebo.

Selegiline: Pharmacology and Relevant Past Experience

Selegiline (also known by the older name of L-deprenyl) is an irreversible inhibitor of MAO-B and has, for many years, been the reference agent of this class of drugs. Originally developed as a possible treatment for depression, the drug in fact exhibits no relevant activity in that condition when used at the low (≤ 10 mg/day) doses effective in the treatment of PD. The inhibition of MAO-B that is the basis of selegiline's efficacy in PD appears to reside in the parent drug and its principal metabolite, desmethylselegiline (DMS). Selegiline has been credited, on the basis of preclinical observations, with a range of effects described under the umbrella term of neuroprotective (Hara *et al.*, 2006; Saravanan *et al.*, 2006; Kim *et al.*, 2004; Magyar & Szende, 2004; Muralikrishnan *et al.*, 2003; Tatton *et al.*, 2003; Matsubara *et al.*, 2001; Szende *et al.*, 2001; Naoi *et al.*, 2000a, b), though the relevance of these actions to its clinical applications in PD remains uncertain, in part because it has proven difficult to differentiate accurately symptomatic and possible neuroprotective effects. It has been conjectured that the metabolism of selegiline to L-methamphetamine (and of DMS to L-amphetamine) may have an adverse influence on the safety of the drug, but observations in humans do not sustain this conjecture (Heinonen, 1995).

Evaluation of selegiline in PD has been extensive and includes a series of 12 controlled trials of efficacy in patients with early PD (excluding MONOCOMB) (Ives *et al.*, 2004). Of these, four were long-term, placebo-controlled studies of selegiline monotherapy (Kirollos *et al.*, 1996; Allain *et al.*, 1993; Parkinson Study Group, 1993; Tetrud & Langston, 1989) and seven were studies of selegiline (with or without levodopa) versus levodopa alone (or with placebo) (Caraceni & Musicco, 2001; Larsen *et al.*, 1999; Przuntek *et al.*, 1999; Pålhagen *et al.*, 1998; Lees, 1995; Myllylä *et al.*, 1995; Olanow *et al.*, 1995). The remaining investigation was a placebo-controlled comparison of selegiline versus selegiline plus bromocriptine as part of a factorial study design (Olanow *et al.*, 1995). Collective insights from these studies were that use of selegiline delayed the need for the introduction of levodopa and reduced levodopa dosage (Ives *et al.*, 2004). Use of selegiline was also associated with a meaningful reduction in the likelihood of motor fluctuations during levodopa therapy, while having no effect on dyskinesias. The same pooled analysis (Ives *et al.*,

2004) appears to refute an earlier report that use of selegiline plus levodopa in early PD was associated with increased overall mortality (Lees, 1995; see also Macleod *et al.*, 2005; Olanow *et al.*, 1998).

Clinical Trial

Subjects

A cohort of 157 previously untreated patients with idiopathic PD were enrolled in the first phase of MONOCOMB at 10 centers in Sweden (Pålhagen *et al.*, 1998). Exclusion criteria included: secondary parkinsonism; dementia; unstable pulmonary, hepatic, renal, or gastrointestinal disease; major psychiatric disorders; evidence of severe heart disease; malignant disease (except for basal cell carcinoma of the skin or treated in situ carcinoma of the uterine cervix); age >75 years at inclusion; known allergy to selegiline or quinine (a component of the placebo tablet); pregnancy or breast feeding; known drug or alcohol abuse; or logistic obstacles to protocol-specified follow-up (Pålhagen *et al.*, 1998).

Trial Methods

The design of the trial is depicted in Figure 1. In the first phase of the study patients were randomized to selegiline 10 mg/day or placebo. Selegiline dosage was maintained at 10 mg/day throughout the study. Monotherapy was continued until the patient's clinical status warranted the introduction of levodopa. At that point, experimental medication was withdrawn for 8 weeks, during which time investigators and patients remained unaware of treatment assignments. Patients were then randomized to levodopa plus either selegiline or placebo. Levodopa was initiated

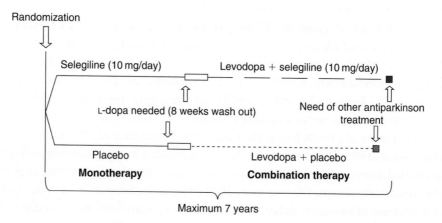

Fig. 1.
The randomized double-blind mono- and combination therapy trial design (MONOCOMB). The length of the combination therapy phase depended on the length of the monotherapy phase so that the maximum length of the trial was 7 years for each patient.

at a dose of 50 mg/day (plus 12.5 mg benserazide), with uptitration in 50 mg/day increments over the next 2 weeks. Levodopa 150 mg/day was then maintained for a further 2 weeks, after which dosage was adjusted as required by the patient's clinical condition. Treatment was then continued until patients needed additional antiparkinsonian therapy or up to a maximum of 7 years from the initial randomization. Additional drugs were introduced when satisfactory disease control required more than eight doses or 1000 mg of standard levodopa within a 24-hour period.

The conduct of the study conformed to the recommendations of the World Medical Assembly Declaration of Helsinki. The study protocol and amendments were submitted to and approved by the local Ethics Committees. Informed consent was obtained from each patient before entry into the trial.

Outcome Measures

The primary efficacy outcome for the monotherapy phase of the study was time to introduction of levodopa. The primary efficacy endpoints of the combined therapy phase were: (1) time to development of fluctuations in disability, defined as wearing-off in the efficacy of levodopa therapy in patients taking levodopa four times a day. This definition had to be fulfilled at two consecutive contacts; (2) time to the addition of supplementary antiparkinsonian treatment. Patients requiring these medications were considered to have reached the termination point of the study and were withdrawn from further evaluation.

Secondary efficacy variables included assessment of the progression of clinical disability using the Unified Parkinson's Disease Rating Scale (UPDRS, total and parts II and III during "ON" phase) (Lang & Fahn, 1989), modified Hoehn and Yahr staging (Hoehn & Yahr, 1967), and patient self-assessment of tremor and motor dysfunction using a 100-mm visual analog scale (VAS) (Ganz, 1990).

From the UPDRS scores, the cardinal symptoms of the disease (rigidity (UPDRS item 22), bradykinesia and hypokinesia (UPDRS item 31), and tremor (combining UPDRS items 16, 20 and 21)) were analyzed separately. Dyskinesias (UPDRS item 32) were considered to be present if a patient had a score of ≥ 1 on a 0–4 scale in which 0 = no dyskinesia and 4 = dyskinesia during most waking hours. The Mini-Mental State Examination (MMSE) (Folstein *et al.*, 1975) and the Hamilton Depression Scale (HDS) (Hamilton, 1960) were used for the determination of cognitive decline and depression.

Secondary endpoints of the combination phase were as for the initial phase of monotherapy.

Adverse reactions, cardiovascular vital signs and standard laboratory investigations were recorded at each follow-up visit.

Analysis

The risks of developing wearing-off fluctuations and dyskinesias or reaching the termination point of the study were compared using Kaplan–Meier methodology, log-rank tests and a Cox proportional hazards regression model (hazard ratio). The daily dose of levodopa, UPDRS total and subscores, VAS subscores, and safety and laboratory variables were tested with ANCOVA for an incomplete, repeated measures design, with treatment group (selegiline or placebo), center and visit as between factors, and time (months 3–78) as the within factor. Additionally, one-way ANCOVAs were performed for the 12-, 48- and 78-month visits, controlling for baseline values. The non-parametric Wilcoxon's rank sum test was used to test between-group differences in the modified Hoehn and Yahr staging, MMSE and HDS. The frequencies of patients with wearing-off fluctuations and dyskinesia, of patients reaching the termination point, and of adverse events (AEs) were tested with chi-square or Fisher's exact test, as appropriate.

Results

Randomization produced two broadly comparable groups of patients during both phases of the study (Table 1). Such differences as existed were mostly small, not statistically significant and tended to favor the placebo group (Table 1). The overall deterioration in patients' PD symptom status is apparent in the changes in scores for the various indices between the start of the study and entry into the phase of combination therapy (Table 1). Patient disposition during the trial is illustrated in Figure 2.

Monotherapy Phase

Mean total UPDRS scores at time of initiation of levodopa were similar in both groups but selegiline therapy was associated with a statistically significant 4-month extension of the median time to start of levodopa therapy (Figure 3); during this interval, moreover, the mean rate of deterioration in total UPDRS score (and several other subindices) was significantly lower in patients who received selegiline (Table 2). At 6 and 12 weeks, use of selegiline was associated with reductions in average scores for all PD symptom indices examined, whereas all scores increased (i.e. worsened) in the placebo group ($p \leq 0.05$ for 9/12 comparisons). Treatment effects on changes in severity of disability during the first 6 months of the study was significantly in favor of selegiline on the UPDRS total score scale and motor scale (both $p < 0.001$) and with complementary but not statistically significant trends in other indices. Scores at 12 months favored selegiline monotherapy but were not statistically robust due to small patient numbers.

MMSE and HDS scores did not alter greatly during the monotherapy phase and no robust inter-group differences were identified.

Inter-Phase Wash-Out

All symptom scores deteriorated in both patient groups during the 8-week wash-out. In most instances the numerical change in the selegiline group exceeded that

Table 1. **Summary (Mean ± SD) of the Baseline Characteristics at the Start of the Trials and at Commencement of the Combination Therapy Phase**

MONOTHERAPY PHASE

VARIABLE	SELEGILINE N = 81	PLACEBO N = 76
Age (years)	63.3 ± 9.1	64.2 ± 6.6
Male/female	49/32	44/32
Duration (years) of PD	1.9 ± 1.6	1.9 ± 1.3
UPDRS total score	23.6 ± 11.1	20.6 ± 10.9
UPDRS motor score	16.7 ± 8.8	14.2 ± 8.6
Schwab and England score	89.1 ± 6.2	89.6 ± 6.4
VAS, motor dysfunction score	30.7 ± 23.1	25.0 ± 19.4
VAS, tremor score	33.5 ± 19.8	30.8 ± 25.1
MMSE score	28.5 ± 1.6	28.7 ± 1.8
HDS score	2.4 ± 3.5	2.6 ± 3.6

COMBINATION PHASE[a]

VARIABLE	SELEGILINE N = 71 (N = 20)	PLACEBO N = 69 (N = 28)
Age (years)[b]	62.7 ± 9.4 (62.0 ± 9.5)	64.2 ± 6.6 (65.5 ± 5.3)
Male/female	43/28 (10/10)	42/27 (16/12)
Duration (years) of PD	3.0 ± 1.6 (2.5 ± 1.3)	2.9 ± 1.3 (2.9 ± 1.0)
UPDRS total score	34.9 ± 11.8 (30.4 ± 11.3)	34.4 ± 13.4 (32.8 ± 13.0)
UPDRS motor score	24.4 ± 9.7 (20.9 ± 8.7)	23.4 ± 10.4 (22.0 ± 10.0)
UPDRS ADL score	9.8 ± 3.3 (8.7 ± 3.6)	9.7 ± 3.6 (9.4 ± 3.3)
VAS, motor dysfunction score	48.7 ± 21.7 (45.3 ± 23.3)	48.3 ± 23.4 (45.8 ± 21.8)
VAS, tremor score	48.0 ± 22.8 (46.6 ± 20.4)	49.6 ± 24.2 (47.0 ± 23.0)
MMSE score	29.2 ± 1.5 (29.6 ± 0.8)	29.2 ± 1.4 (29.1 ± 1.5)
HDS score	2.5 ± 3.7 (3.1 ± 5.1)	2.7 ± 3.5 (3.1 ± 3.4)

[a]Upper figures denote all patients randomized; data in parentheses pertain to those patients still in the study at 60-week follow-up.
[b]At start of the monotherapy phase.

in the placebo group, but the numerical differences were small and not significantly significant. Average progression of UPDRS score from baseline to the *start* of the inter-phase wash-out was significantly slower with selegiline than with placebo (7.5 ± 8.4 versus 10.6 ± 9.6; $p = 0.042$). Average progression of UPDRS scores from baseline to the *end* of the wash-out phase, examined with time to endpoint as

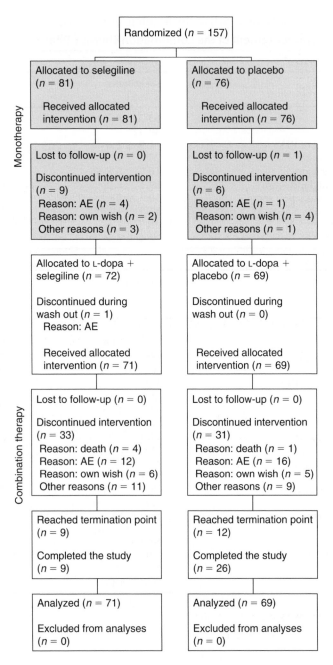

Fig. 2.
Disposition of patients in the monotherapy (lightly shaded) and combination therapy parts of the study.

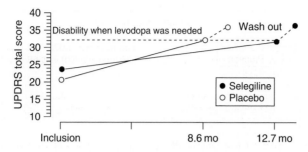

Fig. 3.

The rate of progression of clinical disability in the monotherapy phase of MONOCOMB was significantly lower in patients randomly assigned to selegiline than in placebo-treated peers. Disability scores at time of inception of levodopa therapy were similar in both sets of patients. The clinical condition of the selegiline-treated patients did not deteriorate to the level of the placebo group during the inter-phase washout. Instead the difference in disability in favor of selegiline was maintained during that 8-week period (from Pålhagen *et al.*, 1998).

Table 2. **Semiannual and Annual Rate of Disease Progression in Patients Treated with Selegiline or Placebo. A Negative Score Indicates an Improvement (Except for the MMSE Score)**

MEASURE	6-MONTH INTERVAL (MEAN ± SD)		12-MONTH INTERVAL (MEAN ± SD)	
	SELEGILINE ($N = 57$)	PLACEBO ($N = 39$)	SELEGILINE ($N = 37$)	PLACEBO ($N = 24$)
UPDRS total score	-1.9 ± 6.3	3.5 ± 6.4^a	1.2 ± 7.7	3.8 ± 8.5
UPDRS mental score	-0.4 ± 1.1	0.1 ± 1.1	-0.1 ± 0.9	0.3 ± 1.3
UPDRS ADL score	0.0 ± 2.1	0.9 ± 2.4	0.5 ± 2.4	0.8 ± 2.3
UPDRS motor score	-1.5 ± 4.7	2.5 ± 4.4^a	0.7 ± 6.1	2.6 ± 6.8
VAS, tremor score	-2.3 ± 21.5	5.9 ± 19.3	0.8 ± 20.0	2.9 ± 12.3
VAS, motor dysfunction score	1.0 ± 23.4	3.9 ± 15.0	3.7 ± 20.3	8.5 ± 16.3
MMSE score	0.7 ± 1.4	0.4 ± 1.4	0.5 ± 1.2	0.3 ± 1.8

$^a p < 0.001$.

a covariate, was also significantly slower with selegiline than with placebo (11.3 ± 9.1 versus 14.2 ± 10.9; $p = 0.033$).

Combination Therapy Phase

Fifty-five of the 140 patients (39%) who took part in the combination phase completed 7 years of follow-up. Twenty-one of the other 85 participants reached the prespecified termination point and 64 dropped out prematurely (Figure 2). There was no significant between-group difference in the percentage of patients

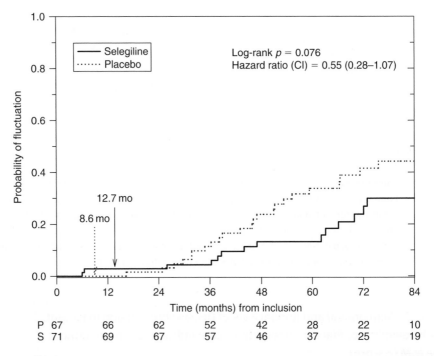

Fig. 4.
Kaplan–Meier curves for the cumulative probability of developing wearing-off fluctuations. The time covers both monotherapy and combination therapy phases (see Methods section). Number of patients at risk at the beginning of each year (P = placebo, S = selegiline) is shown below the x-axis. The arrows point to the median time from inclusion to the end of monotherapy/start of the 8-week washout before combination therapy.

completing 7 years of follow-up or reaching the termination point, nor in the time to termination from the initiation of the study (hazard ratio [95% CI] = 0.41 [0.28–1.69], $p = 0.41$).

Thirty-seven patients experienced fluctuations (placebo 34% versus selegiline 20%; $p = 0.053$). There was a trend for selegiline to delay the start of wearing-off fluctuations ($p = 0.076$, hazard ratio 0.55, 0.28–1.07); the quartile time was 72.0 months with selegiline and 50.9 months with placebo (Figure 4). The median time could not be estimated because fewer than 50% of patients reached this endpoint.

A total of 52 patients (37%) developed dyskinesias. Neither the proportions of patients developing dyskinesias (selegiline 35%, placebo 40%) nor the time to onset differed significantly between the treatment groups ($p > 0.5$).

As anticipated, patients in both treatment groups experienced an initial improvement in measures of PD-related disability following the initiation of levodopa. However, the trajectory of subsequent deterioration was more pronounced in the placebo group than in selegiline-treated patients and the mean total UPDRS

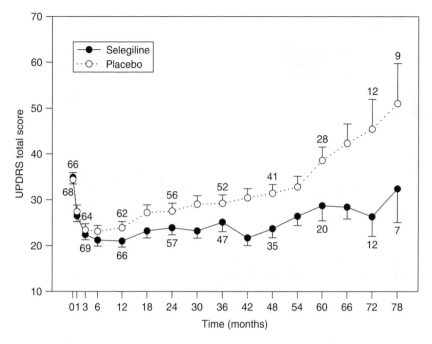

Fig. 5.
Mean (standard error) total UPDRS score ("ON" phase) for patients with PD treated with selegiline or placebo in addition to levodopa during 78 months of follow-up (ANCOVA, controlling for baseline, center and visit, treatment, $p = 0.003$; treatment $\times$ time, $p = 0.12$).

score during follow-up worsened noticeably more in the placebo group than in the selegiline group (Figure 5). In fact, the mean score among selegiline-treated patients at the end of follow-up was lower than at the start of the combination therapy phase whereas the final mean score in the placebo group was some 40% higher than that at the commencement of levodopa therapy.

By year 4 of follow-up the difference in mean total UPDRS score was more than 6 points, in favor of selegiline ($p = 0.003$; Table 3). Between-group comparisons at and beyond 5 years were numerically even larger but not statistically significant because too few patients remained in the study. A similar trend was evident for the UPDRS mean motor score (Figure 6a) and activities of daily living (ADL) (Figure 6b).

Patients treated with selegiline had better mean scores for tremor ($p = 0.0002$ versus placebo), bradykinesia ($p = 0.007$) and rigidity ($p = 0.018$) than those who received placebo. In time point analyses, there was a significant difference between the treatments for tremor and bradykinesia, but not for rigidity (Table 3). For rigidity, the between-group difference increased with time ($p = 0.037$ for time $\times$ treatment interaction). The mean score for the VAS tremor subscale was significantly lower with selegiline than with placebo ($p = 0.005$); mean scores for

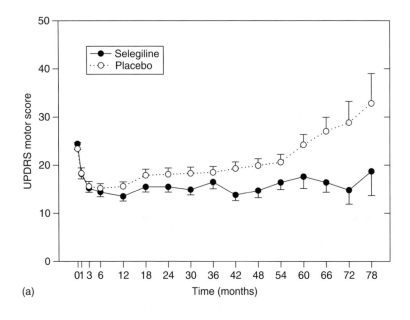

(a)

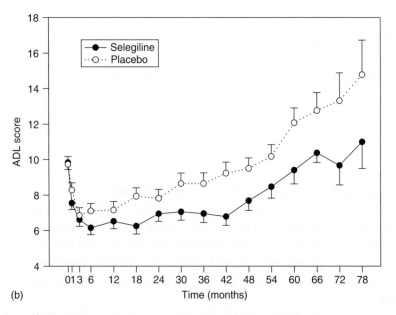

(b)

Fig. 6.
(a) Mean (standard error) motor UPDRS score ("ON" phase) for patients with PD treated with selegiline or placebo in addition to levodopa during 78 months of follow-up (ANCOVA, controlling for baseline, center and visit, treatment, $p = 0.002$; treatment $\times$ time, $p = 0.045$). Number of patients as in Figure 5. (b) Mean (standard error) ADL UPDRS score ("ON" phase) for patients with PD treated with selegiline or placebo in addition to levodopa during 78 months of follow-up (ANCOVA, controlling for baseline, center and visit, treatment, $p = 0.0002$; treatment $\times$ time, $p < 0.0001$). Number of patients as in Figure 5.

Table 3. **Mean ± Standard Deviation for UPDRS and VAS Scores, and Daily Levodopa Dose in Patients Treated with Selegiline Levodopa and Placebo and Levodopa After 12, 48 and 60 Months on Treatment**

	12-MONTH INTERVAL		48-MONTH INTERVAL		60-MONTH INTERVAL	
	SELEGILINE (N = 66)	PLACEBO (N = 62)	SELEGILINE (N = 35)	PLACEBO (N = 41)	SELEGILINE (N = 19)	PLACEBO (N = 28)
UPDRS total score	21.0 ± 10.7	23.9 ± 10.7	23.7 ± 11.6[b]	31.4 ± 12.6	28.7 ± 14.7	38.6 ± 15.5
Tremor (items 16, 20, 21)	2.72 ± 0.26[a]	4.05 ± 0.41	2.58 ± 0.48[a]	3.65 ± 0.46	1.86 ± 0.42[a]	4.03 ± 0.60
Bradykinesia (item 31)	1.16 ± 0.09[b]	1.48 ± 0.09	1.25 ± 0.15[b]	1.58 ± 0.13	1.29 ± 0.21[b]	1.90 ± 0.15
Rigidity (item 22)	2.24 ± 0.24	2.35 ± 0.27	2.61 ± 0.51	3.42 ± 0.39	2.95 ± 0.73	3.97 ± 0.57
UPDRS ADL score	6.52 ± 3.4	7.2 ± 3.8	7.7 ± 3.3[a]	9.5 ± 3.8	9.4 ± 3.4[a]	12.1 ± 4.5
VAS, motor dysfunction score	34.5 ± 22.4	32.6 ± 21.6	37.7 ± 22.5	41.0 ± 19.3	41.2 ± 20.8	49.1 ± 16.8
VAS, tremor score	30.9 ± 21.6	37.3 ± 24.5	29.7 ± 22.2[b]	42.1 ± 25.3	25.7 ± 20.9[a]	39.2 ± 22.7
Levodopa dose (mg/day)	327.6 ± 114.6	343.0 ± 113.0	448.6 ± 150.7[b]	552.3 ± 161.8	529.0 ± 145.6[c]	631.0 ± 186.3

[a] $p < 0.05$, [b] $p < 0.01$, [c] $p < 0.001$.

the motor dysfunction subscale did not differ ($p = 0.86$) (Table 3). There was no difference between treatment groups for effects on the MMSE ($p = 0.74$) but the HDS mean scores were consistently lower for selegiline than for placebo, and this difference increased with time (treatment, $p = 0.016$; treatment × time, $p = 0.0001$).

Daily levodopa requirements were consistently lower in selegiline-treated patients than in those who received placebo, and the difference between groups increased with time, reaching nearly 100 mg/day after 4 years (Table 3).

Tolerability and Safety

AEs most frequently recorded during the monotherapy phase were gastrointestinal, psychiatric or urogenital. Mild gastrointestinal events were significantly more common in the selegiline group (12 versus 3; $p = 0.028$). Other events occurred with similar frequency in both groups. No serious AEs were recorded and no patients died during the monotherapy phase of the trial. Heart rate was approximately 4 beats/min higher in the selegiline group than in the placebo group at 6 weeks and 6 months ($p \leq 0.04$). Arterial blood pressure was similar in both groups during monotherapy; during the subsequent washout, pressures rose 1–2 mmHg more in the selegiline group ($p = 0.002$ for diastolic blood pressure; not significant for systolic blood pressure) but the clinical relevance of these results was considered small.

The overall rates of AEs during the combination therapy phase were 69% in the selegiline group and 54% in the placebo group ($p = 0.053$). Significantly more patients in the selegiline group reported nausea (Table 4). There were no significant between-group differences for other frequently reported AEs (Table 4). Twenty-eight of the 64 patients who dropped out of the study were withdrawn because of an AE (selegiline $n = 12$, placebo $n = 16$). AEs were most usually psychiatric ($n = 9$) or gastrointestinal ($n = 9$).

Table 4. **Number (%) of Patients in the Two Treatment Groups Reporting Frequent Adverse Events (Prevalence ≥5% in One of the Groups) During the Combination Therapy Phase**

	SELEGILINE	PLACEBO	p-VALUE[a]
All AEs	50 (69.4)	37 (53.6)	0.053
Nausea	17 (23.6)	7 (10.1)	0.033
Diarrhea	6 (8.3)	6 (8.7)	0.71
Hallucinations	4 (5.6)	2 (2.9)	0.44

[a]Chi-square test (Fisher's exact test in the case of hallucinations).

Blood pressures did not differ significantly during combination therapy between groups and although both standing and supine heart rates were significantly ($p = 0.008$ and $p < 0.001$) higher in the selegiline group these differences were not considered clinically meaningful. No clinically significant differences in laboratory values were observed between the treatment groups.

Five patients died during the combination therapy phase of the study (selegiline $n = 4$, placebo $n = 1$; $p = 0.37$). All of the patients who died were aged >70 years. None of these deaths was expressly attributed to study medication but the possibility was not definitively excluded for the three deaths attributed to cardiac or cerebral infarction.

Unique Aspects of Trial

The MONOCOMB trial is among the largest and longest-duration placebo-controlled studies to report experience with selegiline monotherapy in early-phase PD. The unique feature of the study is (1) the long wash out period (8 weeks) during which the condition of the selegiline patients did not return to the levels seen in the placebo group, (2) the overall long duration of the study showing that the clinical condition of the patients was maintained significantly better than without the drug. These contradictory data hampered investigation into whether the clinical benefits of selegiline owed anything to neuroprotective effects that delayed the progression of PD or if they were attributable wholly to amelioration of symptoms.

How the Trial Results Fit into the Current and Emerging Treatment Framework

The results of the MONOCOMB study affirm the utility and value of selegiline 10 mg/day as monotherapy in the early stages of PD. Selegiline monotherapy extended significantly the time to initiation of levodopa therapy and was associated with improvements in PD symptom status and disability as reflected in a broad range of well-established indices. Progression of disease to the point of needing levodopa therapy was notably less rapid in patients randomized to selegiline than in those receiving placebo, and took longer.

Levodopa remains the pivotal pharmacological therapy for all stages of PD including early-phase disease, but its usefulness is confounded by toxicity, tardive dyskinesias and motor fluctuations. Interventions that delay the progression of PD-related symptoms and disability, thereby postponing the need for levodopa and minimizing the dosage needed for a worthwhile effect, expand the treatment horizons of PD patients. The evidence of the MONOCOMB study is that selegiline delivers these gains: in the first phase of the study it arrested the progression of PD sufficiently to defer significantly the time when levodopa therapy became necessary (Figure 3); in older patients with more advanced PD, use of selegiline as an adjunct to levodopa enabled a given degree of therapeutic effect to be achieved with a notably lower total consumption of levodopa (Table 3; Figures 3–5). Patients treated with selegiline plus levodopa showed a significant slowing in the anticipated increase in the UPDRS scores over time – in fact the mean scores did not return to the baseline values during the entire 7-year study period (Figures 5 and 6). After 5 years on combination treatment, the mean UPDRS total score in patients on levodopa and placebo was 10 points higher than in patients treated with levodopa and selegiline. This was as great an improvement as that seen after initiating levodopa therapy. Clear-cut differences in the UPDRS scores of all the three cardinal symptoms of the disease (tremor, bradykinesia and rigidity) were also evident, all in favor of selegiline.

The emergence of motor (wearing-off) fluctuations during the second phase of the study was delayed by selegiline and the proportion of patients experiencing these untoward events during the whole course of follow-up was lower than with placebo (20% versus 34%; $p = 0.053$). Similar data, also not meeting formal criteria for statistical significance, have been reported from other studies (Larsen et al., 1999; Pålhagen et al., 1998; Myllylä et al., 1997; 1995). Meta-analysis, including those previous data, is supportive of a significant positive effect of selegiline on the propensity to motor fluctuations (odds ratio 0.75 [95% CI 0.59–0.95]; $p = 0.02$) (Ives et al., 2004), and the results of MONOCOMB are fully consistent with this pooled estimate. MONOCOMB data are likewise in accord with meta-analysis estimates of no overall effect on dyskinesias (Ives et al., 2004).

Rascol, Goetz and colleagues have undertaken two qualitative reviews of therapies for PD (Goetz et al., 2005; Rascol et al., 2002). In the most recent of these they classified selegiline as shown in Table 5. On the basis of experience in MONOCOMB (plus the quantitative data from Ives et al., 2004) it may now be appropriate to revise that classification of efficacy as suggested in the lower row of Table 5.

Some conjectures may be offered on the mechanism(s) underlying these findings, but must be prefaced with the acknowledgement that MONOCOMB was not designed to offer detailed mechanistic insights on this question – the importance of possible distinctions between clinical effects on disease progression and neuronal effects has been remarked upon by other researchers (Parkinson Study Group, 2004a). A starting point for this discussion is the observations during the wash-out phase of MONOCOMB. The deterioration in symptoms of disability was similar in the two study groups during this phase even though there was clear evidence of initial symptomatic benefits from selegiline during the preceding phase of monotherapy. (It should be recalled that the signal for the wash-out phase was a clinical decision to initiate levodopa treatment.) The absence of any statistically significant inter-group differences in disability scores during the wash-out phase

Table 5. **Classification of the Efficacy of Selegiline**

	SLOWING OF PROGRESSION	SYMPTOMATIC MONOTHERAPY	SYMPTOMATIC ADJUNCT TO LEVODOPA	PREVENTION OF MOTOR COMPLICATIONS	TREATMENT OF MOTOR COMPLICATIONS
[a]Goetz *et al.* 2005	Insufficient data	Efficacious	Insufficient data	Insufficient data for fluctuations Not efficacious for dyskinesias	Insufficient data
[b]MONOCOMB	Additional evidence of efficacy (reduced rate of progression)	Confirmed	Additional evidence for efficacy	Additional evidence of efficacy for fluctuations No change for dyskinesias	No change

[a]This row shows the classification of the efficacy of selegiline in PD as proposed by Goetz *et al.* (2005). Drugs could be classified as: likely efficacious, unlikely efficacious, non-efficacious or insufficient evidence. The classification of "insufficient evidence" was offered in any instance where there were conflicting data from controlled trials considered to be of good quality.
[b]This row shows suggested amendments to the Goetz *et al.* efficacy classification, based on observations in MONOCOMB. The safety adjudication by Goetz *et al.* was favorable ("acceptable risk without specialized monitoring") and is not altered materially by MONOCOMB data.

of MONOCOMB supports the proposition that the effects of selegiline involved slowing of disease progression, in addition to initial "wash-in" symptom relief.

Plausible neuroprotective effects, some separate from MAO-B inhibition, have been reported in numerous studies (Hara *et al.*, 2006; Saravanan *et al.*, 2006; Kim *et al.*, 2004; Magyar & Szende, 2004; Muralikrishnan *et al.*, 2003; Tatton *et al.*, 2003; Ebadi *et al.*, 2002; Matsubara *et al.*, 2001; Szende *et al.*, 2001; Brannan & Yahr, 1995; Heinonen, 1995) but demonstrating similar effects unambiguously in a clinical setting has proved to be difficult even with highly sophisticated techniques (Ahlskog, 2003). The results of MONOCOMB are an important contribution to this debate, though given the emphasis on "clinical" outcome measures rather than "neuronal protective" ones and cautionary experience in other studies (Parkinson Study Group, 2004b) it is important not to over-interpret this aspect of the MONOCOMB data.

The safety and tolerability of selegiline in this study was generally satisfactory; the only statistically significant difference between the treatment groups was a higher incidence of nausea reported as an AE, which was more common with selegiline. Nausea is a side effect of levodopa and it is possible that the difference observed arose from potentiation of levodopa rather than as an authentic adverse effect of selegiline, but many patients might reasonably regard this as a distinction without a difference.

Five patients died during the study, four in the selegiline and one in the placebo group (not significant). No definite involvement of study medication was affirmed.

The absence of statistical power to examine effects on mortality is a recurring feature of trials in PD and makes the insights from meta-analysis especially important. The reviews by Ives and colleagues (Macleod *et al.*, 2005; Ives *et al.*, 2004) provided no evidence that use of selegiline for up to 8 years was associated with an increase in mortality in patients with early PD relative to placebo or levodopa comparators; addition of the MONOCOMB deaths to that pooled analysis does not materially affect the published odds ratio or confidence intervals (our calculations). This finding refutes the earlier indication from an interim analysis of the United Kingdom Parkinson's Disease Research Group (Lees, 1995) of a substantial increase in mortality in patients with early-stage PD treated with open-label selegiline plus levodopa (versus levodopa alone) for up to about 5.5 years. A full discussion of the issues raised by that interim analysis is beyond the scope of this commentary (though see Ben-Shlomo *et al.*, 1998; Olanow *et al.*, 1998).

The essence of the clinical challenge facing PD patients and their physicians is to defer for as long as possible the need for levodopa and, once started, to extract maximum net benefit from the lowest possible dose of levodopa for as long as possible. The results of MONOCOMB indicate that selegiline can assist the attainment of these objectives. What remains undetermined is whether selegiline 10 mg/day is the *optimal* means of attaining these goals. Alternative therapies include dopaminergic agents (DAs) and catecholamine O-methyl-transferase (COMT) inhibitors; the second of these classes of drugs is currently restricted to one drug in many countries, entacapone, following the withdrawal of tolcapone due to rare but fatal cases of fulminant liver failure. Both these classes of agents have been shown to be effective to varying degrees in clinical trials (Clark & Moore, 2006; Albin & Frey, 2003; Whone *et al.*, 2003; Albin *et al.*, 2002; Parkinson Study Group, 2000; Rascol *et al.*, 2000; Rinne *et al.*, 1998) and there are indications that some DAs may be superior to MAO-B inhibitors in their effects on functional ability (though not motor function scores), but the limited number and scale of direct comparisons between drugs of different classes means that it is not possible to resolve definitively issues of relative effectiveness.

Within the MAO-B inhibitor class the clinical and economic data favor selegiline over newer agents such as rasagiline. The selegiline clinical database (Ives *et al.*, 2004) is substantially larger than that for rasagiline (Chen & Ly, 2006; Parkinson Study Group, 2005; 2004b; 2002) and includes safety experience accrued over a considerably longer period of time (Anon, 2006). In the absence of direct comparisons – and the sample size needed for a meaningful head-to-head comparison would be very large, especially for patients in the early stages of PD – the quantitative balance of clinical experience favors selegiline. Qualitative differences such as the lack of effect of rasagiline on time to initiation of levodopa in the TEMPO study have also to be considered (Parkinson Study Group, 2002).

Levodopa itself and most exemplars of adjunct therapy have very low acquisition costs: selegiline itself is affordable by even the most austere monetary criteria. The emphasis in cost-effectiveness of PD medications ought therefore ideally to be on "effectiveness" rather than "cost". As noted above, however, conclusive determination of relative effectiveness is not possible at present. Economic influences in healthcare must be acknowledged, moreover, and within the class of MAO-B inhibitors these influences favor conventional selegiline over rasagiline. Conventional presentations of rasagiline are more expensive than comparable forms of selegiline, with no conclusive evidence of commensurate clinical advantages.

These reflections affirm selegiline as one (though not the only) useful and affordable first therapy for patients with early PD; in that setting MONOCOMB data indicate that the drug may exert some beneficial effect on the progression of the disease in addition to alleviating symptoms. Used as an adjunct in patients with more advanced PD, selegiline reduced the levodopa requirement and extended the quartile time to emergence of wearing-off symptoms by 21 months; notwithstanding the lack of effect of selegiline on dyskinesias, this extension represents a substantial clinical benefit to patients.

Conclusion

The results of MONOCOMB confirm that selegiline is effective in retarding the progression of early PD, that it has levodopa-sparing qualities in more advanced disease, and that it is reasonably well tolerated in long-term use.

Acknowledgments

The authors wish to thank the patients who took part in the MONOCOMB trials and the members of the Swedish Parkinson Study Group (K. Dahlbom, Örebro; B. Ekstedt, Örebro; M. Fogelberg, Göteborg; M. Hultgren, Jönköping; J. Hägglund, Eskilstuna; T. Kaugesaar, Linköping; J. Kinnman, Halmstad; H. Kontants, Stockholm; B. Lindvall, Linköping; H. Lundh, Halmstad; S.-H. Munthe, Varberg; O. Mäki-Ikola, Turku; J.-E. Olsson, Linköping; R. Palm, Karlstad; B. Petterson, Karstad; S. Pålhagen, Jönköping; L. Sjöström, Danderyd; N.-G. Svennung, Göteborg; O. Sydow, Danderyd; and E. Öhman, Örnsköldsvik).

References

Ahlskog, J.E. (2003). Slowing Parkinson's disease progression: recent dopamine agonist trials. *Neurology*, 60, 381–389.

Albin, R.L., & Frey, K.A. (2003). Initial agonist treatment of Parkinson disease: a critique. *Neurology*, 60, 390–394.

Albin, R.L., Nichols, T.E., & Frey, K.A. (2002). Brain imaging to assess the effects of dopamine agonists on progression of Parkinson disease. *Journal of the American Medical Association*, 288, 311–312; author reply, 312–313.

Allain, H., Pollak, P., & Neukirch, H.C. (1993). Symptomatic effect of selegiline in *de novo* Parkinsonian patients. The French Selegiline Multicenter Trial. *Movement Disorders*, 8(Suppl. 1), S36–S40.

Anon (2006). Rasagiline. Parkinson's disease: a simple me-too. *Prescrire International*, 15, 220.

Ben-Shlomo, Y., Churchyard, A., Head, J., et al. (1998). Investigation by Parkinson's Disease Research Group of United Kingdom into excess mortality seen with combined levodopa and selegiline treatment in patients with early, mild Parkinson's disease: further results of randomised trial and confidential inquiry. *British Medical Journal*, 316, 1191–1196.

Brannan, T., & Yahr, M.D. (1995). Comparative study of selegiline plus L-dopa-carbidopa versus L-dopa-carbidopa alone in the treatment of Parkinson's disease. *Annals of Neurology*, 37, 95–98.

Caraceni, T., & Musicco, M. (2001). Levodopa or dopamine agonists, or deprenyl as initial treatment for Parkinson's disease. A randomized multicenter study. *Parkinsonism & Related Disorders*, 7, 107–114.

Chen, J.J., & Ly, A.V. (2006). Rasagiline: a second-generation monoamine oxidase type-B inhibitor for the treatment of Parkinson's disease. *American Journal of Health-System Pharmacy*, 63, 915–928.

Clark, C.E., & Moore, A.P. (2006). Parkinson's disease. www.clinicalevidence.com. Last accessed 23 December 2006.

Ebadi, M., Sharma, S., Shavali, S., & El Refaey, H. (2002). Neuroprotective actions of selegiline. *Journal of Neuroscience Research*, 67, 285–289.

Folstein, M.F., Folstein, S.E., & McHugh, P.R. (1975). "Mini-mental state". A practical method for grading the cognitive state of patients for the clinician. *Journal of Psychiatric Research*, 12, 189–198.

Ganz, P.A. (1990). Methods of assessing the effect of drug therapy on quality of life. *Drug Safety*, 5, 233–242.

Goetz, C.G., Poewe, W., Rascol, O., & Sampaio, C. (2005). Evidence-based medical review update: pharmacological and surgical treatments of Parkinson's disease: 2001 to 2004. *Movement Disorders*, 20, 523–539.

Golbe, L.I., & Duvoisin, R.C. (1987). Double-blind trial of R-(−)-deprenyl for the "on-off" effect complicating Parkinson's disease. *Journal of Neural Transmission Supplement*, 25, 123–129.

Golbe, L.I., Lieberman, A.N., Muenter, M.D., et al. (1988). Deprenyl in the treatment of symptom fluctuations in advanced Parkinson's disease. *Clinical Neuropharmacology*, 11, 45–55.

Hamilton, M.A. (1960). Rating scale for depression. *Journal of Neurology, Neurosurgery, and Psychiatry*, 21, 56–62.

Hara, M.R., Thomas, B., Cascio, M.B., et al. (2006). Neuroprotection by pharmacologic blockade of the GAPDH death cascade. *Proceedings of the National Academy of Science of the United States of America*, 103, 3887–3889.

Heinonen, E. (1995). *Selegiline in the Treatment of Parkinson's Disease. Pharmacokinetic and Clinical Studies*, Research Report No. 13, Department of Neurology, University of Turku, Turku, Finland, pp. 30–33.

Hoehn, M.M., & Yahr, M.D. (1967). Parkinsonism: onset, progression and mortality. *Neurology*, 17, 427–442.

Ives, N.J., Stowe, R.L., Marro, J., *et al.* (2004). Monoamine oxidase type B inhibitors in early Parkinson's disease: meta-analysis of 17 randomised trials involving 3525 patients. *British Medical Journal*, 329, 593–599.

Kim, S.G., Lee, C.H., & Park, J.W. (2004). Deprenyl, a therapeutic agent for Parkinson's disease, inhibits arsenic toxicity potentiated by GSH depletion via inhibition of JNK activation. *Journal of Toxicology and Environmental Health: Part A*, 67, 2013–2024.

Kirollos, C., Charlett, A., Bowes, S.G., *et al.* (1996). Time course of physical and psychological responses to selegiline monotherapy in newly diagnosed, idiopathic parkinsonism. *European Journal of Clinical Pharmacology*, 50, 7–18.

Lang, A.E., & Fahn, S. (1989). Assessment of Parkinson's disease. In: Munsat, T.L. (ed.), *Quantification of Neurologic Deficit*. Boston: Butterworths, pp. 285–309.

Larsen, J.P., Boas, J., & Erdal, J.E. (1999). Does selegiline modify the progression of early Parkinson's disease? Results from a five-year study. The Norwegian-Danish Study Group. *European Journal of Neurology*, 6, 539–547.

Lees, A.J., on behalf of the Parkinson's Disease Research Group of the United Kingdom (1995). Comparison of therapeutic effects and mortality data of levodopa and levodopa combined with selegiline in patients with early, mild Parkinson's disease. *British Medical Journal*, 311, 1602–1607.

Macleod, A.D., Counsell, C.E., Ives, N., & Stowe, R. (2005). Monoamine oxidase B inhibitors for early Parkinson's disease. *Cochrane Database of Systemic Reviews*, July 20, (3), CD004898.

Magyar, K., & Szende, B. (2004). (–)-Deprenyl, a selective MAO-B inhibitor, with apoptotic and anti-apoptotic properties. *Neurotoxicology*, 25, 233–242.

Matsubara, K., Senda, T., Uezono, T., *et al.* (2001). L-Deprenyl prevents the cell hypoxia induced by dopaminergic neurotoxins, MPP(+) and beta-carbolinium: a microdialysis study in rats. *Neuroscience Letters*, 302, 65–68.

Muralikrishnan, D., Samantaray, S., & Mohanakumar, K.P. (2003). D-deprenyl protects nigrostriatal neurons against 1-methyl-4-phenyl-1,2,3,6-tetrahydropyridine-induced dopaminergic neurotoxicity. *Synapse*, 5, 7–13.

Myllylä, V.V., Sotaniemi, K.A., Vuorinen, J.A., & Heinonen, E.H. (1992). Selegiline as initial treatment in de novo parkinsonian patients. *Neurology*, 42, 339–343.

Myllylä, V.V., Heinonen, E.H., Vuorinen, J.A., Kilkku, O.I., & Sotaniemi, K.A. (1995). Early selegiline therapy reduces levodopa dose requirement in Parkinson's disease. *Acta Neurological Scandinavica*, 91, 177–182.

Myllylä, V.V., Sotaniemi, K.A., Hakulinen, P., Maki-Ikola, O., & Heinonen, E.H. (1997). Selegiline as the primary treatment of Parkinson's disease – a long-term double-blind study. *Acta Neurological Scandinavica*, 95, 211–218.

Naoi, M., Maruyama, W., Takahashi, T., Akao, Y., & Nakagawa, Y. (2000a). Involvement of endogenous N-methyl(R)salsolinol in Parkinson's disease: induction of apoptosis and protection by (–)deprenyl. *Journal of Neural Transmission Supplement*, 58, 111–121.

Naoi, M., Maruyama, W., Yagi, K., & Youdim, M. (2000b). Anti-apoptotic function of L-(–)deprenyl (selegiline) and related compounds. *Neurobiology (Bp)*, 8, 69–80.

Olanow, C.W., Hauser, R.A., Gauger, L., *et al.* (1995). The effect of deprenyl and levodopa on the progression of Parkinson's disease. *Annals of Neurology*, 38, 771–777.

Olanow, C.W., Myllylä, V.V., Sotaniemi, K.A., *et al.* (1998). Effect of selegiline on mortality in patients with Parkinson's disease: a meta-analysis. *Neurology*, 51, 825–830.

Pålhagen, S., Heinonen, E.H., Hägglund, J., *et al.* (1998). Selegiline delays the onset of disability in de novo Parkinsonian patients. Swedish Parkinson Study Group. *Neurology*, 51, 520–525.

Parkinson Study Group (1993). Effects of tocopherol and deprenyl on the progression of disability in early Parkinson's disease. *New England Journal of Medicine*, 328, 176–183.

Parkinson Study Group (2000). Pramipexole vs levodopa as initial treatment for Parkinson disease: a randomized controlled trial. *Journal of the American Medical Association*, 284, 1931–1938.

Parkinson Study Group (2002). A controlled trial of rasagiline in early Parkinson disease: the TEMPO Study. *Archives of Neurology*, 59, 1937–1943.

Parkinson Study Group (2004a). Levodopa and the progression of Parkinson's disease. *New England Journal of Medicine*, 351, 2498–2508.

Parkinson Study Group (2004b). A controlled, randomized, delayed-start study of rasagiline in early Parkinson disease. *Archives of Neurology*, 61, 561–566.

Parkinson Study Group (2005). A randomized placebo-controlled trial of rasagiline in levodopa-treated patients with Parkinson disease and motor fluctuations: the PRESTO study. *Archives of Neurology*, 62, 241–248.

Presthus, J., & Hajba, A. (1983). Deprenyl (selegiline) combined with levodopa and a decarboxylase inhibitor in the treatment of Parkinson's disease. *Acta Neurological Scandinavica Supplement*, 95, 127–133.

Presthus, J., Berstad, J., & Lien, K. (1987). Selegiline (L-deprenyl) and low-dose levodopa treatment of Parkinson's disease. A double-blind crossover trial. *Acta Neurological Scandinavica*, 76, 200–203.

Przuntek, H., Conrad, B., Dichgans, J., et al. (1999). SELEDO: a 5-year long-term trial on the effect of selegiline in early Parkinsonian patients treated with levodopa. *European Journal of Neurology*, 6, 141–150.

Rascol, O., Brooks, D.J., Korczyn, A.D., De Deyn, P.P., Clarke, C.E., & Lang, A.E. (2000). A five-year study of the incidence of dyskinesia in patients with early Parkinson's disease who were treated with ropinirole or levodopa. 056 Study Group. *New England Journal of Medicine*, 342, 1484–1491.

Rascol, O., Goetz, C., Koller, W., Poewe, W., & Sampaio, C. (2002). Treatment interventions for Parkinson's disease: an evidence based assessment. *The Lancet*, 359, 1589–1598.

Rinne, U.K., Siirtola, T., & Sonninen, V. (1978). L-deprenyl treatment of on–off phenomena in Parkinson's disease. *Journal of Neural Transmission*, 43, 253–262.

Rinne, U.K., Bracco, F., Chouza, C., et al. (1998). Early treatment of Parkinson's disease with cabergoline delays the onset of motor complications. Results of a double-blind levodopa controlled trial. The PKDS009 Study Group. *Drugs*, 55(Suppl. 1), 23–30.

Saravanan, K.S., Sindhu, K.M., Senthilkumar, K.S., & Mohanakumar, K.P. (2006). L-deprenyl protects against rotenone-induced, oxidative stress-mediated dopaminergic neurodegeneration in rats. *Neurochemistry International*, 49, 28–40.

Schachter, M., Marsden, C.D., Parkes, J.D., Jenner, P., & Testa, B. (1980). Deprenyl in the management of response fluctuations in patients with Parkinson's disease on levodopa. *Journal of Neurology, Neurosurgery, and Psychiatry*, 43, 1016–1021.

Shan, D.E., & Yeh, S.I. (1996). An add-on study of selegiline to Madopar in the treatment of parkinsonian patients with dose-related fluctuations: comparison between Jumexal and Parkryl. *Zhonghua Yi Xue Za Zhi (Taipei)*, 58, 264–268.

Shoulson, I., Oakes, D., Fahn, S., et al. (2002). Impact of sustained deprenyl (selegiline) in levodopa-treated Parkinson's disease: a randomized placebo-controlled extension of the deprenyl and tocopherol antioxidative therapy of parkinsonism trial. *Annals of Neurology*, 51, 604–612.

Stern, G.M., Lees, A.J., & Sandler, M. (1978). Recent observations on the clinical pharmacology of (–)deprenyl. *Journal of Neural Transmission*, 43, 245–251.

Szende, B., Bokonyi, G., Bocsi, J., Keri, G., Timar, F., & Magyar, K. (2001). Anti-apoptotic and apoptotic action of (–)-deprenyl and its metabolites. *Journal of Neural Transmission*, 108, 25–33.

Tatton, W., Chalmers-Redman, R., & Tatton, N. (2003). Neuroprotection by deprenyl and other propargylamines: glyceraldehyde-3-phosphate dehydrogenase rather than monoamine oxidase B. *Journal of Neural Transmission*, 110, 509–515.

Tetrud, J.W., & Langston, J.W. (1989). The effect of deprenyl (selegiline) on the natural history of Parkinson's disease. *Science*, 245, 519–522.

Whone, A.L., Watts, R.L., Stoessl, A.J., *et al.* (2003). Slower progression of Parkinson's disease with ropinirole versus levodopa: the REAL-PET study. *Annals of Neurology*, 54, 93–101.

Progress in Neurotherapeutics and Neuropsychopharmacology, 3:1, 73–84 © 2008 Cambridge University Press
DOI: 10.1017/S1748232107000122   Printed in the United Kingdom

Ropinirole 24-h Prolonged Release in Advanced Parkinson Disease: Review of a Randomized, Double-Blind, Placebo-Controlled Study (EASE PD - Adjunct Study)

Kelly E. Lyons*

Department of Neurology, University of Kansas Medical Center, Kansas City, USA; Email: lyons.kelly@att.net

Rajesh Pahwa**

Department of Neurology, University of Kansas Medical Center, Kansas City, USA; Email: rpahwa@kumc.edu

ABSTRACT

This chapter reviews the EASE PD - Adjunct trial which is a double-blind, placebo-controlled, 24-week study of 393 Parkinson disease (PD) subjects with levodopa-induced motor fluctuations randomized to ropinirole 24-h prolonged release or placebo. The objective of the trial was to assess the efficacy and tolerability of once daily ropinirole 24-h prolonged release as an adjunct to levodopa. The primary outcome variable was the reduction in daily "off" time as measured by subject diaries which was significantly reduced by 2.1 h with ropinirole 24-h prolonged release (mean dosage: 18.8 mg/day) compared to 0.3 h with placebo. There were also significant improvements in daily "on" time, "on" time without troublesome dyskinesia, Unified Parkinson's Disease Rating Scale (UPDRS) motor and activities of daily living subscales, depression, quality of life and sleep with ropinirole 24-h prolonged release compared to placebo. The most common adverse events with ropinirole 24-h prolonged release were dyskinesia, nausea, dizziness, somnolence, hallucinations and orthostatic hypotension. Ropinirole 24-h prolonged release was well tolerated and led to improvements in both motor and non-motor symptoms of PD.

Key words: motor complications, Parkinson disease, ropinirole prolonged release.

*Dr. Lyons is a consultant for GlaxoSmithKline, Schwarz, Novartis, Teva, and Valeant.
**Dr. Pahwa is a consultant for GlaxoSmithKline, Schwarz, Novartis, Teva, Valeant, Vernalis, and Boehringer Ingelheim.

Correspondence should be addressed to: Kelly E. Lyons, PhD, Department of Neurology, University of Kansas Medical Center, 3599 Rainbow Blvd, Mailstop 2012, Kansas City, KS 66160, USA; Ph: +1 913 588 7159; Fax: +1 913 588 6920; Email: lyons.kelly@att.net

Introduction and Overview

Parkinson disease (PD) is a neurodegenerative disorder with the primary symptoms of bradykinesia, tremor and rigidity. Initially, PD symptoms are generally well controlled (Miyasaki *et al.*, 2002); however, as the disease progresses, increased dopaminergic treatment is necessary and often leads to the development of motor fluctuations (Pahwa *et al.*, 2006). Motor fluctuations can lead to significant disability and can negatively impact quality of life (Chapuis *et al.*, 2005). Several oral medications currently approved by the Food and Drug Administration (FDA) as treatments for advanced PD have been reported to significantly reduce levodopa-induced motor fluctuations including the monoamine oxidase type B (MAO-B) inhibitors, rasagiline (Parkinsonian Study Group, 2005; Rascol *et al.*, 2005), selegiline (Golbe *et al.*, 1988), and orally disintegrating selegiline (Waters *et al.*, 2004); the catechol-O-methyltransferase (COMT) inhibitors, entacapone (Rinne *et al.*, 1998; Parkinsonian Study Group, 1997) and tolcapone (Baas *et al.*, 1997; Rajput *et al.*, 1997) and the dopamine agonists pramipexole (Guttman, 1997; Lieberman *et al.*, 1997) and ropinirole (Lieberman *et al.*, 1998; Rascol *et al.*, 1996). Although rasagiline and orally disintegrating selegiline are both once daily medications, entacapone, tolcapone, pramipexole and ropinirole all require multiple daily doses.

Multiple daily dosing may lead to decreased medication compliance and unsteady plasma concentrations which can contribute to the occurrence of motor fluctuations. Leopold *et al.* (2004) evaluated compliance in 40 PD patients taking at least one anti-parkinsonian medication at least three times daily. A computerized monitoring system was used to measure compliance. There were four subjects that had 100% compliance during a 4-week period. Only 24% reported missed doses; however, the monitoring system indicated that 51% missed at least one dose each week, 21% missed three or more doses each week and 82% did not take all doses on time. According to the subjects, the most common reasons for non-compliance were that they forgot or they did not have their medication with them. Similarly, Grosset *et al.* (2005) examined medication compliance in 54 PD patients using a computerized monitoring system. Satisfactory compliance was defined as taking at least 80% of the prescribed medications. Forty-three (80%) of the subjects had satisfactory compliance; however, the majority of subjects did not take their medications on time. This was associated with a greater number of daily doses, younger age, depression and reduced quality of life.

Ropinirole 24-h prolonged release was developed with the goal of providing a once per day oral dopamine agonist to increase patient compliance and create a more steady pharmacokinetic profile to reduce levodopa-induced motor fluctuations and improve tolerability. To assess the efficacy and tolerability of prolonged release ropinirole, a multinational, randomized, double-blind, placebo-controlled trial in PD patients with levodopa-induced motor fluctuations, the Efficacy and

Safety Evaluation in Parkinson's Disease-Adjunct (EASE PD - Adjunct) trial was conducted (Pahwa *et al.*, 2007).

Purpose of Trial

The purpose of the EASE PD - Adjunct trial was to examine the efficacy and tolerability of ropinirole 24-h prolonged release in PD patients experiencing levodopa-induced motor fluctuations.

Ropinirole 24-h Prolonged Release

Ropinirole 24-h prolonged release is a 24-h formulation of the FDA approved immediate release dopamine agonist ropinirole. Ropinirole is a non-ergot dopamine agonist with affinity for the D2 family of dopamine receptors. It is rapidly absorbed with less than 10% of the drug excreted in the urine and it is metabolized by the liver primarily by the cytochrome P450 enzyme CYP1A2. In PD patients, ropinirole takes approximately 1.5 h to reach maximum concentration and the half life is approximately 6 h (Pahwa *et al.*, 2004). Immediate release ropinirole is approved for both monotherapy in early PD and also as an adjunct to levodopa in more advanced disease.

In a randomized, double-blind, placebo-controlled, 6-month trial of 149 PD subjects with motor fluctuations (ropinirole $n = 95$; placebo $n = 54$), Lieberman *et al.* (1998) reported a significant reduction in daily "off" time with immediate release ropinirole (11.7%) compared to placebo (5.1%). This translates into a reduction of daily "off" time of a little over an hour per day. In addition, there was a significantly greater reduction of daily levodopa in the ropinirole group (242 mg) compared to the placebo group (51 mg).

The ropinirole component of ropinirole 24-h prolonged release is identical to immediate release ropinirole. The prolonged release formulation uses a Geomatrix® technology with alternating layers of ropinirole and erodible hydroxypropyl methylcellulose polymers. This once a day 24-h formulation allows for a more steady absorption of the drug with the goal of improved efficacy, fewer side effects and reduced motor fluctuations while allowing for a faster titration schedule compared to immediate release ropinirole (8 weeks versus 13 weeks).

Clinical Trial

Subjects

There were 393 men and women with idiopathic PD experiencing levodopa-induced motor fluctuations enrolled in the trial. Patients included in the trial were at least 30 years old, had a modified Hoehn and Yahr stage of II–IV, were on a stable dose of levodopa for at least 1 month and had at least 3 h of daily "off" time confirmed by patient diaries. The anti-parkinsonian medications, amantadine, anti-cholinergics, selegiline and COMT inhibitors, were allowed if they had been stable for at least 1 month; however, subjects with any dopamine agonist use in the past month were not eligible. The use of anti-emetics or neuroleptics was not allowed during the trial. Other exclusion criteria included disabling dyskinesia, dementia, symptomatic postural hypotension, recent or current drug or alcohol abuse and any significant, uncontrolled medical disorders or abnormal laboratory values. Finally, patients with recent initiation, discontinuation or dose adjustment of hormone replacement therapy or any drug known to substantially inhibit or induce cytochrome P450 1A2 were not eligible for the study. All subjects provided written, informed consent.

Trial Methods

The EASE PD - Adjunct trial was a 24-week, randomized, double-blind, parallel-group, placebo-controlled study conducted at 67 centers in Belgium, the Czech Republic, France, Hungary, Italy, Poland, Spain and the United States between July 2003 and December 2004. Subjects completed a 14-day placebo run-in period prior to randomization at which time, if still eligible for the trial, they were assigned to receive either once daily ropinirole 24-h prolonged release or once daily matching placebo in a ratio of 1 : 1 based on a computer-generated randomization schedule.

Evaluations were done at baseline and 1, 2, 3, 4, 6, 8, 10, 12, 16, 20 and 24 weeks thereafter. At study completion or withdrawal, there was a 7-day down-titration phase and a safety visit was conducted within 2 weeks of the last dose of study medication. Study drug was initiated at 2 mg/day and titrated at each visit, until an optimal response or adverse event occurred, with a maximum dose of 24 mg/day. The dose was titrated from 2 to doses of 4, 6, 8, 12, 16, 20 or 24 mg/day. All subjects were titrated to a minimum dose of 6 mg/day. When the optimal dose was reached, that dose was maintained throughout the treatment phase unless further titration was necessary. With each increase in study medication after the 8 mg/day dose, levodopa was reduced by one half or one tablet as was the accompanying entacapone dose if applicable. If the levodopa reduction resulted in a worsening of PD symptoms, the study medication was increased to the next dose and levodopa was not changed. Another increase in study medication to the next dose without changing the levodopa dose could be made if the worsening of PD had not resolved. If PD worsening was not resolved after two increases in study medication, levodopa could be increased but could not exceed the baseline dose.

Instruments/Measures

Subjects completed 2 days of 24-h home diaries before each visit. The diaries measured whether the subject was "on" and PD symptoms were well controlled, "on with troublesome dyskinesia" which interfered with functioning, "off" and medications were not adequately controlling symptoms or asleep for each 30-min interval throughout the 24-h day (Hauser *et al.*, 2000). Other measures included the Unified Parkinson's Disease Rating Scale (UPDRS) to assess motor symptoms and activities of daily living (Fahn *et al.*, 1987), Beck Depression Inventory-II (BDI) to assess depression (Beck *et al.*, 1961), Parkinson's Disease Questionnaire-39 (PDQ-39) to assess quality of life (Peto *et al.*, 1998), Epworth Sleepiness Scale (ESS) to assess daytime sleepiness (Johns, 1991), Parkinson's Disease Sleep Scale (PDSS) to assess changes in sleep (Chaudhuri *et al.*, 2002) and the Clinical Global Impression-Improvement (CGI-I) to assess overall improvement or worsening. Safety measures included laboratory tests, vital signs and electrocardiogram (EKG).

Primary and Secondary Outcomes

The primary outcome variable was the average change in daily hours "off" from baseline to week 24 as measured by subject home diaries.

Secondary outcome variables included the average change in hours and percentage of daily "on" time and "on" time with troublesome dyskinesia as well as change in percentage of daily "off" time from baseline to week 24 as measured by patient home diaries. Changes in UPDRS motor scores a minimum of 2 h after a dose of levodopa, the average of medication "on" and "off" UPDRS activities of daily living scores, BDI, PDQ-39, ESS and PDSS scores were also assessed. The proportion of subjects "very much improved" or "much improved" as measured by the CGI-I and the proportion of subjects who had at least a 20% reduction in "off" time and at least a 20% reduction in levodopa compared to baseline were recorded.

Analysis

The sample size calculations were based on the mean change from baseline to endpoint in daily "off" hours as reported in previous studies of levodopa-induced motor fluctuations that used patient diaries as an outcome measure (Kieburtz & Hubble, 2000; Rinne *et al.*, 1998; Parkinson Study Group, 1997). Based on these studies, a difference of 1.2 h between ropinirole 24-h prolonged release and placebo in the reduction in daily "off" hours was considered clinically significant. The calculations indicated that 133 subjects in each group were necessary to detect a difference of 1.2 h between groups with a standard deviation of 3 h, 90% power and a 5% significance level. Assuming an attrition rate of 27%, at least 368 subjects needed to be randomized.

The change from baseline to week 24 in daily "off" hours, the primary outcome variable, was evaluated by analysis of covariance. The continuous secondary outcome measures were evaluated with normal, linear models. Dichotomous variables were analyzed using logistic regression and time to event data were analyzed using Cox's regression model. For all efficacy measures analyzed at week 24, the last observation carried forward (LOCF) method was used for missing data.

Safety data were based on the safety population which included all subjects who received at least one dose of randomized study medication. Assessments of efficacy were based on the intention-to-treat (ITT) population which included all randomized subjects who received at least one dose of study medication and had at least one post-baseline efficacy assessment.

Results

Efficacy

The efficacy data were based on 391 subjects; 201 that received ropinirole 24-h prolonged release and 190 that received placebo. At baseline, the ropinirole 24-h prolonged release group had an average age of 66.3 years, disease duration of 8.6 years, duration of levodopa use of 6.5 years and daily levodopa dose of 824 mg/day. Similarly, the placebo group had an average age of 66.0 years, disease duration of 8.6 years, duration of levodopa use of 6.6 years and daily levodopa use of 776 mg/day. Both groups had 7.0 h of daily "off" time at baseline. The mean dose of ropinirole 24-h prolonged release at week 24 was 18.8 ± 6.3 mg/day, ranging from 2 to 24 mg/day with 50% of subjects receiving the maximum dose of 24 mg/day.

The mean reduction in hours of daily "off" time from baseline to week 24 as measured by subject diaries was 2.1 h for the ropinirole 24-h prolonged release group and 0.3 h for the placebo group which represented an adjusted treatment effect of 1.7 h (95% CI: $-2.34, -1.09; p < 0.0001$). It should be noted that there was a significant treatment effect of ropinirole 24-h prolonged release at all visits from week 2 to 24 in the reduction of daily "off" time compared to placebo.

Other diary measures including hours of "on" time (increase of 1.6 h with ropinirole 24-h prolonged release; decrease of 0.1 h with placebo) and hours of "on" time without troublesome dyskinesia (increase of 1.6 h with ropinirole 24-h prolonged release; increase of 0.1 h with placebo) were significantly more improved with ropinirole 24-h prolonged release compared to placebo ($p < 0.00001$). In addition, mean daily "on" time with troublesome dyskinesia decreased by 0.04 h in the ropinirole 24-h prolonged release group and by 0.2 h in the placebo group. Percent of daily "off" time, "on" time and "on" time without troublesome dyskinesia were significantly more improved in the ropinirole 24-h prolonged release group compared to placebo (Figure 1).

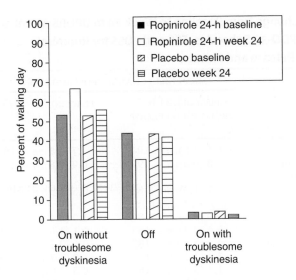

Fig. 1.
Percent of daily "off" time, "on" time without troublesome dyskinesia and "on" time with troublesome dyskinesia from baseline to week 24 for ropinirole 24-h prolonged release and placebo.

The ropinirole 24-h prolonged release group also had significant improvements from baseline to week 24 compared to placebo in UPDRS motor scores, UPDRS activities of daily living scores, BDI, PDSS and PDQ-39 subscales of mobility, activities of daily living, emotional well-being, stigma and communication. There were no significant differences between ropinirole 24-h prolonged release and placebo in the ESS or PDQ-39 subscales of social support, cognition or bodily discomfort (Table 1).

In the ropinirole 24-h group there were 42% that were "much improved" or "very much improved" on the CGI-I assessment scale compared to 14% in the placebo group. There was a reduction of 278 mg in daily levodopa in the ropinirole 24-h prolonged release group compared to a reduction of 164 mg in the placebo group. It was five times more likely for a subject in the placebo group to require a subsequent increase in levodopa dose following a levodopa dose reduction compared to subjects in the ropinirole 24-h prolonged release group (adjusted odds ratio: 0.2; 95% CI: 0.09, 0.34; $p < 0.001$) and the subsequent increase in levodopa dose occurred more quickly in the placebo group (adjusted hazard ratio: 0.2; 95% CI: 0.11, 0.37; $p < 0.0001$). Finally, 52% of subjects in the ropinirole 24-h prolonged release group had at least a 20% reduction in both daily "off" time and levodopa dose compared to 20% in the placebo group.

Table 1. **Mean Change from Baseline to Week 24 in UPDRS Motor and ADL Subscales, BDI, PDQ-39 Subscales, ESS and PDSS for Ropinirole 24-h Prolonged Release and Placebo**

	MEAN (2SE) CHANGE FROM BASELINE		*p*-VALUE
	ROPINIROLE 24-h PROLONGED RELEASE ($n = 201$)	PLACEBO ($n = 190$)	
UPDRS motor	-6.5 (1.8); $n = 194$	-1.7 (1.8); $n = 183$	<0.0001
UPDRS ADL (mean "on" + "off" scores)	-3.5 (0.8); $n = 197$	-0.9 (0.8); $n = 184$	<0.0001
BDI	-2.1 (1.3); $n = 188$	-0.5 (1.3); $n = 179$	0.01
PDQ-39 subscales			
Mobility	-4.9 (3.4); $n = 186$	1.9 (3.4); $n = 172$	<0.0001
ADLs	-5.4 (3.3); $n = 185$	1.1 (3.8); $n = 176$	<0.0001
Emotional well-being	-4.3 (3.1); $n = 182$	-0.6 (3.1); $n = 172$	0.01
Stigma	-3.3 (3.7); $n = 187$	1.2 (3.7); $n = 178$	0.02
Social support	-1.5 (3.0); $n = 185$	-0.3 (3.0); $n = 177$	0.44
Cognition	3.4 (2.7); $n = 188$	2.9 (2.7); $n = 178$	0.72
Communication	-1.4 (3.3); $n = 187$	2.4 (3.3); $n = 176$	0.02
Bodily discomfort	-3.6 (3.4); $n = 189$	-1.5 (3.5); $n = 176$	0.22
ESS	0.5 (0.8); $n = 188$	0.2 (0.8); $n = 173$	0.37
PDSS	1.3 (4.2); $n = 191$	-3.3 (4.2); $n = 178$	0.02

ADL, activities of daily living. (Modified from Pahwa *et al.*, 2007.)

Tolerability and Safety

Ropinirole 24-h prolonged release was well tolerated. Study withdrawal due to adverse events was 5% for both ropinirole 24-h prolonged release and placebo groups. In the ropinirole 24-h prolonged release group, four subjects withdrew due to hallucinations compared to two in the placebo group, two subjects withdrew due to nausea compared to one in the placebo group and one subject withdrew due to syncope compared to none in the placebo group. There were no subjects in the ropinirole 24-h prolonged release group that withdrew due to worsening of PD symptoms but there were two in the placebo group. The most common reason for discontinuation was lack of efficacy which occurred in 3% of the ropinirole 24-h prolonged release group (6/202) and 14% of the placebo group (27/191).

Adverse events were typical of non-ergot dopamine agonists. They occurred in 64% (129/202) of subjects in the ropinirole 24-h prolonged release group and 55% (106/191) of the placebo group. The most common adverse events ($\geqslant 5\%$) with ropinirole 24-h prolonged release compared to placebo were dyskinesia (13% versus 3%), nausea (11% versus 4%), dizziness (8% versus 3%), somnolence (7% versus 4%), hallucinations (6% versus 1%) and orthostatic hypotension (5% versus 1%). The majority of subjects reporting dyskinesia or nausea did so during the up-titration phase of the trial, before the levodopa dose was reduced. In addition, the majority of the subjects reporting dyskinesia also reported that they were not disabling. Only one ropinirole 24-h prolonged release subject and one placebo subject reported an unintended sleep episode which both resolved after 1 day and both subjects completed the study. There were no adverse events suggestive of fibrosis.

Unique Aspects of the Trial

This trial is the first randomized, double-blind, placebo-controlled trial of ropinirole 24-h prolonged release in advanced PD patients with motor fluctuations that has been published. In addition to assessing the effects of ropinirole 24-h prolonged release on the motor symptoms of PD using the UPDRS and subject diaries, this study also assessed effects on non-motor symptoms including various aspects of quality of life, depression, daytime sleepiness and nighttime sleep.

Translation to Clinical Practice

Other Recent Advances

The two most recently approved MAO-B (monoamine oxidase type B) inhibitors, rasagiline and orally disintegrating selegiline, are both once a day preparations approved for advanced PD and both have been shown to significantly reduce levodopa-induced motor fluctuations. In the PRESTO study (Parkinson Study Group, 2005) PD subjects with motor fluctuations were randomized to receive either rasagiline 0.5 mg/day, rasagiline 1.0 mg/day or placebo for 26 weeks. Daily "off" time was decreased by 1.8 h in the 1.0 mg/day group, 1.4 in the 0.5 mg/day group and 0.9 h with placebo. In a similar study (Rascol *et al.*, 2005), PD subjects with motor fluctuations were randomized to receive rasagiline 1.0 mg/day once daily, 200 mg of entacapone with each dose of levodopa or placebo. Daily "off" time was decreased by 1.2 h for both rasagiline and entacapone compared to a decrease of 0.4 h with placebo. In a 12-week study of once daily orally disintegrating selegiline (up to 2.5 mg/day) in PD subjects with motor fluctuations (Waters *et al.*, 2004), daily "off" time was reduced by 2.2 h in the orally disintegrating selegiline group compared to a reduction of 0.6 h with placebo.

There are currently no once a day dopamine agonists approved by the FDA for the treatment of advanced PD; however, a study of the effect of the dopamine agonist, rotigotine 24-h transdermal system, on levodopa-induced motor fluctuations was recently reported (LeWitt *et al.*, 2007). A 24-week, randomized, double-blind, placebo-controlled trial was conducted to assess the efficacy and safety rotigotine in subjects with advanced PD and daily motor fluctuations. Subjects were randomized to receive placebo patches, rotigotine up to 8 mg/24 h (mean 7.16 mg/24 h) or rotigotine up to 12 mg/24 h (mean 9.51 mg/24 h). There were significant reductions in daily "off" time of 2.7 h/day for the rotigotine 8 mg/24-h group, 2.1 h/day for the 12 mg/24-h group and 0.9 h/day for placebo. Adverse events were typical for dopamine agonists except for skin reactions related to the patch.

How This Trial Fits into Emerging Treatment and Research Framework

Ropinirole 24-h prolonged release will add a once daily oral dopamine agonist to the treatment options for levodopa-induced motor fluctuations in advanced PD. This formulation of ropinirole should provide more stable plasma concentrations and greater patient compliance, resulting in a reduction in motor fluctuations and improvement in parkinsonian symptoms and quality of life. In addition, ropinirole 24-h prolonged release was shown to significantly decrease depression which has been increasingly recognized as a common, under-treated problem in PD patients (Miyasaki *et al.*, 2006). There were also significant improvements in nighttime sleep which is an important benefit of this drug as it has been estimated that up to 98% of PD patients experience some type of nocturnal disruption. Sleep disruption can impact not only parkinsonian symptoms but also quality of life in general (Chaudhuri *et al.*, 2006).

The faster, less complicated titration schedule will make the initiation of this drug easier for both patients and physicians compared to immediate release ropinirole. Despite the faster titration of ropinirole prolonged release, when the adverse events are compared to a similar trial of immediate release ropinirole taken three times daily (Lieberman *et al.*, 1998), the 24-h preparation appears to be better tolerated. There were 17% more subjects in the ropinirole 24-h prolonged release study that had at least a 20% reduction in both levodopa dose and daily "off" time (52% versus 35%) compared to the immediate release formulation. The most common adverse events reported in the prolonged release trial were less than those reported in the immediate release trial: dyskinesia (13% versus 34%), nausea (11% versus 20%), dizziness (8% versus 20%), somnolence (7% versus 19%) and postural hypotension (5% versus 17%). Furthermore, 16% of the immediate release study withdrew due to adverse events compared with 5% in the prolonged release study.

Further study of this drug in advanced PD may shed light on the cause and prevention of motor fluctuations and their relationship to depression, sleep problems and other non-motor symptoms associated with PD.

Summary

Ropinirole 24-h prolonged release is efficacious and well tolerated in PD patients with levodopa-induced motor fluctuations. The once daily dosing and less complicated titration schedule should also improve patient compliance. In addition to the reduction of motor fluctuations, parkinsonian symptoms and levodopa dose, ropinirole 24-h prolonged release provides significant improvements in depression, nighttime sleep and quality of life.

References

Baas, H., Beiske, A.G., Ghika, J., Jackson, M., Oertel, W.H., Poewe, W., *et al.* (1997). Catechol-O-methyltransferase inhibition with tolcapone reduces the "wearing off" phenomenon and levodopa requirements in fluctuating parkinsonian patients. *Journal of Neurology Neurosurgery and Psychiatry*, 63(4), 421–428.

Beck, A.T., Ward, C.H., Mendelson, M., Mock, J., & Erbaugh, J. (1961). An inventory for measuring depression. *Archives of General Psychiatry*, 4, 561–571.

Chapuis, S., Ouchchane, L., Metz, O., Gerbaud, L., & Durif, F. (2005). Impact of the motor complications of Parkinson's disease on the quality of life. *Movement Disorders*, 20(2), 224–230.

Chaudhuri, K.R., Pal, S., DiMarco, A., Whately-Smith, C., Bridgman, K., Mathew, R., *et al.* (2002). The Parkinson's disease sleep scale: a new instrument for assessing sleep and nocturnal disability in Parkinson's disease. *Journal of Neurology Neurosurgery Psychiatry*, 73(6), 629–635.

Chaudhuri, K.R., Healy, D.G., & Schapira, A.H. (2006). Non-motor symptoms of Parkinson's disease: diagnosis and management. *Lancet Neurology*, 5(3), 235–245.

Fahn, S., Elton, R.L., & Committee MotUD (1987). Unified Parkinson's disease rating scale. In: Fahn, S., Marsden, C.D., Calne, D.B., & Lieberman, A. (eds.), *Recent Developments in Parkinson's Disease*. Florham Park, New Jersey: Macmillan Health Care Information, pp. 153–163.

Golbe, L.I., Lieberman, A.N., Muenter, M.D., Ahlskog, J.E., Gopinathan, G., Neophytides, A.N., *et al.* (1988). Deprenyl in the treatment of symptom fluctuations in advanced Parkinson's disease. *Clinical Neuropharmacology*, 11(1), 45–55.

Grosset, K.A., Bone, I., & Grosset, D.G. (2005). Suboptimal medication adherence in Parkinson's disease. *Movement Disorders*, 20(11), 1502–1507.

Guttman, M. (1997). Double-blind comparison of pramipexole and bromocriptine treatment with placebo in advanced Parkinson's disease. International Pramipexole–Bromocriptine Study Group. *Neurology*, 49(4), 1060–1065.

Hauser, R.A., Friedlander, J., Zesiewicz, T.A., Adler, C.H., Seeberger, L.C., O'Brien, C.F., *et al.* (2000). A home diary to assess functional status in patients with Parkinson's disease with motor fluctuations and dyskinesia. *Clinical Neuropharmacology*, 23(2), 75–81.

Johns, M.W. (1991). A new method for measuring daytime sleepiness: the Epworth sleepiness scale. *Sleep*, 14(6), 540–545.

Kieburtz, K., & Hubble, J. (2000). Benefits of COMT inhibitors in levodopa-treated parkinsonian patients: results of clinical trials. *Neurology*, 55(11 Suppl. 4), S42–S45; discussion S46–S50.

Leopold, N.A., Polansky, M., & Hurka, M.R. (2004). Drug adherence in Parkinson's disease. *Movement Disorders*, 19(5), 513–517.

LeWitt, P.A., Lyons, K.E., & Pahwa, R. (2007). Advanced Parkinson disease treated with rotigotine transdermal system: PREFER study. *Neurology*, 68(16), 1262–1267.

Lieberman, A., Ranhosky, A., & Korts, D. (1997). Clinical evaluation of pramipexole in advanced Parkinson's disease: results of a double-blind, placebo-controlled, parallel-group study. *Neurology*, 49(1), 162–168.

Lieberman, A., Olanow, C.W., Sethi, K., Swanson, P., Waters, C.H., Fahn, S., *et al.* (1998). A multicenter trial of ropinirole as adjunct treatment for Parkinson's disease. Ropinirole Study Group. *Neurology*, 51(4), 1057–1062.

Miyasaki, J.M., Martin, W., Suchowersky, O., Weiner, W.J., & Lang, A.E. (2002). Practice parameter: initiation of treatment for Parkinson's disease: an evidence-based review: report of the Quality Standards Subcommittee of the American Academy of Neurology. *Neurology*, 58(1), 11–17.

Miyasaki, J.M., Shannon, K., Voon, V., Ravina, B., Kleiner-Fisman, G., Anderson, K., et al. (2006). Practice parameter: evaluation and treatment of depression, psychosis, and dementia in Parkinson disease (an evidence-based review): report of the Quality Standards Subcommittee of the American Academy of Neurology. *Neurology*, 66(7), 996–1002.

Pahwa, R., Lyons, K.E., & Hauser, R.A. (2004). Ropinirole therapy for Parkinson's disease. *Expert Reviews on Neurotherapy*, 4(4), 581–588.

Pahwa, R., Factor, S.A., Lyons, K.E., Ondo, W.G., Gronseth, G., Bronte-Stewart, H., et al. (2006). Practice parameter: treatment of Parkinson disease with motor fluctuations and dyskinesia (an evidence-based review): report of the Quality Standards Subcommittee of the American Academy of Neurology. *Neurology*, 66(7), 983–995.

Pahwa, R., Stacy, M.A., Factor, S.A., Lyons, K.E., Stocchi, F., Hersh, B.P., et al. (2007). Ropinirole 24-hour prolonged release: randomized, controlled study in advanced Parkinson disease. *Neurology*, 68(14), 1108–1115.

Parkinson Study Group (1997). Entacapone improves motor fluctuations in levodopa-treated Parkinson's disease patients. *Annals of Neurology*, 42(5), 747–755.

Parkinson Study Group (2005). A randomized placebo-controlled trial of rasagiline in levodopa-treated patients with Parkinson disease and motor fluctuations: the PRESTO study. *Archives of Neurology*, 62(2), 241–248.

Peto, V., Jenkinson, C., & Fitzpatrick, R. (1998). PDQ-39: a review of the development, validation and application of a Parkinson's disease quality of life questionnaire and its associated measures. *Journal of Neurology*, 245(Suppl. 1), S10–S14.

Rajput, A.H., Martin, W., Saint-Hilaire, M.H., Dorflinger, E., & Pedder, S. (1997). Tolcapone improves motor function in parkinsonian patients with the "wearing-off" phenomenon: a double-blind, placebo-controlled, multicenter trial. *Neurology*, 49(4), 1066–1071.

Rascol, O., Lees, A.J., Senard, J.M., Pirtosek, Z., Montastruc, J.L., & Fuell, D. (1996). Ropinirole in the treatment of levodopa-induced motor fluctuations in patients with Parkinson's disease. *Clinical Neuropharmacology*, 19(3), 234–245.

Rascol, O., Brooks, D.J., Melamed, E., Oertel, W., Poewe, W., Stocchi, F., et al. (2005). Rasagiline as an adjunct to levodopa in patients with Parkinson's disease and motor fluctuations (LARGO, lasting effect in adjunct therapy with rasagiline given once daily, study): a randomised, double-blind, parallel-group trial. *Lancet*, 365(9463), 947–954.

Rinne, U.K., Larsen, J.P., Siden, A., & Worm-Petersen, J. (1998). Entacapone enhances the response to levodopa in parkinsonian patients with motor fluctuations. Nomecomt Study Group. *Neurology*, 51(5), 1309–1314.

Waters, C.H., Sethi, K.D., Hauser, R.A., Molho, E., & Bertoni, J.M. (2004). Zydis selegiline reduces off time in Parkinson's disease patients with motor fluctuations: a 3-month, randomized, placebo-controlled study. *Movement Disorders*, 19(4), 426–432.

Progress in Neurotherapeutics and Neuropsychopharmacology, 3:1, 85–110 © 2008 Cambridge University Press
DOI: 10.1017/S1748232107000031   Printed in the United Kingdom

Insulin Resistance Alzheimer's Disease: Pathophysiology and Treatment

G. Stennis Watson

Geriatric Research, Education, and Clinical Center (GRECC), Veterans Affairs Puget Sound Health Care System;
Department of Psychiatry and Behavioral Sciences, University of Washington School of Medicine, Seattle, WA, USA;
Email: gswatson@u.washington.edu

Suzanne Craft

Geriatric Research, Education, and Clinical Center (GRECC), Veterans Affairs Puget Sound Health Care System;
Department of Psychiatry and Behavioral Sciences, University of Washington School of Medicine, Seattle, WA, USA;
Email: scraft@u.washington.edu

ABSTRACT

Insulin and insulin resistance likely play a significant role in the pathophysiology and cognitive decline associated with Alzheimer's disease (AD). Insulin, insulin receptors, and insulin-sensitive glucose transporters are selectively localized the brain, including medial temporal areas that support memory. Raising brain insulin levels can facilitate memory and increase cerebrospinal fluid levels of β-amyloid (Aβ) and inflammatory markers. Insulin's effects on cognition may reflect normal regulation of glucose metabolism, long-term potentiation, and neurotransmitter levels. Consequently, insulin abnormalities may disrupt normal memory functioning and promote pathophysiological processes observed in patients with neurodegenerative disorders. Conversely, restoring normal insulin activity may exert a beneficial effect on pathophysiological processes. For example, peroxisome proliferator-activated receptor (PPAR)-gamma agonists (insulin sensitizing agents used to treat type 2 diabetes mellitus) modulate neuronal cell survival, inflammatory responses, mitochondrial functioning, and possibly Aβ processing and deposition. One PPAR-gamma agonist, rosiglitazone, facilitates memory and modulates plasma Aβ levels in patients with AD. Likewise, a healthy diet and regular exercise may improve insulin sensitivity and decrease the risk for both AD. Furthermore, intranasal insulin administration rapidly delivers insulin to the brain without altering plasma insulin or glucose levels. Studies to date suggest that this procedure can facilitate memory and modulate plasma Aβ levels in memory-impaired adults. Interestingly, the adverse effects of insulin abnormalities and the beneficial effects of improving

Correspondence should be addressed to: Suzanne Craft, Ph.D., VAPSHCS, S-182-GRECC, 1660 South Columbian Way, Seattle, WA 98108, USA; Ph: +1 206 277 1156; Fax: +1 206 764 2569; Email: scraft@u.washington.edu

insulin sensitivity may differ by apolipoprotein E (*APOE*) genotype, an established risk factor for AD. Patients who do carry lower doses of the *APOE* e4 allele have an enhanced risk for insulin abnormalities and are also more responsive to the memory enhancing effects of both rosiglitazone and intranasal insulin administration, relative to other patients. Therefore, future therapeutic trials should consider the moderating effects of *APOE* genotype.

Key words: apolipoprotein E, β-amyloid, diabetes, exercise, glucose metabolism, inflammation, insulin, memory, mitochondria, PPAR-gamma agonists.

A substantial body of research suggests that insulin and insulin resistance play an important role in the pathophysiology and cognitive decline associated with Alzheimer's disease (AD) and other neurodegenerative disorders. Insulin resistance (reduced effectiveness to stimulate glucose utilization) is an essential feature of type 2 diabetes mellitus (T2DM) and impaired glucose tolerance (IGT), the prodromal state of T2DM. IGT and T2DM increase the risk for declines in memory and other cognitive functions, especially in older adults, and several studies show that improving glucoregulation can attenuate cognitive decline. A decade ago, epidemiologic evidence emerged indicating that diabetes and chronic hyperinsulinemia increase the risk for AD and vascular dementia. Furthermore, it appears that patients with AD are more likely than healthy older adults to have insulin abnormalities. These observations are especially alarming in light of the growing epidemic of IGT and T2DM among older adults in North America and Europe. To the extent that insulin resistance and neurodegenerative disorders are related, the increasing prevalence of insulin resistance could eventuate in an increasing prevalence of dementia.

Several factors likely contribute to the influence of insulin resistance on the pathophysiology of AD. For example, insulin modulates levels of β-amyloid (Aβ, the principal constituent of the senile plaques that are a hallmark of AD), neurotransmitters, and hormones. Furthermore, insulin has a complex relationship with the inflammatory network: low levels of insulin are anti-inflammatory, and high levels or chronic elevations of insulin are proinflammatory. Thus, low levels of insulin may be beneficial, and high levels may be detrimental in the chronic inflammatory states that characterize AD and other neurodegenerative disorders. Finally, the deleterious pathophysiologic and cognitive effects of insulin resistance may relate to altered cerebral glucose metabolism or metabolic syndrome, which comprises hypertension, dyslipidemia (elevated low density lipoprotein (LDL) and/or low high density lipoprotein (HDL) levels), hyperglycemia, and obesity.

Both increasing insulin activity and attenuating insulin resistance can offer novel therapeutic approaches for treating AD. First, acute intravenous administration of insulin can facilitate memory for patients with AD; however, this procedure requires glucose supplementation and careful monitoring to prevent hypoglycemia.

Intranasal administration rapidly delivers insulin to the brain and avoids the risk of hypoglycemia, and has been shown to facilitate memory in a subgroup of patients with AD. Second, the peroxisome proliferator-activated receptor-gamma (PPAR-gamma) agonists rosiglitazone and pioglitazone are insulin sensitizing agents that have been approved to treat T2DM. At least two studies support the therapeutic efficacy of these agents for AD. Third, diet and exercise are powerful interventions for IGT and T2DM. Therefore, these lifestyle modifications may provide non-pharmacologic strategies for attenuating the pathophysiologic processes and cognitive dysfunction associated with AD.

In this chapter, we will review the evidence that supports this connection between insulin resistance and AD and that supports novel therapeutic strategies for AD. We review the results of several clinical trials including those of oral hypoglycemic agents and exercise programs that address issues relevant to insulin resistance and AD.

Insulin and Insulin Resistance in the Central Nervous System

Insulin Resistance and Neurodegenerative Disease

In healthy humans, peripheral glucose metabolism is a tightly regulated process that ensures a constant supply of fuel to the body. In contrast, insulin resistant individuals have a reduction in insulin-mediated glucose disposal, resulting in a compensatory increase in insulin secretion. Consequently, persons with IGT or early T2DM often have both hyperglycemia and hyperinsulinemia (Ramlo-Halsted & Edelman, 1999). The complications of diabetes are well known and include metabolic syndrome, renal dysfunction, macular degeneration, and peripheral neuropathy. Age is a primary risk factor for insulin resistant conditions. In the US, the prevalence of diabetes rises from 1–2% among young adults to about 20% among adults aged 60 and older (Harris *et al.*, 1998), and the prevalence of either IGT or diabetes rises to about 34% among this older age group (MMWR, 2003). Aging is also the primary risk factor for AD, doubling the incidence of late onset AD for every 5 years. Therefore, aging increases the risk for both AD and insulin resistant conditions in older adults.

Converging evidence supports the notion that insulin resistance and AD may be reciprocal risk factors. In comparison with healthy older adults, patients with AD are at greater risk for hyperinsulinemia and hyperglycemia (Luchsinger *et al.*, 2004; Razay & Wilcock, 1994; Meneilly *et al.*, 1993). We have reported that patients with moderate AD have increased insulin levels in plasma and reduced levels of insulin in cerebrospinal fluid (CSF) (Craft *et al.*, 1998). Furthermore, this relationship between insulin resistance and AD is supported by several epidemiological studies. In the Honolulu-Asia Aging Study, Japanese-American men with T2DM had an increased incidence of dementia, including AD and vascular dementia (Peila *et al.*,

2002). Other investigators have reported that T2DM is a risk factor for AD, independent of vascular dementia (Ott *et al.*, 1999; Leibson *et al.*, 1997). Collectively, these observations argue in favor of an association between AD and insulin resistance (Messier, 2003). Additional support comes from work demonstrating that insulin is active in the central nervous system (CNS), where it may contribute to the pathophysiology and cognitive dysfunction found in patients with AD.

Insulin in the Central Nervous System

A plethora of evidence proves that the brain is insulin sensitive. Notably, insulin and insulin receptors are expressed in the brains of rats (Havrankova *et al.*, 1978a, b) and humans (Rivera *et al.*, 2005; Frolich *et al.*, 1998). Insulin receptors are found on synapses of neurons and astroglial cells (Abbott *et al.*, 1999), and insulin binding is greatest in the olfactory bulb, cortex, hippocampus, hypothalamus, amygdala, and septum (Unger *et al.*, 1991; Baskin *et al.*, 1987; Havrankova *et al.*, 1978a, b). Insulin is secreted by pancreatic β cells and subsequently transported across the blood–brain barrier via a saturable receptor-mediated transport system (Banks *et al.*, 1997a, b; Baura *et al.*, 1993). Although controversial, brain insulin may also be produced locally in the adult human brain (de la Monte & Wands, 2005). We have shown an acute intravenous infusion of insulin raises levels of insulin in both blood and CSF in less than 2 h in healthy older adults (Watson & Craft, 2003); however, this transport process may be compromised in patients with AD (Watson *et al.*, 2006a). Paradoxically, chronic hyperinsulinemia associated with insulin resistance may down-regulate the rate of insulin transport across the blood–brain barrier (Schwartz *et al.*, 1990), and we observed that patients with moderate AD have lower CSF-to-plasma insulin ratios than do healthy older adults (Craft *et al.*, 1998), consistent with reduced blood-to-brain transport in these patients. Thus, biological mechanisms exist through which peripherally-secreted insulin is transported into the brain where it can affect insulin signaling in areas that are disturbed in patients with AD.

Brain insulin signaling contributes to normal memory processing (Watson & Craft, 2004). We have reported that raising peripheral insulin levels, while maintaining normal blood glucose levels, facilitates verbal memory and complex attention in both patients with AD and healthy older adults (Craft *et al.*, 2003; 1999a, b; 1996). Other studies have shown that insulin-induced hypoglycemia can impair cognitive performance in humans and in non-human animals (Watson & Craft, 2004), suggesting that adequate glucose levels are crucial to insulin-induced memory facilitation; however, when we administered glucose and suppressed the endogenous insulin response to glucose, we failed to observe memory facilitation (Craft *et al.*, 1999a). Collectively, these observations support our hypothesis that blood-borne insulin is transported across the blood–brain barrier where, in the presence of adequate glucose levels, it facilitates cognitive performance.

Animal studies employing administration of insulin directly to CNS corroborate this hypothesis. In rats, intracerebroventricular injection of insulin improves performance on a passive avoidance task (Park *et al.*, 2000). In humans, intracerebroventricular insulin administration would be an extremely invasive procedure and therefore, inappropriate as an experimental means of exploring memory.

Intranasal drug administration can provide direct access to the CNS via a minimally invasive procedure. When Thorne and Frey applied insulin-like growth factor-1 (IGF-1) to the cribriform plate in rats, they observed rapid IGF-1 transport along two different bulk-flow channels: (1) the olfactory system that projects to rostral brain regions, including the hippocampus and amygdala (2) the peripheral trigeminal system that projects to the brain stem and spinal cord (Thorne *et al.*, 2004). When healthy young adult humans received intranasal insulin administration, CSF insulin levels rose within 10 min and reached peak levels within 30 min. In contrast, intranasal insulin administration did not alter serum glucose or insulin levels, demonstrating that insulin was not transported into peripheral circulation (Kern *et al.*, 1999) . Furthermore, intranasal insulin administration has been shown to produce functional, cognitive, and affective changes consistent with transport into the CNS. Acute intranasal insulin administration modulates auditory-evoked brain potentials (Kern *et al.*, 1999) and facilitates verbal memory in patients with AD (Reger *et al.*, 2006). Chronic administration enhances verbal memory and mood in young healthy adults (Benedict *et al.*, 2004), and decreases body fat and weight (Hallschmid *et al.*, 2004). Thus, insulin plays a role in memory and other CNS functions, a role that may be mediated through divergent mechanisms, including cerebral glucose metabolism, molecular events, and neurotransmitter modulation (Craft & Watson, 2004; Watson & Craft, 2003).

Mechanisms for Insulin's Effects on Memory

In the periphery, a principal function of insulin is to mediate glucose utilization. Since glucose is the primary brain energy substrate, it is important to consider whether insulin mediates glucose utilization in the brain as well as in the periphery. Glucose is transported across the blood–brain barrier by glucose transporters expressed on the vascular endothelial cells, astrocytes, and neurons (Schulingkamp *et al.*, 2000). Although low doses of exogenously applied insulin can raise cerebral glucose metabolism, it appears unlikely that insulin modulates the normal transport of glucose into the brain (Bingham *et al.*, 2002). Thus, the cognitive effects of insulin do not reflect global changes in cerebral glucose metabolism; however, insulin likely exerts an influence on glucose metabolism in selective brain regions. Insulin-sensitive glucose transporters are normally located within the cell and translocated to the cell membrane in the presence of insulin, so that they provide a mechanism by which insulin increases glucose uptake. In rats, insulin-sensitive glucose transporters are selectively expressed in areas that include the hippocampus, hypothalamus, pituitary, cerebellum, and sensorimotor cortex (Reagan *et al.*, 2001; Apelt *et al.*, 1999). Furthermore, this distribution of insulin-sensitive glucose transporters over-laps with insulin-containing neurons and insulin receptors (Apelt *et al.*, 1999), suggesting that insulin-sensitive glucose transporters, insulin, and insulin recep-tors work in concert to regulate local glucose disposal in such regions as the hip-pocampus, a brain structure that is essential for the formation of declarative memory. Consistent with this notion, rat studies have shown local changes in cerebral glucose metabolism in response to hyperinsulinemia (Doyle *et al.*, 1995; Marfaing *et al.*, 1990). The cognitive facilitation associated with intranasal insulin administration described above (Reger *et al.*, 2006; Benedict *et al.*, 2004) may be attributable, in part, to increased local glucose metabolism, since insulin is delivered rapidly to the medial temporal lobe (Thorne *et al.*, 2004).

In addition to cerebral glucose metabolism, insulin regulates other events that influence cognitive function. For example, molecular components of the insulin signaling cascade are altered during the acquisition phase of a spatial memory task in rats (Zhao *et al.*, 1999). The investigators reported that spatial learning was associated with increased insulin receptor messenger RNA expression in the CA1 region of the hippocampus and in the dentate gyrus, increased insulin receptor pro-tein in the crude synaptic membrane fraction, and altered tyrosine phosphoryla-tion levels in membrane and cytosolic proteins. Interestingly, different phases of spatial memory acquisition have opposite effects on insulin receptor substrate-1 (IRS-1) levels in hippocampal synaptic membranes. IRS-1 levels are increased shortly following task acquisition but decreased when the task has been well learned. Thus, behaviors associated with learning and memory can alter the insulin receptor and insulin signaling cascade.

Insulin also has been shown to modulate long-term potentiation (LTP) and long-term depression (LTD) (van der Heide *et al.*, 2005). These persistent changes in strength of synaptic association are thought to describe events that subserve learning and memory at a cellular level. In hippocampal CA1 neurons, introduction of insulin reduces the electrical stimulation frequency required for the induction of LTP and LTD. Furthermore, inhibition of the PI3K insulin signaling pathway reduces induction of LTD (van der Heide *et al.*, 2005). Other investigators have shown that membrane expression of *N*-methyl-D-aspartate (NMDA) receptors is promoted by insulin (Skeberdis *et al.*, 2001) which increases the influx of Ca^{++} into neurons, which likely activates α-calcium-calmodulin-dependent-kinase II (αCaMKII) and strengthens synaptic associations (Byrne, 2003). In contrast, streptozotocin administration causes hypoinsulinemia and lowers α-CaMKII-dependent activity in NMDA receptors (Di Luca *et al.*, 1999). Thus, insulin may contribute to cognitive functions through effects on synaptic plasticity.

Insulin regulates levels of neurotransmitters, such as acetylcholine and norep-inephrine, which modulate cognitive functions. It is well known that cholinergic transmission is disrupted in AD, and drugs that attenuate cholinergic disruption (cholinesterase inhibitors) are first line agents in the treatment of AD. Cholinergic receptor antagonists such as scopolamine have a deleterious effect on memory (Kopf & Baratti, 1996; Ragozzino *et al.*, 1994). Notably, a dose of insulin that does not induce hypoglycemia can attenuate scopolamine-induced memory impairment, even though the same dose of insulin fails to influence memory when administered without scopolamine (Blanchard & Duncan, 1997). This finding suggests that a low dose of insulin can improve disruptions in cholinergic transmission. Similarly, insulin can modulate catecholamine signaling. In rats, insulin reduces norepinephrine uptake in primary neuronal cultures (Boyd *et al.*, 1985) and hypothalamic slices (Figlewicz *et al.*, 1993a), and reduces norepinephrine transporter mRNA in the locus coeruleus *in vivo* (Figlewicz *et al.*, 1993b). Thus, physiological levels of insulin may increase synaptic concentrations of norepinephrine via reduced uptake. We have reported that a 105-min intravenous insulin infusion increases CSF norepinephrine levels in healthy older adults (Watson *et al.*, 2006a).

Insulin, Insulin Resistance, and AD Pathophysiology

Thus, insulin can modulate cognitive functions through a variety of normal mechanisms including cerebral glucose metabolism, molecular events, and neurotransmitter regulation. Consequently, insulin abnormalities may produce dysfunction in the healthy processes that contribute to normal memory. Furthermore, insulin abnormalities may contribute to the pathophysiology seen in patients with neurodegenerative diseases, in particular via effects on inflammation and beta-amyloid (Aβ). Finally, the deleterious effects of insulin resistance may be related to metabolic syndrome, which comprises hypertension, dyslipidemia (elevated LDL and/or low HDL levels), hyperglycemia, and obesity.

Insulin Resistance and Inflammation

In the periphery, insulin has a complex relationship with the inflammatory network. On the one hand, low doses of insulin have an anti-inflammatory effect (Dandona, 2002). In contrast, chronically high levels of insulin provoke a proinflammatory response (Krogh-Madsen *et al.*, 2004). In humans, insulin administration can exacerbate the proinflammatory response to an endotoxic stimulus, such as lipopolysaccharide (Soop *et al.*, 2002). We have recently shown that a brief (105 min) intravenous infusion of insulin produces a dramatic CNS proinflammatory response in healthy older humans. Relative to a baseline (saline) infusion condition, levels of interleukin (IL)-1β and tumor necrosis factor (TNF)-alpha approximately doubled, IL-6 increased several fold, and F_2-isoprostane increased by about 35% during the insulin infusion. It is not surprising, therefore, that insulin resistance is characterized by increased markers of inflammation (Hak *et al.*, 2001; Pickup *et al.*, 1997). AD is also a chronic inflammatory condition. Patients with AD have plasma and CSF elevations of proinflammatory biomarkers (Akiyama *et al.*, 2000), including CSF elevations of IL-6 and F_2-isoprostane (Cacquevel *et al.*, 2004; Montine *et al.*, 2001; Rosler *et al.*, 2001). It has been proposed that cytokines influence the pathophysiology of AD (Hull *et al.*, 1996), possibly in part through a reciprocal interaction with Aβ (Fishel *et al.*, 2005).

Insulin Resistance, Inflammation, and Aβ

Aβ is the principal constituent of senile plaques that are a hallmark of AD, and changes in Aβ levels in both plasma and CSF have been associated with AD. CSF Aβ levels are lower in patients with AD than in healthy older adults (Andreasen & Blennow, 2002). In contrast, patients with AD appear to have higher than normal plasma Aβ levels, which decline with disease progression (Mayeux *et al.*, 2003). Our work has shown that Aβ levels in CSF and plasma are modulated by insulin. Notably, CSF levels of Aβ increase and plasma Aβ levels decrease when healthy older humans receive a 2-h infusion of insulin (Kulstad *et al.*, 2006; Watson *et al.*, 2003). In contrast, patients with AD show an increase in plasma Aβ levels in response to insulin (Kulstad *et al.*, 2006). These phenomena may reflect insulin's promotion intracellular release of Aβ from neurons (Gasparini *et al.*, 2001) and/or modulation of Aβ degradation by insulin-degrading enzyme, a metalloprotease with a preferential affinity for insulin (Qiu *et al.*, 1998).

Proinflammatory reactants and activated microglia have been associated with amyloid plaques (Landreth & Heneka, 2001). Furthermore, Aβ increases the secretion of neurotoxic products, promotes astrocytic activation, and stimulates both monocyte differentiation into macrophages and expression of cytokine genes and COX-2 (Combs *et al.*, 2000). IL-1β levels are increased when Aβ42 is administered to rats, an effect that is down-regulated by the neuromodulator norepinephrine (Heneka *et al.*, 2002). Peripheral insulin administration can raise CSF norepinephrine levels in healthy older humans (Watson *et al.*, 2006a), suggesting that insulin can attenuate Aβ toxicity through effects on norepinephrine. We recently reported that an insulin-induced increase in CSF norepinephrine was associated with lower CSF levels of Aβ42 and IL-1β in healthy older humans (Fishel *et al.*, 2005). Furthermore, insulin may modulate Aβ levels through effects on transthyretin, an Aβ-binding protein produced in the liver. Raising transthyretin levels may increase the transport of Aβ out of the CNS into the periphery (Carro *et al.*, 2002), where Aβ can be degraded in a peripheral sink. Consistent with CNS-to-blood transport, insulin-induced elevations of transthyretin were associated with a decrease in CSF Aβ42 levels and an increase in plasma Aβ42 levels (Fishel *et al.*, 2005). Since patients with AD have reduced transthyretin levels (Carro *et al.*, 2002), neuroinflammation could potentially reflect, in part, decreased Aβ42 transport out of the CNS.

Further support for the notion that insulin modulates Aβ levels comes from observations that Aβ levels are modulated by body mass index (BMI), an anthropomorphic measure that is highly related to insulin resistance. Plasma Aβ42 levels were significantly correlated with both BMI ($r = 0.55$) and fat mass ($r = 0.60$) in a group of healthy young-to-older human adults (Balakrishnan *et al.*, 2005). Furthermore, BMI can modulate the relationship between insulin and plasma Aβ42 levels; specifically, during induced hyperinsulinemia, BMI was correlated with plasma Aβ42 levels ($r = 0.49$) in healthy older humans (Fishel *et al.*, 2005). Thus, Aβ42 levels are related to two correlates of insulin resistance, hyperinsulinemia and to BMI. These findings are consistent with longitudinal data from Gustafson and colleagues who followed 392 Swedish adults from age 70 to age 88 and found that a higher BMI predicted an increase in incident AD (Gustafson *et al.*, 2003). Thus, insulin and insulin resistance may contribute to the risk for AD through effects on the inflammatory network or Aβ42, and furthermore, insulin's effects on these two systems are likely interdependent.

Insulin Resistance and Dyslipidemia

The risk for AD may also be modified by dyslipidemia, since insulin resistance and hyperinsulinemia are often accompanied by elevated free fatty acid levels. These are unesterified fatty acids that can be stored as triglycerides for future energy use. Normally, insulin attenuates free fatty acid release from adipocytes by regulating adipocyte hormone-sensitive lipase activity (Ruan & Lodish, 2003); however, obesity and insulin resistance disrupt regulation of adipocyte hormone-sensitive lipase activity, yielding chronic elevations of triglycerides and free fatty acids (Boden *et al.*, 2001; Brechtel *et al.*, 2001; Reaven *et al.*, 1988; Gordon, 1968). Interestingly, normalizing elevated free fatty acid levels produces a 50% increase in insulin sensitivity in obese individuals (Santomauro, 1999). Lowering free fatty acids could improve insulin sensitivity, and thus, potentially reduce the risk for developing AD.

Insulin, Apolipoprotein E Genotype, and AD

Interestingly, apolipoprotein E (*APOE*) genotype, an established genetic risk factor for AD, appears to modulate the metabolic effects of insulin and insulin resistance on the risk for AD, cognitive functions, and amyloid proteins associated with AD. There are three *APOE* alleles (e2, e3, e4). Possession of the e4 allele dose-dependently increases an individual's risk for developing AD, possibly by lowering the age of onset. In the Kuopio study, investigators observed that hyperinsulinemia (an indicator of insulin resistance) was associated with an increased risk for AD only in persons without the e4 allele. This finding suggests that *APOE* genotype can modify the risk for AD related to insulin resistance

(Kuusisto *et al.*, 1997), a notion corroborated by our clinical findings: non-homozygous e4 patients with AD have decreased insulin-mediated glucose disposal rates, increased plasma insulin concentrations, and decreased CSF-to-plasma insulin ratios, relative to e4 homozygous patients (Craft *et al.*, 1998). Furthermore, our work supports the notion that these metabolic differences translate into functional differences. Relative to AD patients with two copies of the e4 allele, non-homozygous patients require higher insulin doses to facilitate memory and selective attention, as well as to decrease plasma levels of the amyloid precursor protein (Craft *et al.*, 2003). These findings support the notion that *APOE* genotype modulates the cognitive and pathophysiological effects of insulin activity in patients with AD.

Brain Insulin Resistance and AD: A Case for Type 3 Diabetes

In a recent review, de la Monte and Wards presented a compelling case for impaired insulin signaling to AD (de la Monte & Wands, 2005), which they later termed "type 3 diabetes" (Rivera *et al.*, 2005). For example, AD is associated with changes in the insulin signaling cascade, including reduced tyrosine kinase activity, decreased concentrations of insulin, IRS mRNA, IRS-associated phosphotidyl-inositol 3-kinase, and activated phosphor-Akt (Steen *et al.*, 2005; Frolich *et al.*, 1999; 1998), and these brain insulin abnormalities impair cholinergic transmission (Rivera *et al.*, 2005). These findings are consistent with a profound disruption in insulin signal transduction, which potentially could influence energy production, oxidative stress, cell survival, GSK-3β activation, and advanced glycation of proteins (de la Monte & Wands, 2005), and support the notion that insulin resistance contributes to the pathophysiological hallmarks of AD. Insulin promotes intracellular release of Aβ from neurons (Gasparini *et al.*, 2001) and modulates of Aβ degradation (Qiu *et al.*, 1998); therefore, impaired insulin signaling could also influence amyloid deposition. Furthermore, increased oxidative stress and glycogen synthase kinase (GSK)-3β activation have been associated with hyper-phosphorylation of tau. De la Monte and colleagues have used intracerebral streptozotocin administration as a rodent model for type 3 diabetes (Lester-Coll *et al.*, 2006). Streptozotocin-treated animals are similar to controls with regard to blood glucose concentration, peripheral insulin immunoreactivity, and pancreatic architecture; however, intracerebral streptozotocin administration produces marked AD-like brain changes including atrophy; increased levels of activated GSK-3β phospho-tau, and Aβ; and decreased expression of genes associated with neurons, glia, choline acetyltransferase, insulin, insulin receptor, and IRS-1 (Lester-Coll *et al.*, 2006). Notably, PPAR agonist administration rescues treated-streptozotocin rats from AD-like neurodegenerative changes, likely via increased insulin binding and choline acetyltransferase levels and decreased levels of tau phosphorylation and oxidative stress (de la Monte *et al.*, 2006).

In summary, insulin contributes to normal memory processing, and insulin resistant conditions such as chronic hyperinsulinemia, IGT, T2DM, and obesity increase the risk for developing both AD and memory impairment independent of AD. The relationship between AD and insulin resistance may be explained, in part, by the relationships among insulin, insulin resistance, Aβ, inflammation, free fatty acids, and *APOE* genotype. In the following sections, we will review evidence demonstrating that increasing insulin activity, either by improving insulin sensitivity or by selectively increasing brain insulin levels, may constitute novel therapeutic strategies for persons with AD. First, we will examine the effects of insulin sensitizing agents currently used to treat T2DM. Next, we will characterize the effects of intranasal insulin administration. Finally, we will explore the preventative or treatment potential of diet and exercise.

PPAR-gamma Agonists and Treatment of AD

PPAR-gamma Actions in the Periphery and CNS

The ligand-activated nuclear transcription factor PPAR-gamma is an exciting target for improving insulin sensitivity in both the periphery and the CNS. PPAR-gamma is densely expressed in peripheral adipocytes, where it regulates adipogenesis, increases fatty acid influx and thus reduces fatty acid availability for muscles, decreases TNF-alpha expression, and shifts fat from visceral to subcutaneous depots (Ferre, 2004). Additionally, PPAR-gamma agonists exert anti-inflammatory actions in the periphery in both rats (Cuzzocrea *et al.*, 2004) and humans (Sidhu *et al.*, 2003). Notably, the potency of a PPAR-gamma agonist predicts the compound's anti-diabetic action; in contrast, insulin resistance, early onset T2DM, and dyslipidemia have been associated with heterozygous loss of function mutations within the PPAR-gamma ligand binding domain (Gurnell, 2003). PPAR-gamma agonists improve peripheral insulin sensitivity with minimal direct influence on endogenous insulin secretion or gluconeogenesis; however, by reducing insulin resistance, PPAR-gamma agonists effective reduce both hyperinsulinemia and hyperglycemia (Malinowski & Blesta, 2000). Currently, two PPAR-gamma agonists, rosiglitazone, and pioglitazone, are approved to treat T2DM.

PPAR-gamma is expressed on neurons and astrocytes in the brain (Moreno *et al.*, 2004), where it modulates the survival of cells and inflammatory responses. It has been shown that PPAR-gamma agonists decrease both microglial activation (Bernard *et al.*, 2003) and iNOS expression in neurons and glia (Uryu *et al.*, 2002; Heneka *et al.*, 2000; Kitamura *et al.*, 1999a). As previously noted, Aβ, the principal constituent of senile plaques, is proinflammatory. PPAR-gamma agonists appear to modulate Aβ-stimulated proinflammatory responses such as monocyte differentiation into macrophages, activation of microglia, and cytokine gene expression (Combs *et al.*, 2000). Interestingly, patients with AD have increased PPAR-gamma expression in the temporal cortex (Kitamura *et al.*, 1999b), suggestive of an endogenous anti-inflammatory response. Although controversial, there is some evidence suggesting that PPAR-gamma can influence Aβ processing and deposition, partially by increasing β-secretase activity or inhibiting proinflammatory effects on β-secretase activity and Aβ production (Sastre *et al.*, 2003).

Recently, it has been shown that PPAR-gamma agonists belonging to the thiazolidinedione class of anti-diabetic agents, which includes rosiglitazone, can modulate astrocytic glucose metabolism and may have direct effects on mitochondrial function (Dello Russo *et al.*, 2003). As reviewed by Feinstein and colleagues (Feinstein *et al.*, 2005), the thiazolidinediones modulate mitochondrial respiration, thereby increasing glucose consumption and lactate production in astrocytes. Since AD is associated with glucose hypometabolism, thiazolidinediones may enhance cognitive functions by beneficial effects on energy metabolism. Furthermore, thiazolidinediones appear to promote anti-inflammatory and cytoprotective responses by acting on mitochondrial function. In brief, thiazolidinediones provoke the heat shock response, activate the enzyme adenosine 5′-monophosphate-activated protein kinase (AMPK), and increase reactive oxygen species (ROS, which can also activate AMPK). The heat shock response increases IκB expression, which inhibits NF kappa B expression and reduces inflammation. AMPK activation can attenuate inflammatory gene expression and possibly to regulate cell proliferation. Taken together, these observations suggest that thiazolidinediones contribute to cell health through regulation of glucose metabolism and mitochondrial function (Feinstein *et al.*, 2005).

Thus, PPAR-gamma agonists regulate central and peripheral insulin sensitivity, energy metabolism, mitochondrial function, and inflammatory responses. These properties raise the intriguing possibility that these agents may have beneficial effects in neuroinflammatory conditions, such as AD and multiple sclerosis. For example, in animal models of multiple sclerosis, the PPAR-gamma agonist pioglitazone significantly improves disease severity and even can lead to remission (Diab *et al.*, 2002; Feinstein *et al.*, 2002), and pioglitazone has been suggested as a novel treatment for multiple sclerosis (Pershadsingh *et al.*, 2004). Two published studies have support the notion that that the PPAR-gamma agonist rosiglitazone may have therapeutic potential in the treatment of patients with AD.

PPAR-gamma Agonists and Treatment of Patients with AD

We recently reported the results of a pilot trial that investigated the effects of a 6-month course of the PPAR-gamma agonist rosiglitazone in patients with early stage AD or with amnestic mild cognitive impairment, the prodromal phase of AD (Watson *et al.*, 2005). Patients were randomly assigned to receive rosiglitazone (4 mg daily; $n = 20$) or matched placebo ($n = 10$). The primary endpoints were performance on measures of declarative memory and changes plasma Aβ levels. At baseline, the two groups were not significantly different with respect to demographic characteristics, disease severity, or percentage of persons taking cholinesterase inhibitors. On a delayed word list memory task, subjects receiving placebo showed the expected (non-significant) decline over the 6-month treatment period; however, subjects receiving the rosiglitazone did not decline. The net effect was that the two groups recalled an equivalent number of words at 2 months of treatment, and the rosiglitazone group had improved recall, relative to the placebo group, at months 4 and 6. Then we looked at the relationship between plasma insulin levels and delayed recall in the rosiglitazone group. Lower insulin levels reflect enhanced treatment efficacy. After 6 months of rosiglitazone treatment, better recall was associated with lower insulin levels, consistent with the notion that delayed word list recall improved was associated with enhanced treatment efficacy. Similar patterns were observed on a measure of selective attention: the rosiglitazone group remained stable over time, whereas the placebo group showed a decline in performance, and furthermore, better selective attention was associated with lower plasma insulin levels, indicative of an enhanced response to rosiglitazone treatment. Thus, both memory and selective attention were better in the rosiglitazone group than in the placebo group, and cognitive performance was associated with enhanced metabolic response to treatment.

Next, we examined the effect of rosiglitazone on plasma levels of Aβ40 and Aβ42. It has been reported that patients with early AD have an increase in plasma Aβ42 levels, which declines as the disease progresses (Mayeux *et al.*, 2003). In our sample, the pattern of changes in plasma Aβ levels did not differ by species, and so data were collapsed for Aβ40 and Aβ42. For the placebo group, plasma Aβ levels decreased over the 6-month treatment period. In contrast, plasma Aβ levels were stable over time in the rosiglitazone group.

One of the suggested mechanisms for Aβ clearance is a peripheral "sink." In this model, Aβ is transported across the blood–brain barrier into the periphery and degraded (Morgan, 2005). For example, peripheral administration of compounds with a high affinity for Aβ can reduce brain concentrations of Aβ (Matsuoka *et al.*, 2003). Although speculative, the decrease in Aβ levels in the placebo group may have reflected reduced efflux out of the CNS into the periphery, and that rosiglitazone prevented the reduction in transport, possibly by its anti-inflammatory actions. For example, Aβ transport is facilitated by carrier proteins such as albumin and transthyretin, and impeded by TNF-alpha through effects on carrier proteins (Carro *et al.*, 2002). In support of this notion, insulin-induced increases in CSF Aβ42 levels were associated with increases in the CSF levels of the inflammatory markers IL-6 and F_2-isoprostane and a decrease in the CSF level of the Aβ carrier protein transthyretin (Fishel *et al.*, 2005). Rosiglitazone has been shown to reduce TNF-alpha in diabetic humans (Marfella *et al.*, 2006), which, in turn, could modulate Aβ efflux into the periphery.

In this study, we observed effects for rosiglitazone on memory and on plasma Aβ levels. These two effects may be related. We have previously demonstrated that induced hyperinsulinemia increases CSF levels of Aβ42 and that these increases in Aβ42 have a deleterious effect on memory (Watson *et al.*, 2003). If lower plasma Aβ levels in the placebo group reflect greater Aβ sequestration in the brain, then one might hypothesize an association between lower plasma Aβ levels and poorer memory scores.

PPAR-gamma Effects Moderated by APOE Genotype

In a separate intention-to-treat study, Risner and colleagues investigated the cognitive effects of three doses of rosiglitazone (2, 4, 8 mg once per day) and placebo in a sample of 511 patients with a clinical diagnosis of mild-to-moderate probable AD (Risner *et al.*, 2006). *APOE* genotyping was acquired on 322 of 511 subjects. The primary endpoint was performance on the AD Assessment Scale-Cognitive (ADAS-Cog), without respect to *APOE* genotype. In secondary analyses, the sample was stratified by genotype. Contrary to prediction, the investigators failed to observe a cognitive effect for rosiglitazone over the 24-week course of the trial, suggesting that patients with AD as a whole do not benefit from treatment with rosiglitazone. Secondary analyses revealed a beneficial effect for rosiglitazone when the sample was stratified by *APOE* genotype. Subjects without the e4 allele who were taking the highest rosiglitazone dose (8 mg) showed a significant improvement on the ADAS-Cog; however, patients with an e4 allele failed to show improvement. The magnitude of improvement was commensurate with the cognitive effects attributed to cholinesterase inhibitor therapy, the current standard pharmacologic treatment for AD (Risner *et al.*, 2006).

It is well established that insulin and insulin receptors are expressed in the brain, and several investigators have demonstrated that brain insulin signaling is impaired in AD (de Rivera *et al.*, 2006; Schubert *et al.*, 2004; Hoyer & Lannert, 1999). These two rosiglitazone studies support the notion that strategies that improve insulin sensitivity can be used effectively to treat AD. Furthermore, accruing evidence raises the intriguing possibility that *APOE* genotype influences the effects of insulin resistance on pathophysiology and cognitive functions in patients with AD. The observation by Risner and colleagues that *APOE* genotype modulated rosiglitazone's effects on cognition is supported by our prior reports that *APOE* genotype modulates CSF insulin levels, CSF-to-plasma insulin ratios, insulin-mediated glucose disposal, and insulin-induced changes in cognitive functions and plasma levels of the amyloid precursor protein (Craft *et al.*, 2003; 1998). Taken together, these reports demonstrate that *APOE* genotype can influence the effects of insulin on CNS functions. Of course, additional studies are needed to confirm the beneficial effects of PPAR-gamma agonist therapy for the treatment of AD and other memory and neurodegenerative disorders; however, it is clear that these studies should consider the role of *APOE* genotype.

Exercise and Diet and Treatment of AD

Diet, Exercise, and Insulin Resistance

We have examined the evidence showing that improving insulin sensitivity with PPAR-gamma agonists can facilitate memory for patients with AD. Now, we turn briefly to a non-pharmacologic strategy that exerts a powerful and beneficial effect on insulin resistance. Two large-scale studies, the Diabetes Prevention Program (Knowler *et al.*, 2002) and the Finnish Diabetes Prevention Study (Tuomilehto *et al.*, 2001), have examined the impact of lifestyle modification on the risk of converting from IGT (prodromal diabetes) to clinical diabetes. Both studies demonstrated conclusively that a program of physical exercise and good nutrition significantly decrease the incidence of diabetes. Two observations from these studies deserve special attention. First, the Diabetes Prevention Program was designed to compare the effects of two active interventions: metformin, a standard pharmacologic treatment for diabetes, and lifestyle modification. Relative to the control group, both active interventions improved the risk for incident diabetes; however, lifestyle modification produced a larger effect than did metformin. Second, investigators in the Finnish Diabetes Prevention Study reported that participants who showed the most successful lifestyle interventions had the lowest risk of incident diabetes. These findings illustrate the exceptional efficacy of diet and exercise to improve insulin sensitivity. Together with studies showing that insulin resistant conditions impair memory in humans (Luchsinger *et al.*, 2004; Vanhanen *et al.*, 1998; Strachan *et al.*, 1997) and animals (Ho *et al.*, 2004), findings from the Diabetes Prevention Project and the Finnish Diabetes Prevention Study suggest that exercise and dietary interventions may have a positive effect on memory.

Diet, Exercise, and Memory

Recently, we examined the cognitive effects of exercise and nutrition in a sample of Japanese-American adults with IGT (Watson *et al.*, 2006b). The active intervention consisted of an American Heart Association (AHA) step 2 diet (total calories: <30% fat, 55% carbohydrate, balance as protein) and walking or jogging on a treadmill three times weekly for 1 h. The control intervention consisted of an AHA step 1 diet (total calories: 30% fat, 50% carbohydrate, 20% protein) and stretching exercise three times a week for 1 h. After 6 months, BMI was reduced in the active group relative to the control group, demonstrating that the lifestyle modification was effective. Notably, strenuous exercise and dietary restriction improved delayed memory in that the active group retained a greater proportion of delayed story recall information, relative to the control group. Finally, we examined the relationship between plasma insulin levels following a glucose challenge and the effect of diet and exercise on delayed story recall. For participants in the active condition, lower glucose-stimulated insulin levels were correlated with greater improvement in delayed recall, suggesting that improved delayed memory was associated with improved insulin sensitivity in the active group. Thus, lifestyle modification improved both a metabolic index of insulin sensitivity (BMI) and delayed memory, and these changes were correlated in the hypothesized direction.

Diet, Exercise, and AD

Of special relevance to AD, it has been shown that diet-induced insulin resistance can exacerbate amyloid-related pathophysiology in a transgenic murine model of AD. Pasinetti and colleagues used a high-fat diet to promote insulin resistance in Tg2576 mice (Ho *et al.*, 2004). They reported that insulin resistance altered the brain insulin signaling cascade and promoted the generation of Aβ40 and Aβ42. Increased Aβ generation was associated with increased activity of β-secretase (an enzyme that is essential in the production of the amyloidogenic species of Aβ) and reduced levels of insulin-degrading enzyme (a metalloprotease that degrades Aβ). Thus, insulin resistance appears to contribute to impaired insulin signaling and amyloid-related pathophysiology that characterize AD. In contrast, caloric restriction in Tg2576 mice reduce cortical and hippocampal Aβ40 and Aβ42 burden, possibly by increasing β-secretase activity (Wang *et al.*, 2005). Collectively, these findings suggest the nutrition-related changes in insulin resistance may modulate the amyloidogenic processes in patients with AD.

A recent prospective cohort study provides evidence for the beneficial effects of exercise on the incidence of dementia (Larson *et al.*, 2006). A large sample of cognitively intact older adults was followed to determine the relationship between incident dementia and frequent exercise (defined as three or more times per week). Participants who exercised frequently had a lower rate of incident dementia (13.0/1000 person-years) than did participants who exercised fewer than three times per week (19.7/1000 person-years). The authors concluded that regular exercise delayed the onset of both dementia in general and specifically AD. A limitation of this study is that mechanisms must be inferred from the cognitive effects of exercise. Animal work points to several potential mechanisms for the beneficial effects of exercise on the risk for AD. Fo example, exercise enhances protein and mRNA levels of brain-derived neurotrophic factor (BDNF) in the hippocampus and increases cell proliferation in the dentate gyrus (Molteni *et al.*, 2004). Another neurotrophic factor, IGF-1 likely contributes to the effects of exercise on hippocampal plasticity and cell proliferation (Kim *et al.*, 2004; Trejo *et al.*, 2001). Therefore, exercise may induce the expression of neurotrophic factors that promote cell survival and plasticity.

We have considered evidence demonstrating that improving insulin sensitivity with diet and exercise can preserve memory and retard the pathophysiologic processes associated with impaired insulin signaling and amyloidogenesis in patients with AD. These findings corroborate and extend the evidence showing that improving insulin sensitivity with PPAR-gamma agonists may have therapeutic efficacy in the treatment of AD. Thus, strategies that improve insulin's activity by reducing insulin resistance show therapeutic promise for patients with AD. Raising brain insulin levels is an alternative approach to increasing brain insulin activity. In the next section, we will turn to another potential therapeutic strategy for AD, intranasal administration of insulin.

Intranasal Insulin Administration and Treatment of AD

A plethora of evidence has demonstrated that brain insulin signaling contributes to normal memory functions and that insulin abnormalities are present in neurodegenerative disorders such as AD (Craft & Watson, 2004). We have shown that peripheral insulin administration raises CNS insulin levels and facilitates memory in adults with AD and in cognitively intact older adults (Watson & Craft, 2004). Based on studies showing abnormal brain insulin signaling in patients with AD (111–113), we have hypothesized that raising peripheral insulin levels facilitates memory by increasing brain insulin levels and thus restoring brain insulin signaling. In AD patients, the increased risk for peripheral insulin abnormalities may exacerbate brain insulin impairments (Craft & Watson, 2004).

Insulin Resistance and Brain Insulin

Insulin resistance can reduce the rate of transport of insulin from the periphery into the CNS (Kaiyala *et al.*, 2000), a defect that could result in reduced the CNS insulin levels or reduced CSF-to-plasma insulin ratios observed in patients with moderate AD (Craft *et al.*, 1998). Thus, insulin resistance could contribute to impaired brain insulin signaling through absolute or relative reductions in brain insulin levels; increasing insulin sensitivity (with medications or lifestyle modification) may improve memory, in part, by increasing the rate of insulin transport into the CNS. Reduced insulin transport across the blood–brain barrier would also explain, in part, insulin-induced memory facilitation: acute peripheral insulin administration would overcome the reduced rate of transport, elevate CNS insulin levels, and thereby produce a transient increase in brain insulin levels and activity. Furthermore, impaired rates of insulin transport could also account for the *APOE* genotypic effects in response to insulin or rosiglitazone administration. As previously noted, *APOE* genotype has been shown to modulate the effects of insulin on cognitive functions and on plasma levels of the amyloid precursor protein, such that the presence of one or two e4 alleles is associated with greater insulin sensitivity than is the absence of an e4 allele (Watson & Craft, 2004). These observations suggest a model in which insulin is transported from the periphery into the brain where it participates in normal memory and amyloid processing. Insulin resistant conditions reduce insulin transport into the CNS, disrupting normal memory. AD is associated with reduced insulin transport and impaired insulin signaling, and the *APOE* e4 negative genotype further increases the risk for abnormal insulin transport and brain insulin signaling. Acute insulin administration transiently increases brain insulin levels, which restores insulin signaling and facilitates memory. Relative to patients without an e4 positive genotype, AD patients with an e4 genotype show these effects at a lower insulin dose due to greater insulin sensitivity.

This model predicts that reduced brain insulin levels and impaired brain insulin signaling are appropriate therapeutic targets for persons with AD. Indeed, we have shown that transient peripheral hyperinsulinemia effectively facilitates memory and modulates amyloid precursor protein and Aβ levels in AD (Fishel *et al.*, 2005; Craft *et al.*, 2003); however, peripheral insulin administration is not a practical long-term therapeutic strategy because it requires careful monitoring to prevent hypoglycemic episodes and over chronic use it may induce or exacerbate peripheral insulin resistance. Fortunately, there is an alternative strategy for delivering insulin to the brain without altering plasma insulin or glucose levels.

Intranasal Insulin Administration and AD

As previously noted, many small molecule neuropeptides, such as insulin and IGF-1, can be transported directly from the nasal cavity into the CNS, bypassing the periphery (Thorne *et al.*, 2004; Born *et al.*, 2002). We recently examined the cognitive effects of intranasal insulin administration in a sample comprising memory impaired patients (i.e., patients with AD or amnestic mild cognitive impairment) and cognitively intact older adults, for whom *APOE* genotyping had been acquired (Reger *et al.*, 2006). Participants made three study visits on separate days. For each visit, they received one of three insulin doses (20 IU, 40 IU, saline) in randomized order, rested for 15 min, and then completed a brief cognitive test battery. Blood was acquired prior to and 45 min after insulin administration. Testing revealed insulin-induced memory facilitation on two measures (story recall and word list recall) for memory impaired patients without and *APOE* e4 allele. In contrast, insulin failed to enhance story recall in memory impaired patients possessing at least one e4 allele, and the higher insulin dose impaired word list recall in this group. Intranasal insulin administration did not affect memory in the cognitively intact group, nor did it affect selective attention or working memory for either memory impaired or intact participants. Neither insulin dose altered blood glucose or insulin levels (Reger *et al.*, 2006).

As predicted, insulin influenced cognitive functioning without altering peripheral glucose metabolism. Although unexpected, the observation that *APOE* genotype modulated insulin's effects on memory in the memory impaired group corroborates earlier studies revealing genotypic effects of intravenous insulin administration on memory and plasma amyloid precursor protein levels (Craft *et al.*, 2003), as well as genotypic modulation of rosiglitazone's effects on memory (Risner *et al.*, 2006). Collectively, these studies support the notion that *APOE* genotype modulates insulin signaling in patients with AD. One speculative possibility is that CNS insulin resistance is more severe in AD patients who do not carry the e4 allele, due to reduced CSF insulin levels and reduced CSF-to-plasma insulin ratios (Craft *et al.*, 1998). It is possible that a lower intranasal insulin dose may have facilitated memory in patients with the e4 allele. Finally, this study supports further investigation of the therapeutic potential of intranasal insulin administration for patients with AD. Several important questions should be addressed, including the effects of chronic versus acute administration on cognitive, neuroendocrine, amyloid, and inflammatory endpoints that are relevant to AD. Furthermore, extensive investigation is needed to determine whether *APOE* genotype modulates treatment response.

Summary

A growing body of literature has identified perturbations in CNS insulin levels and signaling that may contribute to the pathophysiology and cognitive dysfunction observed in AD. Insulin resistant conditions such as IGT, T2DM, and hyperinsulinemia increase the risk for AD, and experimental models have shown that inducing insulin resistance exacerbates amyloid pathology and increases inflammatory markers. Several human studies support the further investigation of insulin resistance as a potential therapeutic target in the treatment of AD. For example, the insulin sensitizing agent rosiglitazone appears to stabilize cognitive decline and the decline in peripheral amyloid levels in patients with early AD, and frequent physical activity may reduce the incidence of AD among older adults. Furthermore, strategies that increase brain insulin activity may also yield beneficial cognitive effects for AD patients. As we have shown, intranasal insulin administration facilitates cognition while bypassing systemic metabolic effects of insulin. Therefore, these three strategies (PPAR-gamma agonists, diet and exercise, intranasal insulin administration) merit further investigation as potential novel therapies for AD.

Several questions should be considered. A looming issue concerns the moderating role of *APOE* genotype in the relationship of AD and insulin resistance. As we have seen, *APOE* genotype may alter the risk for insulin resistance, peripheral and central insulin perturbations, and treatment response to both rosiglitazone and to intranasal insulin administration. These data raise the intriguing possibility of genotypic differences in response to treatment strategies that target insulin resistance. At a more basic level, these data emphasize the broad role that *APOE* genotype appears to play in the development of AD. Additionally, insulin has been shown to influence both the amyloidogenic and neuroinflammatory processes that have been implicated in the pathophysiology of AD. Therefore, studies that target insulin resistance should examine the effects of increasing insulin activity on AD in the light of these processes.

In conclusion, we believe that improving insulin sensitivity will contribute to a reduction in the pathophysiology and cognitive dysfunction associated with AD, as well as to general health.

References

Abbott, M.A., Wells, D.G., & Fallon, J.R. (1999). The insulin receptor tyrosine kinase substrate p58/53 and the insulin receptor are components of CNS synapses. *Journal of Neurosciences*, 19, 7300–7308.

Akiyama, H., Barger, S., Barnum, S., et al. (2000). Inflammation and Alzheimer's disease. *Neurobiology of Aging*, 21, 383–421.

Andreasen, N., & Blennow, K. (2002). Beta-amyloid (Abeta) protein in cerebrospinal fluid as a biomarker for Alzheimer's disease. *Peptides*, 23, 1205–1214.

Apelt, J., Mehlhorn, G., & Schliebs, R. (1999). Insulin-sensitive GLUT4 glucose transporters are colocalized with GLUT3-expressing cells and demonstrate a chemically distinct neuron-specific localization in rat brain. *Journal of Neuroscience Research*, 57, 693–705.

Balakrishnan, K., Verdile, G., Mehta, P.D., et al. (2005). Plasma Abeta42 correlates positively with increased body fat in healthy individuals. *Journal of Alzheimers Disease*, 8, 269–282.

Banks, W.A., Jaspan, J.B., Huang, W., & Kastin, A.J. (1997a). Transport of insulin across the blood–brain barrier: saturability at euglycemic doses of insulin. *Peptides*, 18, 1423–1429.

Banks, W.A., Jaspan, J.B., & Kastin, A.J. (1997b). Selective, physiological transport of insulin across the blood–brain barrier: novel demonstration by species-specific radioimmunoassays. *Peptides*, 18, 1257–1262.

Baskin, D.G., Figlewicz, D.P., Woods, S.C., Porte Jr, D., & Dorsa, D.M. (1987). Insulin in the brain. *Annual Review of Physiology*, 49, 335–347.

Baura, G.D., Foster, D.M., Porte Jr, D., et al. (1993). Saturable transport of insulin from plasma into the central nervous system of dogs *in vivo*. A mechanism for regulated insulin delivery to the brain. *Journal of Clinical Investigation*, 92, 1824–1830.

Benedict, C., Hallschmid, M., Hatke, A., et al. (2004). Intranasal insulin improves memory in humans. *Psychoneuroendocrinology*, 29, 1326–1334.

Bernard, N., Kitabgi, P., & Rovere-Jovene, C. (2003). The Arg617-Arg618 cleavage site in the C-terminal domain of PC1 plays a major role in the processing and targeting of the enzyme within the regulated secretory pathway. *Journal of Neurochemistry*, 85, 1592–1603.

Bingham, E.M., Hopkins, D., Smith, D., et al. (2002). The role of insulin in human brain glucose metabolism: an 18fluoro-deoxyglucose positron emission tomography study. *Diabetes*, 51, 3384–3390.

Blanchard, J.G., & Duncan, P.M. (1997). Effect of combinations of insulin, glucose and scopolamine on radial arm maze performance. *Pharmacology, Biochemistry and Behavior*, 58, 209–214.

Boden, G., Lebed, B., Schatz, M., Homko, C., & Lemieux, S. (2001). Effects of acute changes of plasma free fatty acids on intramyocellular fat content and insulin resistance in healthy subjects. *Diabetes*, 50, 1612–1617.

Born, J., Lange, T., Kern, W., McGregor, G.P., Bickel, U., & Fehm, H.L. (2002). Sniffing neuropeptides: a transnasal approach to the human brain. *Nature Neuroscience*, 5, 514–516.

Boyd Jr, F.T., Clarke, D.W., Muther, T.F., & Raizada, M.K. (1985). Insulin receptors and insulin modulation of norepinephrine uptake in neuronal cultures from rat brain. *Journal of Biological Chemistry*, 260, 15880–15884.

Brechtel, K., Dahl, D.B., Machann, J., *et al.* (2001). Fast elevation of the intramyocellular lipid content in the presence of circulating free fatty acids and hyperinsulinemia: a dynamic 1H-MRS study. *Magnetic Resonance Medicine*, 45, 179–183.

Byrne, J.H. (2003). Learning and memory: basic mechanisms. In: Squire, L.R., Bloom, F.E., McConnell, S.K., Roberts, J.L., Spitzer, N.C., & Zigmond, M.J. (eds.), *Fundamental Neuroscience* (2nd ed.). San Diego, CA: Academic Press, pp. 1276–1298.

Cacquevel, M., Lebeurrier, N., Cheenne, S., & Vivien, D. (2004). Cytokines in neuroinflammation and Alzheimer's disease. *Current Drug Targets*, 5, 529–534.

Carro, E., Trejo, J.L., Gomez-Isla, T., LeRoith, D., & Torres-Aleman, I. (2002). Serum insulin-like growth factor I regulates brain amyloid-beta levels. *Nature Medicine*, 8, 1390–1397.

Combs, C.K., Johnson, D.E., Karlo, J.C., Cannady, S.B., & Landreth, G.E. (2000). Inflammatory mechanisms in Alzheimer's disease: inhibition of beta-amyloid-stimulated proinflammatory responses and neurotoxicity by PPARgamma agonists. *Journal of Neuroscience*, 20, 558–567.

Craft, S., & Watson, G.S. (2004). Insulin and neurodegenerative disease: shared and specific mechanisms. *Lancet Neurology*, 3, 169–178.

Craft, S., Newcomer, J., Kanne, S., *et al.* (1996) Memory improvement following induced hyperinsulinemia in Alzheimer's disease. *Neurobiology of Aging*, 17, 123–130.

Craft, S., Peskind, E., Schwartz, M.W., Schellenberg, G.D., Raskind, M., & Porte Jr, D. (1998). Cerebrospinal fluid and plasma insulin levels in Alzheimer's disease: relationship to severity of dementia and apolipoprotein E genotype. *Neurology*, 50, 164–168.

Craft, S., Asthana, S., Newcomer, J.W., *et al.* (1999a). Enhancement of memory in Alzheimer disease with insulin and somatostatin, but not glucose. *The Archives of General Psychiatry*, 56, 1135–1140.

Craft, S., Asthana, S., Schellenberg, G., *et al.* (1999b). Insulin metabolism in Alzheimer's disease differs according to apolipoprotein E genotype and gender. *Neuroendocrinology*, 70, 146–152.

Craft, S., Asthana, S., Cook, D.G., *et al.* (2003). Insulin dose-response effects on memory and plasma amyloid precursor protein in Alzheimer's disease: interactions with apolipoprotein E genotype. *Psychoneuroendocrinology*, 28, 809–822.

Cuzzocrea, S., Pisano, B., Dugo, L., *et al.* (2004). Rosiglitazone, a ligand of the peroxisome proliferator-activated receptor-gamma, reduces acute inflammation. *European Journal of Pharmacology*, 483, 79–93.

Dandona, P. (2002). Endothelium, inflammation, and diabetes. *Current Diabetes Reports*, 2, 311–315.

de la Monte, S.M., & Wands, J.R. (2005). Review of insulin and insulin-like growth factor expression, signaling, and malfunction in the central nervous system: relevance to Alzheimer's disease. *Journal of Alzheimers Disease*, 7, 45–61.

de la Monte, S.M., Tong, M., Lester-Coll, N., Plater Jr, M., & Wands, J.R. (2006). Therapeutic rescue of neurodegeneration in experimental type 3 diabetes: relevance to Alzheimer's disease. *Journal of Alzheimers Disease*, 10, 89–109.

de Rivera, C., Shukitt-Hale, B., Joseph, J.A., & Mendelson, J.R. (2006). The effects of antioxidants in the senescent auditory cortex. *Neurobiology of Aging*, 27, 1035–1044.

Dello Russo, C., Gavrilyuk, V., Weinberg, G., *et al.* (2003). Peroxisome proliferator-activated receptor gamma thiazolidinedione agonists increase glucose metabolism in astrocytes. *Journal of Biological Chemistry*, 278, 5828–5836.

Di Luca, M., Ruts, L., Gardoni, F., Cattabeni, F., Biessels, G.J., & Gispen, W.H. (1999). NMDA receptor subunits are modified transcriptionally and post-translationally in the brain of streptozotocin-diabetic rats. *Diabetologia*, 42, 693–701.

Diab, A., Deng, C., Smith, J.D., et al. (2002). Peroxisome proliferator-activated receptor-gamma agonist 15-deoxy-Delta(12,14)-prostaglandin J(2) ameliorates experimental autoimmune encephalomyelitis. *Journal of Immunology*, 168, 2508–2515.

Doyle, P., Cusin, I., Rohner-Jeanrenaud, F., & Jeanrenaud, B. (1995). Four-day hyperinsulinemia in euglycemic conditions alters local cerebral glucose utilization in specific brain nuclei of freely moving rats. *Brain Research*, 684, 47–55.

Feinstein, D.L., Galea, E., Gavrilyuk, V., et al. (2002). Peroxisome proliferator-activated receptor-gamma agonists prevent experimental autoimmune encephalomyelitis. *Annals of Neurology*, 51, 694–702.

Feinstein, D.L., Spagnolo, A., Akar, C., et al. (2005). Receptor-independent actions of PPAR thiazolidinedione agonists: is mitochondrial function the key? *Biochemical Pharmacology*, 70, 177–188.

Ferre, P. (2004). The biology of peroxisome proliferator-activated receptors: relationship with lipid metabolism and insulin sensitivity. *Diabetes*, 53(Suppl. 1), S43–S50.

Figlewicz, D.P., Bentson, K., & Ocrant, I. (1993a). The effect of insulin on norepinephrine uptake by PC12 cells. *Brain Research Bulletin*, 32, 425–431.

Figlewicz, D.P., Szot, P., Israel, P.A., Payne, C., & Dorsa, D.M. (1993b). Insulin reduces norepinephrine transporter mRNA *in vivo* in rat locus coeruleus. *Brain Research*, 602, 161–164.

Fishel, M.A., Watson, G.S., Montine, T.J., et al. (2005). Hyperinsulinemia provokes synchronous increases in central inflammation and beta-amyloid in normal adults. *Archives of Neurology*, 62, 1539–1544.

Frolich, L., Blum-Degen, D., Bernstein, H.G., et al. (1998). Brain insulin and insulin receptors in aging and sporadic Alzheimer's disease. *Journal of Neural Transmission*, 105, 423–438.

Frolich, L, Blum-Degen, D., Riederer, P., & Hoyer, S. (1999). A disturbance in the neuronal insulin receptor signal transduction in sporadic Alzheimer's disease. *Annals of the New York Academic Sciences*, 893, 290–293.

Gasparini, L., Gouras, G.K., Wang, R., et al. (2001). Stimulation of beta-amyloid precursor protein trafficking by insulin reduces intraneuronal beta-amyloid and requires mitogen-activated protein kinase signaling. *Journal of Neuroscience*, 21, 2561–2570.

Gordon, E.S. (1968). Efficiency of energy metabolism in obesity. *American Journal of Clinical Nutrition*, 21, 1480–1485.

Gurnell, M. (2003). PPARgamma and metabolism: insights from the study of human genetic variants. *Clinical Endocrinology (Oxf)*, 59, 267–277.

Gustafson, D., Rothenberg, E., Blennow, K., Steen, B., & Skoog, I. (2003). An 18-year follow-up of overweight and risk of Alzheimer disease. *Archives of Internal Medicine*, 163, 1524–1528.

Hak, A.E., Pols, H.A., Stehouwer, C.D., et al. (2001). Markers of inflammation and cellular adhesion molecules in relation to insulin resistance in nondiabetic elderly: the Rotterdam study. *Journal of Clinical Endocrinology and Metabolism*, 86, 4398–4405.

Hallschmid, M., Benedict, C., Schultes, B., Fehm, H.L., Born, J., & Kern, W. (2004). Intranasal insulin reduces body fat in men but not in women. *Diabetes*, 53, 3024–3029.

Harris, M.I., Flegal, K.M., Cowie, C.C., et al. (1998). Prevalence of diabetes, impaired fasting glucose, and impaired glucose tolerance in US adults. The Third National Health and Nutrition Examination Survey, 1988–1994. *Diabetes Care*, 21, 518–524.

Havrankova, J., Roth, J., & Brownstein, M. (1978a). Insulin receptors are widely distributed in the central nervous system of the rat. *Nature*, 272, 827–829.

Havrankova, J., Schmechel, D., Roth, J., & Brownstein, M. (1978b). Identification of insulin in rat brain. *Proceedings of the National Academy of Sciences of the United States of America*, 75, 5737–5741.

Heneka, M.T., Klockgether, T., & Feinstein, D.L. (2000). Peroxisome proliferator-activated receptor-gamma ligands reduce neuronal inducible nitric oxide synthase expression and cell death *in vivo*. *Journal of Neuroscience*, 20, 6862–6867.

Heneka, M.T., Galea, E., Gavriluyk, V., *et al.* (2002). Noradrenergic depletion potentiates beta -amyloid-induced cortical inflammation: implications for Alzheimer's disease. *Journal of Neuroscience, 22*, 2434–2442.

Ho, L., Qin, W., Pompl, P.N., *et al.* (2004). Diet-induced insulin resistance promotes amyloidosis in a transgenic mouse model of Alzheimer's disease. *FASEB Journal, 18*, 902–904.

Hoyer, S., & Lannert, H. (1999). Inhibition of the neuronal insulin receptor causes Alzheimer-like disturbances in oxidative/energy brain metabolism and in behavior in adult rats. *Annals of the New York Academic Sciences, 893*, 301–303.

Hull, M., Strauss, S., Berger, M., Volk, B., & Bauer, J. (1996). The participation of interleukin-6, a stress-inducible cytokine, in the pathogenesis of Alzheimer's disease. *Behavioral Brain Research, 78*, 37–41.

Kaiyala, K.J., Prigeon, R.L., Kahn, S.E., Woods, S.C., & Schwartz, M.W. (2000). Obesity induced by a high-fat diet is associated with reduced brain insulin transport in dogs. *Diabetes, 49*, 1525–1533.

Kern, W., Born, J., Schreiber, H., & Fehm, H.L. (1999). Central nervous system effects of intranasally administered insulin during euglycemia in men. *Diabetes, 48*, 557–563.

Kim, Y.P., Kim, H., Shin, M.S., *et al.* (2004). Age-dependence of the effect of treadmill exercise on cell proliferation in the dentate gyrus of rats. *Neuroscience Letters, 355*, 152–154.

Kitamura, Y., Kakimura, J., Matsuoka, Y., Nomura, Y., Gebicke-Haerter, P.J., & Taniguchi, T. (1999a). Activators of peroxisome proliferator-activated receptor-gamma (PPARgamma) inhibit inducible nitric oxide synthase expression but increase heme oxygenase-1 expression in rat glial cells. *Neuroscience Letters, 262*, 129–132.

Kitamura, Y., Shimohama, S., Koike, H., *et al.* (1999b). Increased expression of cyclooxygenases and peroxisome proliferator-activated receptor-gamma in Alzheimer's disease brains. *Biochemical and Biophysical Research Communications, 254*, 582–586.

Knowler, W.C., Barrett-Connor, E., Fowler, S.E., *et al.* (2002). Reduction in the incidence of type 2 diabetes with lifestyle intervention or metformin. *TheNew England Journal of Medicine, 346*, 393–403.

Kopf, S.R., & Baratti, C.M. (1996). Effects of post-training administration of glucose on retention of a habituation response in mice: participation of a central cholinergic mechanism. *Neurobiology of Learning and Memory, 65*, 253–260.

Krogh-Madsen, R., Plomgaard, P., Keller, P., Keller, C., & Pedersen, B.K. (2004). Insulin stimulates interleukin-6 and tumor necrosis factor-alpha gene expression in human subcutaneous adipose tissue. *American Journal of Physiology, Endocrinology and Metabolism, 286*, E234–E238.

Kulstad, J.J., Green, P.S., Cook, D.G., *et al.* (2006). Differential modulation of plasma beta-amyloid by insulin in patients with Alzheimer disease. *Neurology, 66*, 1506–1510.

Kuusisto, J., Koivisto, K., Mykkanen, L., *et al.* (1997). Association between features of the insulin resistance syndrome and Alzheimer's disease independently of apolipoprotein E4 phenotype: cross sectional population based study. *British Medical Journal, 315*, 1045–1049.

Landreth, G.E., & Heneka, M.T. (2001). Anti-inflammatory actions of peroxisome proliferator-activated receptor gamma agonists in Alzheimer's disease. *Neurobiology of Aging, 22*, 937–944.

Larson, E.B., Wang, L., Bowen, J.D., *et al.* (2006). Exercise is associated with reduced risk for incident dementia among persons 65 years of age and older. *Annals of Internal Medicine, 144*, 73–81.

Leibson, C.L, Rocca, W.A., & Hanson, V.A., *et al.* (1997). The risk of dementia among persons with diabetes mellitus: a population-based cohort study. *Annals of the New York Academy of Sciences, 826*, 422–427.

Lester-Coll, N., Rivera, E.J., Soscia, S.J., Doiron, K., Wands, J.R., & de la Monte, S.M. (2006). Intracerebral streptozotocin model of type 3 diabetes: relevance to sporadic Alzheimer's disease. *Journal of Alzheimers Disease, 9*, 13–33.

Luchsinger, J.A., Tang, M.X., Shea, S., & Mayeux, R. (2004). Hyperinsulinemia and risk of Alzheimer disease. *Neurology*, 63, 1187–1192.

Malinowski, J.M., & Bolesta, S. (2000). Rosiglitazone in the treatment of type 2 diabetes mellitus: a critical review. *Clinical Therapeutics*, 22, 1151–1168; discussion 1149–1150.

Marfaing, P., Penicaud, L., Broer, Y., Mraovitch, S., Calando, Y., & Picon, L. (1990). Effects of hyperinsulinemia on local cerebral insulin binding and glucose utilization in normoglycemic awake rats. *Neuroscience Letters*, 115, 279–285.

Marfella, R., D'Amico, M., Esposito, K., et al. (2006). The ubiquitin-proteasome system and inflammatory activity in diabetic atherosclerotic plaques: effects of rosiglitazone treatment. *Diabetes*, 55, 622–632.

Matsuoka, Y., Saito, M., LaFrancois, J., et al. (2003). Novel therapeutic approach for the treatment of Alzheimer's disease by peripheral administration of agents with an affinity to beta-amyloid. *Journal of Neuroscience*, 23, 29–33.

Mayeux, R., Honig, L.S., Tang, M.X., et al. (2003). Plasma A[beta]40 and A[beta]42 and Alzheimer's disease: relation to age, mortality, and risk. *Neurology*, 61, 1185–1190.

Meneilly, G.S., Cheung, E., Tessier, D., Yakura, C., & Tuokko, H. (1993). The effect of improved glycemic control on cognitive functions in the elderly patient with diabetes. *Journal of Gerontology*, 48, M117–M121.

Messier, C. (2003). Diabetes, Alzheimer's disease and apolipoprotein genotype. *Experimental Gerontology*, 38, 941–946.

MMWR Report (2003). Prevalence of diabetes and impaired fasting glucose in adults – United States, 1999–2000. *Morbidity Mortality Weekly Report*, 52, 833–837.

Molteni, R., Wu, A., Vaynman, S., Ying, Z., Barnard, R.J., & Gomez-Pinilla, F. (2004). Exercise reverses the harmful effects of consumption of a high-fat diet on synaptic and behavioral plasticity associated to the action of brain-derived neurotrophic factor. *Neuroscience*, 123, 429–440.

Montine, T.J., Kaye, J.A., Montine, K.S., McFarland, L., Morrow, J.D., & Quinn, J.F. (2001). Cerebrospinal fluid abeta42, tau, and F_2-isoprostane concentrations in patients with Alzheimer disease, other dementias, and in age-matched controls. *Archives of Pathology and Laboratory Medicine*, 125, 510–512.

Moreno, S., Farioli-Vecchioli, S., & Ceru, M.P. (2004). Immunolocalization of peroxisome proliferator-activated receptors and retinoid X receptors in the adult rat CNS. *Neuroscience*, 123, 131–145.

Morgan, D. (2005). Mechanisms of A beta plaque clearance following passive A beta immunization. *Neurodegenerative Diseases*, 2, 261–266.

Ott, A., Stolk, R.P., van Harskamp, F., Pols, H.A., Hofman, A., & Breteler, M.M. (1999). Diabetes mellitus and the risk of dementia: The Rotterdam Study. *Neurology*, 53, 1937–1942.

Park, C.R., Seeley, R.J., Craft, S., & Woods, S.C. (2000). Intracerebroventricular insulin enhances memory in a passive-avoidance task. *Physiology & Behavior*, 68, 509–514.

Peila, R., Rodriguez, B.L., & Launer, L.J. (2002). Type 2 diabetes, APOE gene, and the risk for dementia and related pathologies: The Honolulu-Asia Aging Study. *Diabetes*, 51, 1256–1262.

Pershadsingh, H.A., Heneka, M.T., Saini, R., Amin, N.M., Broeske, D.J., & Feinstein, D.L. (2004). Effect of pioglitazone treatment in a patient with secondary multiple sclerosis. *Journal of Neuroinflammation*, 1, 3.

Pickup, J.C., Mattock, M.B., Chusney, G.D., & Burt, D. (1997). NIDDM as a disease of the innate immune system: association of acute-phase reactants and interleukin-6 with metabolic syndrome X. *Diabetologia*, 40, 1286–1292.

Qiu, W.Q., Walsh, D.M., Ye, Z., et al. (1998). Insulin-degrading enzyme regulates extracellular levels of amyloid beta-protein by degradation. *Journal of Biological Chemistry*, 273, 32730–32738.

Ragozzino, M.E., Arankowsky-Sandoval, G., & Gold, P.E. (1994). Glucose attenuates the effect of combined muscarinic-nicotinic receptor blockade on spontaneous alternation. *European Journal of Pharmacology*, 256, 31–36.

Ramlo-Halsted, B.A., & Edelman, S.V. (1999). The natural history of type 2 diabetes. Implications for clinical practice. *Primary Care*, 26, 771–789.

Razay, G., & Wilcock, G.K. (1994). Hyperinsulinaemia and Alzheimer's disease. *Age and Ageing*, 23, 396–399.

Reagan, L.P., Gorovits, N., Hoskin, E.K., *et al.* (2001). Localization and regulation of GLUTx1 glucose transporter in the hippocampus of streptozotocin diabetic rats. *Proceedings of the National Academy of Sciences of United States America*, 98, 2820–2825.

Reaven, G.M., Chang, H., & Hoffman, B.B. (1988). Additive hypoglycemic effects of drugs that modify free-fatty acid metabolism by different mechanisms in rats with streptozocin-induced diabetes. *Diabetes*, 37, 28–32.

Reger, M.A., Watson, G.S., Frey 2nd, W.H., *et al.* (2006). Effects of intranasal insulin on cognition in memory-impaired older adults: modulation by APOE genotype. *Neurobiology of Aging*, 27, 451–458.

Risner, M.E., Saunders, A.M., Altman, J.F., *et al.* (2006). Efficacy of rosiglitazone in a genetically defined population with mild-to-moderate Alzheimer's disease. *Pharmacogenomics Journal*, 6, 246–254.

Rivera, E.J., Goldin, A., Fulmer, N., Tavares, R., Wands, J.R., & de la Monte, S.M. (2005). Insulin and insulin-like growth factor expression and function deteriorate with progression of Alzheimer's disease: link to brain reductions in acetylcholine. *Journal of Alzheimers Disease*, 8, 247–268.

Rosler, N., Wichart, I., & Jellinger, K.A. (2001). Intra vitam lumbar and post mortem ventricular cerebrospinal fluid immunoreactive interleukin-6 in Alzheimer's disease patients. *Acta Neurologica Scandinavica*, 103, 126–130.

Ruan, H., & Lodish, H.F. (2003). Insulin resistance in adipose tissue: direct and indirect effects of tumor necrosis factor-alpha. *Cytokine & Growth Factor Reviews*, 14, 447–455.

Santomauro, A.T., Boden, G., Silva, M.E., *et al.* (1999). Overnight lowering of free fatty acids with Acipimox improves insulin resistance and glucose tolerance in obese diabetic and nondiabetic subjects. *Diabetes*, 48, 1836–1841.

Sastre, M., Dewachter, I., Landreth, G.E., *et al.* (2003). Nonsteroidal anti-inflammatory drugs and peroxisome proliferator-activated receptor-gamma agonists modulate immunostimulated processing of amyloid precursor protein through regulation of beta-secretase. *Journal of Neuroscience*, 23, 9796–9804.

Schubert, M., Gautam, D., Surjo, D., *et al.* (2004). Role for neuronal insulin resistance in neurodegenerative diseases. *Proceedings of the National Academy of Sciences of the United States of America*, 101, 3100–3105.

Schulingkamp, R.J., Pagano, T.C., Hung, D., & Raffa, R.B. (2000). Insulin receptors and insulin action in the brain: review and clinical implications. *Neuroscience and Biobehavioral Reviews*, 24, 855–872.

Schwartz, M.W., Figlewicz, D.F., Kahn, S.E., Baskin, D.G., Greenwood, M.R., & Porte Jr, D. (1990). Insulin binding to brain capillaries is reduced in genetically obese, hyperinsulinemic Zucker rats. *Peptides*, 11, 467–472.

Sidhu, J.S., Cowan, D., & Kaski, J.C. (2003). The effects of rosiglitazone, a peroxisome proliferator-activated receptor-gamma agonist, on markers of endothelial cell activation, C-reactive protein, and fibrinogen levels in non-diabetic coronary artery disease patients. *Journal of the American College of Cardiology*, 42, 1757–1763.

Skeberdis, V.A., Lan, J., Zheng, X., Zukin, R.S., & Bennett, M.V. (2001). Insulin promotes rapid delivery of N-methyl-D-aspartate receptors to the cell surface by exocytosis. *Proceedings of the National Academy of Sciences of United States of America*, 98, 3561–3566.

Soop, M., Duxbury, H., Agwunobi, A.O., *et al.* (2002). Euglycemic hyperinsulinemia augments the cytokine and endocrine responses to endotoxin in humans. *American Journal of Physiology, Endocrinology and Metabolism*, 282, E1276–E1285.

Steen, E., Terry, B.M., Rivera, E.J., *et al.* (2005). Impaired insulin and insulin-like growth factor expression and signaling mechanisms in Alzheimer's disease – is this type 3 diabetes? *Journal of Alzheimers Disease*, 7, 63–80.

Strachan, M.W., Deary, I.J., Ewing, F.M., & Frier, B.M. (1997). Is type II diabetes associated with an increased risk of cognitive dysfunction? A critical review of published studies. *Diabetes Care*, 20, 438–445.

Thorne, R.G., Pronk, G.J., Padmanabhan, V., & Frey 2nd, W.H. (2004). Delivery of insulin-like growth factor-I to the rat brain and spinal cord along olfactory and trigeminal pathways following intranasal administration. *Neuroscience*, 127, 481–496.

Trejo, J.L., Carro, E., & Torres-Aleman, I. (2001). Circulating insulin-like growth factor I mediates exercise-induced increases in the number of new neurons in the adult hippocampus. *Journal of Neuroscience*, 21, 1628–1634.

Tuomilehto, J., Lindstrom, J., Eriksson, J.G., *et al.* (2001). Prevention of type 2 diabetes mellitus by changes in lifestyle among subjects with impaired glucose tolerance. *The New England Journal of Medicine*, 344, 1343–1350.

Unger, J.W., Livingston, J.N., & Moss, A.M. (1991). Insulin receptors in the central nervous system: localization, signalling mechanisms and functional aspects. *Progress in Neurobiology*, 36, 343–362.

Uryu, S., Harada, J., Hisamoto, M., & Oda, T. (2002). Troglitazone inhibits both post-glutamate neurotoxicity and low-potassium-induced apoptosis in cerebellar granule neurons. *Brain Research*, 924, 229–236.

van der Heide, L.P., Kamal, A., Artola, A., Gispen, W.H., & Ramakers, G.M. (2005). Insulin modulates hippocampal activity-dependent synaptic plasticity in a N-methyl-D-aspartate receptor and phosphatidyl-inositol-3-kinase-dependent manner. *Journal of Neurochemistry*, 94, 1158–1166.

Vanhanen, M., Koivisto, K., Kuusisto, J., *et al.* (1998). Cognitive function in an elderly population with persistent impaired glucose tolerance. *Diabetes Care*, 21, 398–402.

Wang, J., Ho, L., Qin, W., *et al.* (2005). Caloric restriction attenuates beta-amyloid neuropathology in a mouse model of Alzheimer's disease. *FASEB Journal*, 19, 659–661.

Watson, G.S., & Craft, S. (2003). The role of insulin resistance in the pathogenesis of Alzheimer's disease: implications for treatment. *CNS Drugs*, 17, 27–45.

Watson, G.S., & Craft, S. (2004). Modulation of memory by insulin and glucose: neuropsychological observations in Alzheimer's disease. *European Journal of Pharmacology*, 490, 97–113.

Watson, G.S., Peskind, E.R., Asthana, S., *et al.* (2003). Insulin increases CSF Abeta42 levels in normal older adults. *Neurology*, 60, 1899–1903.

Watson, G.S., Cholerton, B.A., Reger, M.A., *et al.* (2005). Preserved cognition in patients with early Alzheimer disease and amnestic mild cognitive impairment during treatment with rosiglitazone: a preliminary study. *American Journal of Geriatric Psychiatry*, 13, 950–958.

Watson, G.S., Bernhardt, T., Reger, M.A., *et al.* (2006a). Insulin effects on CSF norepinephrine and cognition in Alzheimer's disease. *Neurobiology of Aging*, 27, 38–41.

Watson, G.S., Reger, M.A., Baker, L.D., *et al.* (2006b). Effects of exercise and nutrition on memory in Japanese-Americans with impaired glucose tolerance. *Diabetes Care*, 29, 135–136.

Zhao, W., Chen, H., Xu, H., *et al.* (1999). Brain insulin receptors and spatial memory. Correlated changes in gene expression, tyrosine phosphorylation, and signaling molecules in the hippocampus of water maze trained rats. *Journal of Biological Chemistry*, 274, 34893–34902.

Progress in Neurotherapeutics and Neuropsychopharmacology, 3:1, 111–125 © 2008 Cambridge University Press
DOI: 10.1017/S1748232107000171   Printed in the United Kingdom

Targeting Amyloid with Tramiprosate in Patients with Mild-to-Moderate Alzheimer Disease[*]

P.S. Aisen

Department of Neurology, Georgetown University Medical Center, Washington DC, USA; Email: psa@georgetown.edu

R. Briand

Neurochem Inc., Laval, Quebec, Canada; Email: rbriand@neurochem.com

D. Saumier

Neurochem Inc., Laval, Quebec, Canada; Email: dsaumier@neurochem.com

J. Laurin

Neurochem Inc., Laval, Quebec, Canada; Email: jlaurin@neurochem.com

A. Duong

Neurochem Inc., Laval, Quebec, Canada; Email: aduong@neurochem.com

D. Garceau

Neurochem Inc., Laval, Quebec, Canada; Email: dgarceau@neurochem.com

ABSTRACT

Background: Tramiprosate (3-amino-1-propanesulfonic acid, 3APS, ALZHEMED™) is an investigational product candidate that is believed to reduce amyloid deposition in the brain by binding to soluble Aβ, thereby slowing or halting the progression of Alzheimer Disease (AD). *Design and Methods*: We assessed the safety, tolerability, and pharmacokinetic/pharmacodynamic profiles of tramiprosate in a randomized, double-blind, placebo-controlled Phase II study in which 58 subjects with mild-to-moderate AD were randomly assigned to receive placebo or tramiprosate 50, 100, or 150 mg BID for 3 months. At the end of the double-blind study, 42 of these patients entered an open-label extension study in which they received tramiprosate 150 mg BID for an additional 17 months. Assessments included plasma and CSF tramiprosate concentrations, CSF Aβ_{42} concentrations, and psychometric tests (Alzheimer's

---

[*]Trial data adapted and Figure 2 reproduced with permission from Aisen *et al.* (2007). A phase II study targeting amyloid-B with 3APS in mild-to-moderate Alzheimer disease. *Neurology*, 67, 1757–1763.

Correspondence should be addressed to: Daniel Saumier, PhD, Neurochem Inc., 275 boul. Armand Frappier, Laval, QC, Canada, H7V 4A7; Ph: +1 450-680-4500; Fax: +1 450-680-4505; Email: dsaumier@neurochem.com

Disease Assessment Scale – cognitive subscale, Mini-Mental State Examination, and Clinical Dementia Rating Scale – Sum of Boxes). *Results*: Tramiprosate had no significant impact on vital signs or laboratory test values. The most frequent side effects were nausea, vomiting, and diarrhea, which were intermittent and mild-to-moderate in severity. Overall, six tramiprosate-treated patients discontinued because of side effects (all causalities) and there were no drug-related serious adverse events. Tramiprosate crossed the blood–brain barrier and dose-dependently reduced CSF $A\beta_{42}$ levels after 3 months of treatment. There were no psychometric score differences between treatment groups after 3 months of double-blind treatment. However, psychometric score changes over the 17-month open-label extension study are consistent with a slowing of cognitive and clinical decline, particularly in mild subjects. *Interpretation*: Long-term administration of tramiprosate is safe and tolerated in patients with mild-to-moderate AD. The short-term reduction of CSF $A\beta_{42}$ levels and the long-term open-label cognitive and clinical assessments are consistent with disease-modification.

Key words: Alzheimer's Disease, amyloid beta, biomarker, clinical trial, cognition, CSF, disease modification.

Introduction and Overview

While symptomatic treatments for Alzheimer's Disease (AD) have been the main focus of investigations in this therapeutic area, recent research efforts have targeted beta-amyloid ($A\beta$) peptides to modify the underlying pathophysiology of the disease. According to the "amyloid hypothesis", the pathogenesis of AD is linked to the generation of $A\beta$ by enzymatic cleavage of the amyloid precursor protein (APP) with subsequent formation of $A\beta$ oligomers and amyloid fibrils, which are ultimately deposited as amyloid plaques in the brain (Gandy, 2005). These conformational changes of the $A\beta$ peptide are hypothesized to induce neuronal dysfunction and neuronal death (Canevari *et al.*, 2004), events underlying the progressive cognitive and behavioral decline in individuals with AD. Supportive evidence for the causal role of $A\beta$ in AD has come mainly from genetic studies. Notably, individuals with Down syndrome develop AD in parallel with heightened levels of brain $A\beta$ due to an extra copy of the APP gene (Giaccone *et al.*, 1989). Mutations in either the APP (chromosome 21) (Citron *et al.*, 1992; Goate *et al.*, 1991), presenilin 1 (chromosome 14) (Sherrington *et al.*, 1995), or presenilin 2 (chromosome 1) (Levy-Lahad *et al.*, 1995) genes are related to early onset AD and increased $A\beta$ burden. $A\beta$ has also been found to play an early role in the disease process (Naslund *et al.*, 2000).

The importance of brain $A\beta$ as a key element in the pathogenesis of AD is reflected in the increased interest in developing anti-amyloid strategies for the treatment of the disease. Several approaches for the treatment of AD are being evaluated at both the pre-clinical and clinical levels (Citron, 2004). Some of these treatment strategies are focused on reducing the brain concentrations of $A\beta$ by inhibiting the pro-amyloidogenic γ- and β-secretase enzymes, by stimulating the non-amyloidogenic α-secretase cleavage of APP, by reducing Aβ deposition using first- (Ritchie *et al.*, 2003) and second-generation (Christensen, 2007) metal chelators, or by enhancing the clearance of Aβ from the brain (Tanzi *et al.*, 2004). Moreover, active or passive immunotherapy (Solomon, 2007) against Aβ in animal models of AD has shown that reducing amyloid load may have an impact on cognition, tau pathology, and amyloid-associated dystrophic neurites. Clinical trial data from a vaccination study suggest that immunotherapy against Aβ may have a positive effect by decreasing CSF tau, with accompanying improvements on cognition (Gilman *et al.*, 2005). A small pilot study showed an improvement in Alzheimer's Disease Assessment Scale – cognitive subscale (ADAS-cog) (Mohs & Cohen, 1988) following intravenous injection of human immunoglobulin against Aβ (Dodel *et al.*, 2004).

Drugs that can protect against Aβ-induced neurotoxicity have obvious therapeutic value for the treatment of AD (Citron, 2004). Tramiprosate (3-amino-1-propanesulfonic acid, 3APS, ALZHEMED™) represents one such drug. Tramiprosate is a novel therapeutic investigational compound that is believed to reduce the deposition of amyloid in the brain by binding to soluble Aβ, thereby slowing the progression of AD.

Purpose of the Trial

In this Phase II study, we tested the feasibility of tramiprosate in the treatment of AD. We sought to assess the safety, tolerability, and pharmacokinetic/pharmacodynamic profiles of tramiprosate in patients with mild-to-moderate AD, using a 3-month double-blind, randomized, parallel-group trial design. Tramiprosate's long-term safety, tolerability, and efficacy were further evaluated in a 17-month open-label extension study.

Agent

Tramiprosate is a small, orally administered molecule known as an amyloid-β antagonist. Tramiprosate was selected based on mass spectroscopy studies (Gervais *et al.*, 2007) showing that it binds to soluble amyloid-β_{1-40} (Aβ_{40}) and amyloid-β_{1-42} (Aβ_{42}) peptides but not to fibrillar Aβ structures. By preferentially binding to soluble Aβ_{40} and Aβ_{42}, tramiprosate is designed to prevent conformational transitions that lead to the assembly of oligomers, protofibrils, and fibrils, which ultimately lead to plaque deposition.

In vitro, tramiprosate has been shown to provide neuroprotection against Aβ-induced neurotoxicity in neuronal cell cultures and in mouse organotypic hippocampal cultures (Gervais *et al.*, 2007), and to reverse Aβ_{42}-induced LTP inhibition in rat hippocampal slices (Krzywkowski *et al.*, 2007). The mechanism underlying the neuroprotective activities of tramiprosate may involve, in part, binding to γ-aminobutyric acid A (GABA$_A$) receptors (Azzi *et al.*, 2007). *In vivo*, when administered to an aggressive early onset brain amyloidosis transgenic mouse model of AD (hAPP-TgCRND8), tramiprosate produced a dose-dependent reduction of both soluble and insoluble Aβ$_{40}$ and Aβ$_{42}$ fractions in the brain and plasma (Gervais *et al.*, 2007). Importantly, the administration of tramiprosate in these animals yielded a 25–30% reduction in soluble and insoluble Aβ$_{40}$ and Aβ$_{42}$ fractions in the brain, an approximate 30% plaque deposition reduction in the cerebral cortex, as well as a 61% lowering of plasma Aβ$_{40}$ levels, and a 66% lowering of plasma Aβ$_{42}$ levels (Gervais *et al.*, 2007).

Tramiprosate has been found to have a good safety and tolerability profile in pre-clinical toxicity studies as well as in clinical Phase I studies involving healthy young adult and elderly subjects. The pharmacokinetic profile of tramiprosate has been well documented in a number of Phase I studies. Overall, tramiprosate was found to be safe and well tolerated at the anticipated therapeutic doses (50–150 mg BID) by both young and elderly healthy subjects.

Clinical Trial

Subjects

Patients were recruited at six US centers between October 2002 and March 2003. Eligible patients were aged 50 years and older and had a diagnosis of probable AD by standard criteria (DSM-IV-TR (American Psychiatric Association, 2000) and NINCDS-ADRDA (McKhann *et al.*, 1984)). Their level of severity was mild-to-moderate as reflected by a score of 13–25 (inclusive) on the Mini-Mental State Examination (MMSE) (Folstein *et al.*, 1975). Evidence of diffuse atrophy, as revealed by CT or MRI scanning within 2 years of screening, was acceptable, as was the presence of one lacune (subcortical hypodensity less than 1.5 mm diameter) in a non-strategic area such as the thalamus. ECG and clinical laboratory assessments (hematology, biochemistry, urinalysis, serum B12 and folate, T3, T4, and thyrotropin) were required to be within normal limits. Stable use of the following medications was allowed: Cholinesterase inhibitors (ChEIs, at least 3 months of use at study entry), vitamin E, anxiolytics, sedatives, hypnotics, antidepressants, antipsychotics, estrogen, statins, and non-steroidal anti-inflammatory drugs. Patients were required to live in the community and to have a reliable caregiver. Patients with any other cause of dementia by medical history or by a general physical and neurological examination were excluded. Also excluded were subjects with a body mass index less than 19 or greater than 28, a life expectancy less than 1 year, or a clinically significant and uncontrolled medical condition. Written informed consent was obtained from each patient or legally authorized representative prior to study entry. The institutional review boards at participating sites approved of the study.

Trial Method

This study was a multi-center, randomized, double-blind, placebo-controlled, and parallel-design trial designed to compare tramiprosate with placebo. Fifty-eight patients were randomized to receive in 1:1:1:1 ratio tramiprosate 50, 100, 150 mg BID or placebo BID for 12 weeks. Patients were stratified at randomization based on disease severity as determined by their MMSE score (mild: 19–25 and moderate: 13–18). Study medication was allocated according to a computerized randomization list prepared by an independent biostatistical group. Safety assessments were conducted at screening, baseline, and weeks 2, 4, 8, and 12. CSF Aβ_{42} measurement and psychometric tests were carried out at baseline and at week 12.

During the course of the 3-month double-blind study, all subjects were offered entry into an open-label extension study in which they would receive tramiprosate 150 mg BID for an additional 17 months (for a total study period of 20 months) to assess the long-term safety, tolerability, and efficacy of tramiprosate. Forty-two of the 58 patients elected to take part in the open-label study. Administration of open-label tramiprosate began the day after each subject completed the final double-blind assessment visit. Safety and psychometric efficacy assessments during the open-label study were performed at months 6, 9, 12, 16, and 20.

Instruments/Measures

Safety measures: These included physical examinations, measurements of vital signs, ECGs, laboratory tests (hematology, biochemistry, urinalysis), and AE reporting.

Plasma measures of tramiprosate: Blood samples (5 ml) were collected from each patient prior to dosing (0 h) and at specified times through 12 h post-dose (0.5, 1, 2, 3, 4, 5, 6, 7, 8, 9, 10, and 12 h) after the first dose (week 0) and last dose (week 12). These samples were collected in potassium ethylenediaminetetraacetic acid vacutainers and centrifuged at approximately 1500g for 10 min at 4°C. The resulting plasma was transferred into polypropylene tubes and stored at −80°C until analysis. Plasma concentrations of tramiprosate were determined by a liquid chromatography – tandem mass spectrometry (LC-MS/MS) method previously validated over a concentration range of 5 to 1300 ng/ml.

CSF measures of tramiprosate and Aβ_{42}: CSF samples were obtained by lumbar puncture in the L3/L4 or L4/L5 interspace at baseline (week 0) and at week 12. A total of 5 ml CSF was extracted from each subject after discarding the first milliliter. CSF samples were centrifuged at approximately 1500g for 10 min at 4°C. The resulting CSF was aliquoted into polypropylene tubes and stored at −80°C until the analyses were performed. CSF concentrations of tramiprosate were determined by an LC-MS/MS method previously validated over a concentration range of 2.5–1000 ng/ml. CSF concentrations of Aβ_{42} were quantified using an

Aβ enrichment procedure. Briefly, CSF samples were first treated with formic acid and fractionated on fast protein liquid chromatography (FPLC) using size-exclusion chromatography. An AKTA FPLC apparatus (Amersham Biosciences, Baie D'Urfé, Quebec, Canada) and four Pharmacia LCC-500 apparatuses (Amersham Pharmacia Biotech) were used to recover the Aβ-enriched fractions of CSF samples, which were dried, frozen, and stored at $-80°C$ until assayed using a colorimetric ELISA kit (BioSource International Inc., Camarillo, CA). At the time of assay, dried samples were resuspended with one volume of $0.5\,M$ guanidine/$5\,mM$ Tris-HCl pH 8.0/0.2% Triton X-100 solution and one volume of ELISA diluent containing protease inhibitor.

Psychometric and clinical measures: These included the MMSE scale (Folstein *et al.*, 1975), the ADAS-cog scale (Mohs & Cohen, 1988), and Clinical Dementia Rating Scale – Sum of Boxes (CDR-SB) (Morris, 1993).

Outcome Measures

Changes from baseline in CSF $A\beta_{42}$ were used as secondary outcome measures to assess the pharmacologic effects of tramiprosate on a potential biomarker for AD (Thal *et al.*, 2006). Other secondary outcome measures were changes from baseline in ADAS-cog, MMSE, and CDR-SB, which were performed to monitor the cognitive and clinical progression of AD.

Analysis

As a Phase II study seeking to assess the feasibility of tramiprosate in the treatment of AD, no formal sample size calculation was performed. However, the number of subjects recruited was chosen to provide sufficient preliminary safety, tolerability, and pharmacokinetic/pharmacodynamic data to facilitate the development of definitive Phase III studies of tramiprosate for the treatment of mild-to-moderate AD.

AEs and SAEs were summarized using descriptive statistics. Pharmacokinetic parameters at baseline and week 12 (month 3) were determined using a non-compartmental analysis. CSF $A\beta_{42}$ results were screened for outliers using the Grubbs test[1] and compared using repeated t-tests. A regression analysis (with 95% CI) was performed on the CSF $A\beta_{42}$ concentration changes (from baseline to week 12) as a function of tramiprosate dosage. CSF $A\beta_{42}$ and psychometric measures were analyzed by treatment group and separately for mild (MMSE $= 19–25$) and moderate (MMSE $= 13–18$) AD patients. Because the study was not powered to demonstrate the efficacy of tramiprosate on psychometric tests, ADAS-cog, MMSE, and CDR-SB data were analyzed using descriptive statistics. All data are presented using the observed case approach.

---

[1] Grubbs' Test. www.graphpad.com/quickcalcs/grubbs2.cfm.

Table 1. **Demographic and Baseline Characteristics**

| | TRAMIPROSATE | | | | |
	50 mg BID $n = 15$	100 mg BID $n = 16$	150 mg BID $n = 14$	ACTIVE $n = 45$	PLACEBO $n = 13$
Demographics					
Sex					
Male:female	10:5	4:12	7:7	21:24	7:6
Age (years)					
Mean (SD)	74.3 (8.8)	76.6 (6.6)	74.2 (9.8)	75.1 (8.3)	72.5 (10.4)
Baseline characteristics					
Use of ChEIs (months)					
n (%)	11 (73.3)	11 (68.8)	9 (64.2)	31 (68.9)	7 (53.9)
Mean (SD)	15.1 (13.8)	26.5 (23.0)	25.0 (20.0)	21.9 (19.3)	13.5 (17.5)
MMSE					
n	15	15	12	42	12
Mean (SD)	20.0 (3.8)	18.5 (3.1)	19.8 (3.8)	19.4 (3.5)	20.7 (3.7)
ADAS-cog					
n	15	15	12	42	12
Mean (SD)	23.7 (8.8)	23.8 (9.2)	22.8 (10.1)	23.5 (9.1)	19.8 (10.0)
CDR-SB					
n	15	15	12	42	12
Mean (SD)	5.5 (2.8)	5.3 (2.7)	5.8 (1.7)	5.5 (2.4)	4.2 (3.3)

n: number of subjects; SD: standard deviation; ChEIs: cholinesterase inhibitors; MMSE: Mini-Mental State Examination; ADAS-cog: Alzheimer's Disease Assessment Scale – cognitive subscale; CDR-SB: Clinical Dementia Rating Scale – Sum of Boxes; psychometric scores based on intent-to-treat population.

Results

DEMOGRAPHICS AND BASELINE CHARACTERISTICS

Demographic and baseline characteristics (Table 1) prior to the start of study treatment indicated an equivalent distribution of patients randomized to the tramiprosate or placebo arms. There were no statistically significant differences in mean baseline psychometric scores between the treatment groups.

SAFETY AND TOLERABILITY

Double-blind study: Of the 58 patients randomized, 45 patients received tramiprosate and 13 received placebo. Fifty-two (52) patients completed the study and 6 patients withdrew prematurely (4 patients were on tramiprosate and 2 patients were on placebo). Three patients withdrew because of treatment emergent adverse events: one because of nausea and vomiting (100 mg BID), one because of vomiting (150 mg BID), and one because of weakness and weight loss (150 mg BID). A fourth patient withdrew consent (150 mg BID). In the placebo group, one patient withdrew because of pancreatitis related to alcohol consumption and one patient was withdrawn by the investigator because of treatment non-compliance. The blind was not broken for any of the subjects at the time of discontinuation. The most frequent AEs reported in tramiprosate-treated

Table 2. **Most Common (⩾10%) Adverse Events, All Causalities, over the Course of the Double-Blind Study, Classified by System Organ Class and Preferred Term**

SYSTEM ORGAN CLASS PREFERRED TERM	TRAMIPROSATE				
	50 mg BID n = 15	100 mg BID n = 16	150 mg BID n = 14	ACTIVE n = 45	PLACEBO n = 13
Gastrointestinal disorders					
Nausea	2 (13.3%)	4 (25.0%)	5 (35.7%)	11 (24.4%)	1 (7.7%)
Vomiting	2 (13.3%)	3 (18.8%)	5 (35.7%)	10 (22.2%)	0
Diarrhea	1 (6.7%)	3 (18.8%)	2 (14.3%)	6 (13.3%)	0
General disorders and administration site conditions					
Fall	1 (6.7%)	2 (12.5%)	1 (7.1%)	4 (8.9%)	1 (7.7%)
Infections and infestations					
Urinary tract infection	2 (13.3%)	0	1 (7.1%)	3 (6.7%)	1 (7.7%)
Upper respiratory tract infection	2 (13.3%)	1 (6.3%)	0	3 (6.7%)	0
Nervous system disorders					
Dizziness	2 (13.3%)	2 (12.5%)	1 (7.1%)	5 (11.1%)	1 (7.7%)
Headache	4 (26.7%)	4 (25.0%)	3 (21.4%)	11 (24.4%)	4 (30.8%)
Psychiatric disorders					
Agitation aggravated	2 (13.3%)	0	0	2 (4.4%)	0

AEs are coded using the MedDRA Dictionary, Version 5.0. Percentages are based on the number of patients in the safety population for each treatment group. Patients are counted once per preferred term.

patients were nausea, vomiting, and diarrhea (Table 2). The majority of these events were rated mild-to-moderate in severity. In general, nausea and vomiting were dose related, started during the first 2–4 weeks of treatment and resolved spontaneously. Diarrhea occurred most often after the 2nd week of the study, usually lasted 1 or 2 days, and was not related to dose. Six SAEs were reported by 4 patients (3 on tramiprosate and 1 on placebo). None of the SAEs was reported as treatment related by the investigators. No death was reported during this double-blind study. Laboratory tests, vital signs, and ECG assessments were generally unremarkable. Figure 1 depicts the disposition of patients in each treatment group.

Open-label study: Following the 3-month double-blind study, 24 subjects completed the 17-month open-label follow-up and 18 subjects discontinued prematurely. One subject discontinued because of a drug-related AE (nausea/vomiting), and 3 withdrew because of non-drug-related AEs (increased agitation/delusions [n = 2] and hemorrhagic stroke [n = 1]). Other reasons for early discontinuation included withdrawal of consent (n = 11), loss to follow-up (n = 1), concurrent illness (n = 1), and treatment non-compliance (n = 1). Nausea (n = 9), falling (n = 7), dizziness (n = 5), and headache (n = 5) were the most frequent AEs (all causalities) reported during the open-label extension study. These events were intermittent and mild-to-moderate in severity. Fourteen SAEs were reported

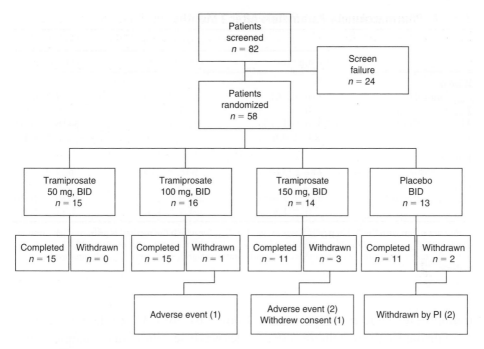

Fig. 1.
Patient disposition in the double-blind study.

by 10 subjects. There was one death due to hemorrhagic stroke. None of these SAEs, including death, were considered by the site investigators to be related to tramiprosate.

PHARMACOKINETICS

Plasma: Following the initial dose of tramiprosate at 50, 100, and 150 mg, C_{max} value was generally attained between 4.5 and 6 h post-dose, consistent with the effect of the enteric-coating formulation. The extent of exposure appeared to increase in a dose-proportional manner between 50 and 100 mg but there was minimal increase between 100 and 150 mg. After dosing on week 12, C_{max} values were generally attained between 3.0 and 3.5 h post-dose and the extent of exposure increased with increasing doses but in a less than dose-proportional manner over the range of 50–150 mg. Mean estimates of $T_{1/2}$ varied approximately between 1.9 and 3.5 h. Neither T_{max} nor $T_{1/2}$ was dependent upon dose. Mean plasma concentrations after 12 weeks of dosing were comparable to those after the initial dose, suggesting no appreciable accumulation of tramiprosate in plasma during repeated dosing. Pharmacokinetic parameters for tramiprosate in plasma are displayed in Table 3.

   CSF: Thirty-six patients treated with tramiprosate volunteered for a lumbar puncture. Tramiprosate was quantifiable in 21 of the 36 CSF samples, indicating that the compound crossed the blood–brain barrier. In these patients, CSF

Table 3. **Pharmacokinetic Parameters After 3 Months**

	TRAMIPROSATE		
	50 mg BID	100 mg BID	150 mg BID
Week 0			
C_{max} (ng/ml)	310 ± 261	618 ± 353	624 ± 627
T_{max} (h)	6.0	4.5	6.0
AUC_∞ (ng*h/ml)	1398 ± 1415	2569 ± 1435	3418 ± 2851
$T_{1/2}$	2.0 ± 0.6	1.9 ± 0.5	2.5 ± 1.1
Week 12			
C_{max} (ng/ml)	451 ± 348	538 ± 213	639 ± 216
T_{max} (h)	3.0	3.5	3.0
AUC_{s-s} (ng*h/ml)	1975 ± 1568	2590 ± 1037	3570 ± 1636
$T_{1/2}$	2.8 ± 1.8	3.4 ± 1.4	3.53 ± 1.8

Values are mean with the SD in parentheses except for T_{max} for which the median is presented; *n*: number of patients; C_{max}: maximum plasma concentration; T_{max}: time of maximal concentration; AUC_∞: area under the curve from zero to infinity; AUC_{s-s}: steady-state area under the curve; $T_{1/2}$: elimination half-life.

tramiprosate concentrations ranged from 2.61 to 7.33 ng/ml. The level of tramiprosate in the remaining CSF samples was below the limit of quantitation of the assay.

EFFICACY

CSF $A\beta_{42}$: Quantitation of $A\beta_{42}$ was performed on CSF samples obtained from 36 tramiprosate-treated patients and 11 placebo-treated patients. Overall, there was a dose-related trend in the reduction of $A\beta_{42}$ levels in the CSF, with the highest reduction (up to 70%) seen in patients receiving 100 and 150 mg BID tramiprosate. A *post hoc* regression analysis revealed a significant linear relationship ($p = 0.041$) between the decreases in CSF $A\beta_{42}$ concentrations and dose (Figure 2), suggesting that tramiprosate significantly reduced the concentration of CSF $A\beta_{42}$ in a dose-dependent manner.

Psychometric measures: Table 4 displays the changes from baseline through month 20 in ADAS-cog, MMSE, and CDR-SB. There were no significant differences in changes from baseline to week 12 (month 3) in the mean ADAS-cog, MMSE, and CDR-SB scores among treatment groups or between each tramiprosate-treated group and placebo. There was a gradual decline in the psychometric scores for subjects remaining in the study over the course of the cumulative 20-month follow-up period. The mean annualized rates of change for the ADAS-cog, MMSE, and CDR-SB assessments were 4.5, 1.7, and 1.5 points, respectively. By 20 months, the mean (SEM) change from baseline in psychometric scores for the mild and moderate groups were as follows: ADAS-cog: mild 3.1 (2.3), moderate 12.7 (2.6); MMSE: mild -2.0 (1.6), moderate -4.1 (1.5); CDR-SB: mild 2.3 (0.9), moderate 2.8 (0.8).

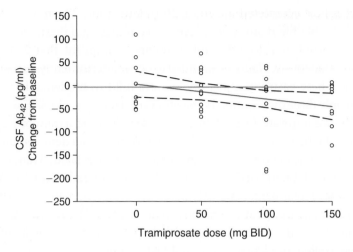

Fig. 2.

Aβ_{42} level changes in the CSF of subjects treated with placebo or tramiprosate at 50, 100, or 150 mg BID after 3 months of double-blind treatment. One patient treated with 3APS 150 mg BID was excluded from the statistical evaluation, because the patient was confirmed as an outlier using the Grubbs test.[1] Markers represent individual subject values; solid line represents best-fit curve ($Y = 2.53 - 0.320X$; $R = 0.306$; $F = 4.4$, $p = 0.041$); dotted lines represent 95% CI limits. Reproduced with permission from **Aisen *et al.*,** *Neurology,* 67, 1757–1763.

Table 4. **Changes from DB Baseline Psychometric Scores through 20 Months, Entire Cohort**

SCALE	MONTHS					
	3	6	9	12	16	20
ADAS-cog						
n	42	41	34	30	26	24
Mean change	1.5	2.2	3.5	4.5	5.4	7.5
SEM	0.8	1.0	1.3	1.4	1.3	1.9
MMSE						
n	42	41	34	31	26	23
Mean change	−0.6	−1.1	−1.6	−1.8	−2.4	−2.9
SEM	0.4	0.5	0.7	0.8	0.8	1.1
CDR-SB						
n	42	41	34	31	26	24
Mean change	0.8	1.5	1.8	2.2	2.0	2.5
SEM	0.3	0.4	0.4	0.5	0.5	0.6

n: number of subjects, observed cases; SEM: standard error of the mean.

UNIQUE ASPECTS OF TRIAL

This study was performed to assess the feasibility of tramiprosate in the treatment of mild-to-moderate AD. Forty-two (81%) of the 52 subjects who completed the double-blind study participated in the open-label study and 24 (41%) of the initial

58-subject cohort completed the entire 20-month study. The most frequent AEs during the double-blind study were nausea, vomiting, and diarrhea. Nausea and vomiting occurred in a dose-dependent manner within the first 2–4 weeks and resolved spontaneously. Nausea continued to occur intermittently during the open-label study. These gastrointestinal events were mild-to-moderate in severity and resulted in only three discontinued subjects over 20 months. No SAE was judged to be related to tramiprosate. Overall, there was no evidence that tramiprosate affected vital signs and laboratory test values. Pharmacokinetic data demonstrated that the increase in systemic exposure to tramiprosate was dose related. Tramiprosate also crossed the blood–brain barrier, and dose-dependently reduced CSF $A\beta_{42}$ levels after 3 months of treatment. Although there were no psychometric score differences between treatment groups after 3 months of double-blind treatment, psychometric score changes over the 17-month open-label study suggest a slowing of cognitive and clinical decline, particularly in the mild AD patients.

Findings of the present study indicate that the long-term administration of tramiprosate is safe and tolerated in individuals with mild-to-moderate AD. They also indicate a significant effect of tramiprosate on CSF $A\beta_{42}$ which is consistent with our earlier *in vitro* and animal data (Gervais *et al.*, 2007). The lack of significant differences between tramiprosate- and placebo-treated groups on cognitive and clinical assessments over a 3-month period is also in agreement with tramiprosate's postulated mechanism of action. As a putative amyloid-β antagonist, tramiprosate is believed to interrupt an early pathological event, thereby potentially halting or slowing the course of the disease. In the present double-blind and open-label studies, the short-term effect of tramiprosate on a clinically significant CSF biomarker and its long-term effect consistent with the stabilization of cognitive and clinical decline provide support to the hypothesis that the treatment is disease modifying. These findings have contributed to the design of two Phase III clinical trials aimed at fully investigating the long-term safety, tolerability, and clinical efficacy of tramiprosate in a larger AD population.

Implication for Current Research Framework and Emerging Treatment

CSF $A\beta$ concentrations may represent one of the best available biomarkers for demonstrating the pharmacological effects of drugs that target $A\beta$. There is indeed evidence from animal studies suggesting that a reduction in CSF $A\beta$ concentration reflects a lowering of $A\beta$ in the brain tissue (Barten *et al.*, 2005; Best *et al.*, 2005; Lemere *et al.*, 2004). For instance, injections of a gamma-secretase inhibitor in transgenic mice over-expressing $A\beta$ have been shown to significantly reduce both brain and CSF $A\beta$ levels (Barten *et al.*, 2005). Similar findings have been obtained with non-transgenic rats (Best *et al.*, 2005). In aged Vervet monkeys, $A\beta$ vaccination by protein immunotherapy significantly reduces both cerebral and CSF $A\beta$ levels.

Taken together, these studies reinforce the relevance of measuring CSF Aβ levels in patients as a means of assessing the effects of anti-amyloid drugs and suggest that lowering CSF Aβ may reflect an Aβ reduction in the brain. The dose-dependent reduction in CSF Aβ$_{42}$ observed after a 3-month treatment with tramiprosate provides support for its intended effects against the amyloid cascade. Reduction in CSF Aβ has already been shown to produce beneficial clinical effects. A correlation between brain Aβ levels and disease severity has been reported (Naslund *et al.*, 2000). Immunization against soluble Aβ has also been shown to reverse memory impairment in transgenic mice (Dodart *et al.*, 2002). While our open-label results are consistent with cognitive and clinical stabilization, a reduction in soluble Aβ peptides coupled with a symptomatic benefit in long-term randomized, double-blind, placebo-controlled studies would provide further convincing support for this causal relationship in humans.

It is conceivable that individuals such as those with mild cognitive impairment or those who are negative for symptoms but positive for AD risk factors could also benefit from treatment with tramiprosate. Finally, other patients such as early onset AD or Down syndrome patients who exhibit clear amyloid pathology could potentially benefit from treatment with tramiprosate.

Progress in the field of biomarker development has been substantial over the past few years. While CSF Aβ biomarkers have been most extensively studied, other biochemical markers may be also relevant at targeting other pathological events such as tau phosphorylation, oxidative stress, or inflammatory processes. Imaging biomarkers such as PIB-ligands that bind to amyloid plaques, or MRI and PET that assess the integrity of neuronal structure and function could also be used to detect treatment response. Certainly a combination of biomarkers will increase the power to detect the effect of disease-modifying agents and their effects on various pathological events. As their mechanism of action and clinical effects become better characterized, these putative treatment agents will contribute to further validate our current understanding of the pathogenesis of AD and increase the number of treatment options available to AD patients.

Summary of How to Treat the Disorder Incorporating the Results of the New Trial Data

Disease-modifying drugs hold many enticing promises, notably, the potential to alter the course of the disease. Combination therapy using both symptomatic and disease-modification interventions will likely become standard for AD. Indeed, traditional symptomatic treatments may be prescribed to achieve symptomatic relief over the short-term. This relief may in turn be sustained over the long-term when the effects of disease-modifying treatments become evident. The concurrent use of different therapeutic classes will hopefully maximize clinical benefit and substantially improve the outlook for individuals with AD.

References

American Psychiatric Association (2000). *Diagnostic and statistical manual of mental disorder* (4th ed.), Text Revision. Washington, DC: American Psychiatric Association.

Azzi, M., Morissette, C., Fallon, L., Martin, R., Galarneau, A., Sebastiani, G., *et al.* (2007). Involvement of both GABA-dependent and -independent pathways in tramiprosate neuroprotective effects against amyloid-beta toxicity. *8th International Conference AD/PD*, 14–18 March, Salzburg, Austria.

Barten, D.M., Guss, V.L., Corsa, J.A., Loo, A., Hansel, S.B., Zheng, M., *et al.* (2005). Dynamics of {beta}-amyloid reductions in brain, cerebrospinal fluid, and plasma of {beta}-amyloid precursor protein transgenic mice treated with a {gamma}-secretase inhibitor. *Journal of Pharmacology and Experimental Therapeutics*, 312(2), 635–643.

Best, J.D., Jay, M.T., Otu, F., Ma, J., Nadin, A., Ellis, S., *et al.* (2005). Quantitative measurement of changes in amyloid-beta(40) in the rat brain and cerebrospinal fluid following treatment with the gamma-secretase inhibitor LY-411575 [N2-[(2S)-2-(3,5-difluorophenyl)-2-hydroxyethanoyl]-N1-[(7S)-5-methyl-6-oxo-6,7-dihydro-5H-dibenzo[b,d]azepin-7-yl]-L-alaninamide]. *Journal of Pharmacology and Experimental Therapeutics*, 313(2), 902–908.

Canevari, L., Abramov, A.Y., & Duchen, M.R. (2004). Toxicity of amyloid beta peptide: tales of calcium, mitochondria, and oxidative stress. *Neurochemical Research*, 29(3), 637–650.

Christensen, D.D. (2007). Changing the course of Alzheimer's disease: anti-amyloid disease-modifying treatments on the horizon. *Primary Care Companion Journal of Clinical Psychiatry*, 9(1), 32–41.

Citron, M. (2004). Strategies for disease modification in Alzheimer's disease. *Nature Reviews Neuroscience*, 5(9), 677–685.

Citron, M., Oltersdorf, T., Haass, C., McConlogue, L., Hung, A.Y., Seubert, P., *et al.* (1992). Mutation of the beta-amyloid precursor protein in familial Alzheimer's disease increases beta-protein production. *Nature*, 360(6405), 672–674.

Dodart, J.C., Bales, K.R., Gannon, K.S., Greene, S.J., DeMattos, R.B., Mathis, C., *et al.* (2002). Immunization reverses memory deficits without reducing brain abeta burden in Alzheimer's disease model. *Nature Neuroscience*, 5(5), 452–457.

Dodel, R.C., Du, Y., Depboylu, C., Hampel, H., Frolich, L., Haag, A., *et al.* (2004). Intravenous immunoglobulins containing antibodies against beta-amyloid for the treatment of Alzheimer's disease. *Journal of Neurology Neurosurgery and Psychiatry*, 75(10), 1472–1474.

Folstein, M.F., Folstein, S.E., & McHugh, P.R. (1975). "Mini-mental state". A practical method for grading the cognitive state of patients for the clinician. *Journal of Psychiatric Research*, 12(3), 189–198.

Gandy, S. (2005). The role of cerebral amyloid beta accumulation in common forms of Alzheimer disease. *Journal of Clinical Investigation*, 115(5), 1121–1129.

Gervais, F., Paquette, J., Morissette, C., Krzywkowski, P., Yu, M., Azzi, M., *et al.* (2007). Targeting soluble abeta peptide with tramiprosate for the treatment of brain amyloidosis. *Neurobiology of Aging*, 28(4), 537–547.

Giaccone, G., Tagliavini, F., Linoli, G., Bouras, C., Frigerio, L., Frangione, B., *et al.* (1989). Down patients: extracellular preamyloid deposits precede neuritic degeneration and senile plaques. *Neuroscience Letters*, 97(1–2), 232–238.

Gilman, S., Koller, M., Black, R.S., Jenkins, L., Griffith, S.G., Fox, N.C., *et al.* (2005). Clinical effects of abeta immunization (AN1792) in patients with AD in an interrupted trial. *Neurology*, 64(9), 1553–1562.

Goate, A., Chartier-Harlin, M.C., Mullan, M., Brown, J., Crawford, F., Fidani, L., *et al.* (1991). Segregation of a missense mutation in the amyloid precursor protein gene with familial Alzheimer's disease. *Nature*, 349(6311), 704–706.

Krzywkowski, P., Sebastiani, G., Williams, S., Delorme, D., & Greenberg, B.G. (2007). Tramiprosate prevents amyloid beta-induced inhibition of long-term potentiation in rat hippocampal slices. *8th International Conference AD/PD*, 14–18 March, Salzburg, Austria.

Lemere, C.A., Beierschmitt, A., Iglesias, M., Spooner, E.T., Bloom, J.K., Leverone, J.F., *et al.* (2004). Alzheimer's disease abeta vaccine reduces central nervous system abeta levels in a non-human primate, the Caribbean vervet. *American Journal of Pathology*, 165(1), 283–297.

Levy-Lahad, E., Wijsman, E.M., Nemens, E., Anderson, L., Goddard, K.A., Weber, J.L., *et al.* (1995). A familial Alzheimer's disease locus on chromosome 1. *Science*, 269(5226), 970–973.

McKhann, G., Drachman, D., Folstein, M., Katzman, R., Price, D., & Stadlan, E.M. (1984). Clinical diagnosis of Alzheimer's disease: report of the NINCDS-ADRDA Work Group under the auspices of Department of Health and Human Services Task Force on Alzheimer's Disease. *Neurology*, 34(7), 939–944.

Mohs, R.C., & Cohen, L. (1988). Alzheimer's disease assessment scale (ADAS). *Psychopharmacology Bulletin*, 24(4), 627–628.

Morris, J.C. (1993). The clinical dementia rating (CDR): current version and scoring rules. *Neurology*, 43(11), 2412–2414.

Naslund, J., Haroutunian, V., Mohs, R., Davis, K.L., Davies, P., Greengard, P., *et al.* (2000). Correlation between elevated levels of amyloid beta-peptide in the brain and cognitive decline (In Process Citation). *JAMA*, 283(12), 1571–1577.

Ritchie, C.W., Bush, A.I., Mackinnon, A., Macfarlane, S., Mastwyk, M., MacGregor, L., *et al.* (2003). Metal-Protein attenuation with iodochlorhydroxyquin (clioquinol) targeting A{beta} amyloid deposition and toxicity in Alzheimer disease: a pilot phase 2 clinical trial. *Archives of Neurology*, 60(12), 1685–1691.

Sherrington, R., Rogaev, E.I., Liang, Y., Rogaeva, E.A., Levesque, G., Ikeda, K., *et al.* (1995). Cloning of a gene bearing missense mutations in early-onset familial Alzheimer's disease. *Nature*, 375, 754–760.

Solomon, B. (2007). Beta-amyloid-based immunotherapy as a treatment of Alzheimers disease. *Drugs Today (Barc)*, 43(5), 333–342.

Tanzi, R.E., Moir, R.D., & Wagner, S.L. (2004). Clearance of Alzheimer's abeta peptide; the many roads to perdition. *Neuron*, 43(5), 605–608.

Thal, L.J., Kantarci, K., Reiman, E.M., Klunk, W.E., Weiner, M.W., Zetterberg, H., *et al.* (2006). The role of biomarkers in clinical trials for Alzheimer disease. *Alzheimer Disease and Associated Disorders*, 20(1), 6–15.

Progress in Neurotherapeutics and Neuropsychopharmacology, 3:1, 127–135 © 2008 Cambridge University Press
DOI: 10.1017/S174823210700016X   Printed in the United Kingdom

Intranasal Zolmitriptan Is Effective and Well Tolerated in Acute Cluster Headache: A Randomized Placebo-Controlled Double-Blind Crossover Study*

E. Cittadini

Headache Group, Institute of Neurology, The National Hospital for Neurology and Neurosurgery, Queen Square, London, UK; Email: e.cittadini@ion.ucl.ac.uk

P.J. Goadsby

Headache Group, Institute of Neurology, The National Hospital for Neurology and Neurosurgery, Queen Square, London, UK
Department of Neurology, University of California, San Francisco, CA, USA; Email: goadsbyp@neurology.ucsf.edu

ABSTRACT

Background: Cluster headache is a form of primary headache characterized by short-lasting, excruciating unilateral head pains, associated with cranial autonomic features. The current gold-standard treatments of acute cluster headache are inhaled oxygen and sumatriptan by injection. The aim of the study was to evaluate zolmitriptan nasal spray (ZNS) in the acute treatment of cluster headache. *Design/Methods*: Ninety-two patients, aged 42 ± 10 years, 80 males and 12 females, with International Headache Society defined cluster headache were randomized into a placebo-controlled double-blind crossover study. One attack was treated with each of placebo, zolmitriptan nasal spray 5 and 10 mg (ZNS5, ZNS10). The primary endpoint was headache relief at 30 min: reduction from moderate, severe or very severe pain to nil or mild. The study was multi-center and multi-national, and was approved by the appropriate Ethics Committees. *Results*: Sixty-nine patients were available for an intention-to-treat analysis. The 30 min headache relief rates were: placebo 21%, ZNS5 40% and ZNS10 62%. Modeling the response as a binary outcome with regression methods, the Wald test was significant for the overall regression ($\chi^2 = 29.4$, $p < 0.001$), with both ZNS5 and ZNS10 giving significant effects against placebo. Headache relief rates for patients with episodic cluster headache were 30% for placebo, 47% for ZNS5 and 80% for ZNS10 while corresponding rates for patients with chronic cluster headache were 14%,

*This chapter is based on the full publication of these data (Cittadini *et al.*, 2006).

Correspondence should be addressed to: Peter J. Goadsby, Department of Neurology, University of California, San Francisco, CA, USA; Email: goadsbyp@neurology.ucsf.edu

28% and 36%, respectively. Zolmitriptan intranasal was well tolerated. *Interpretation*: Zolmitriptan 5 and 10 mg intranasal is effective within 30 min and well tolerated in the treatment of acute cluster headache.

Key words: cluster headache, randomized controlled trial, zolmitriptan.

Introduction and Overview

Cluster headache (CH) is the most painful form of primary headache, typically characterized by attacks lasting between 15 and 180 min (Headache Classification Committee of The International Headache Society, 2004). Because of the rapid onset and short time to peak intensity, fast acting symptomatic therapy is necessary (Bahra *et al.*, 2002). In the treatment of acute CH there is placebo-controlled evidence for sumatriptan by intranasal spray (van Vliet *et al.*, 2003) and subcutaneous injection (Ekbom *et al.*, 1993; Ekbom & The Sumatriptan Cluster Headache Study Group, 1991) and recently for inhaled oxygen (Cohen *et al.*, 2007b). Evidence for the use of intranasal lidocaine (Robbins, 1995) and intranasal dihydroergotamine mesylate (Andersson & Jespersen, 1986) in acute CH is less robust. Oral zolmitriptan has been demonstrated to be effective in acute episodic CH (Bahra *et al.*, 2000), although at higher doses than usually used in migraine. Given the extremely severe nature of acute CH, more data from placebo-controlled trials is desirable so that options for treatment, based on evidence, are increased.

Purpose of the Trial

The aim of the study was to assess the efficacy of zolmitriptan intranasal spray in the acute treatment of CH attacks.

Agent

Zolmitriptan nasal spray.

Relevant Past Clinical Experience

Zolmitriptan is a so-called second generation triptan, serotonin 5-HT$_{1B/1D}$ receptor agonist (Goadsby, 2000), developed to provide improved pharmacokinetics and optimized trigeminovascular targeting of both the peripheral and central trigeminal terminals (Goadsby & Edvinsson, 1994). As a result, zolmitriptan has a relatively high oral bioavailability, significant lipophilicity and the generation of an active hepatic metabolite, 183C91 (Goadsby & Yates, 2006). Zolmitriptan orally and intranasal spray are effective and well tolerated treatments of acute migraine (Palmer & Spencer, 1997).

Zolmitriptan intranasal formulation has faster onset of action than oral formulation (Charlesworth *et al.*, 2003), with clear evidence of intranasal absorption

(Zingmark *et al.*, 2003). A comparison of the pharmacokinetics of intranasal zolmitriptan and intranasal sumatriptan suggests that intranasal zolmitriptan should be effective in acute CH (Goadsby & Yates, 2006). A preliminary, single-blind study of zolmitriptan nasal spray in patients with episodic and chronic CH has showed that this formulation may be effective in CH patients (Mathew *et al.*, 2004).

Clinical Trial

Subjects

At total of 92 patients were recruited, 80 men and 12 women, with a mean $\pm$ SD age of 40 $\pm$ 10 years, between June 2003 and May 2005.

Trial Methods

Patients between 18 and 65 years of age, with diagnosis of CH according to the International Headache Society criteria (Headache Classification Committee of The International Headache Society, 2004), were recruited in five European centers (three in Germany, one in Italy and one in the UK). We included patients with untreated attacks lasting at least 45 min, patients that used zolmitriptan in the past and zolmitriptan-naïve patients were included if, in the opinion of the investigator, it was safe to do so. We excluded patients unsuitable for use of zolmitriptan tablet or nasal spray in the country where the study was performed according to the drug label or regulatory approved use in that country. We also excluded patients with more than two risk factors for cardiovascular disease, patients using regular ergotamine derivatives or analgesic, and patients with an ear, nose and throat disorder that would preclude the use of intranasal zolmitriptan.

The study was a randomized, double-blind, three attack crossover study of 5 mg and 10 mg zolmitriptan, and matching placebo.

Measures

Headache intensity was rated on a five point scale: none, mild, moderate, severe and very severe.

Primary and Secondary Outcome

The primary outcome variable of the study was headache response at 30 min, defined as a reduction in headache from moderate, severe or very severe to mild or no pain. Secondary outcome measures included the percentage of patients headache free at 30 min and rate of relief of associated symptoms. The associated symptoms such as vomiting, nausea, photophobia, phonophobia, lacrimation, nasal congestion, other autonomic features and restlessness and agitation, were recorded immediately prior the treatment and at 30 min.

Statistical Analysis

Based on the result of sumatriptan nasal spray study (van Vliet *et al.*, 2003) and our clinical experience of what would be a meaningful effect, we considered that the difference between placebo and active treatment should be 20%. The outcome data were to be treated as binary, that is, response or no response at 30 min, and using the results of a crossover study of subcutaneous sumatriptan versus placebo (Ekbom & The Sumatriptan Cluster Headache Study Group, 1991) and allowing for some difference in therapeutic responses seen between sumatriptan injections and the nasal spray in migraine (Tfelt-Hansen, 1998), we sized the study for an α of 0.05 and a β of 0.8. Our planned analysis specifically allowed for the dichotomous outcome and used a generalized linear model and logistic regression approach to determinate the effect of active treatment, including modeling terms for treatment order, sex, site and CH type, episodic versus chronic CH. We used a multilevel multivariate analysis approach (Snijders & Bosker, 1999) as the three attacks were not strictly independent (MLwiN 1.1, Yang *et al.*, 2000). Finally, we did not test the effect of the zolmitriptan nasal spray on associated symptoms in order to avoid multiple comparisons, preferring to report the numerical outcome.

Results

Efficacy

The primary endpoint of the study was the combined (attacks 1, 2 and 3) headache response rate at 30 min compared with placebo. The Wald test was significant for the overall regression ($\chi^2 = 29.4; p < 0.001$) with the treatment term and CH type being significantly different from zero. Treatment order and patient sex were not significant.

Efficacy of Whole Cohort

In total, 65 attacks were treated with 5 mg of zolmitriptan nasal spray; 63 attacks, with 10 mg of zolmitriptan nasal spray; and 61 attacks, with placebo. Considering the primary endpoint, in the attacks treated with 5 mg of zolmitriptan nasal spray, 27 patients (42%) reported headache relief at 30 min, and in the attacks treated with 10 mg of zolmitriptan nasal spray, 38 patients (61%) reported headache relief at 30 min, compared with 14 patients (23%) who treated an attack with placebo ($p = 0.002$; Figure 1).

Eighteen patients (28%) were pain free at 30 min when treated with 5 mg of zolmitriptan nasal spray and 31 patients (50%) were pain free at 30 min when treated with 10 mg of zolmitriptan nasal spray, compared with 10 patients (16%) who treated an attack with placebo ($p = 0.0003$). At 15 min after treatment, 2% of patients using placebo, 9% using 5 mg zolmitriptan nasal spray and 19% using 10 mg zolmitriptan nasal spray reported pain relief.

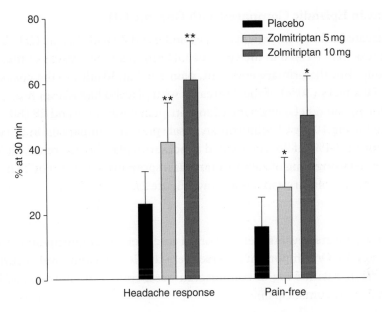

Fig. 1.
Efficacy: headache response, a reduction of headache intensity from very severe, severe or moderate to mild or no pain, and pain-free rates (no pain) at 30 min after treatment with zolmitriptan versus placebo. **$p < 0.002$; *$p < 0.003$ (after Cittadini *et al.*, 2006).

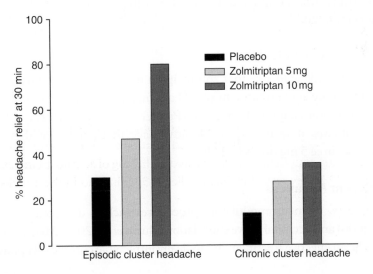

Fig. 2.
Comparison of headache relief rates, moderate, severe or very severe pain going to nil or mild pain, at 30 min after treatment (ordinate %), for placebo zolmitriptan 5 and 10 mg by nasal spray, between episodic and chronic CH (after Cittadini *et al.*, 2006).

Efficacy in Episodic Compared with Chronic CH

Of the treated cohort, 40 patients had episodic and 29 had chronic CH. A total of 104 attacks were treated in the episodic CH group and 85 attacks in the chronic CH group. For the primary endpoint, pain relief at 30 min, in the episodic CH group, 10 attacks (30%) of the 33 treated with placebo had a response, while 17 (47%) of 36 had relief using 5 mg of zolmitriptan nasal spray and 28 (80%) of 35 had relief using 10 mg of zolmitriptan nasal spray. In comparison in the chronic CH group, 4 (14%) of 28 who treated attacks with placebo had relief, 8 (28%) of 29 had relief using 5 mg of zolmitriptan nasal spray and 10 (36%) of 28 had relief using 10 mg of zolmitriptan nasal spray (Figure 2).

Safety

No serious adverse events were reported in either the zolmitriptan or placebo treated attacks. One important adverse event that led to withdrawal occurred in a patient treated with 5 mg of zolmitriptan nasal spray was shortness of breath, vomiting and rheumatic pain.

Unique Aspect of Trial

The study was the first controlled trial of zolmitriptan nasal spray in patients with CH and showed that both 5 and 10 mg of zolmitriptan nasal spray are effective as acute treatments of CH at the primary endpoint of 30 min. Recently, an almost identical study was conducted in the US with a similar positive outcome (Rapoport et al., 2007).

Translation into Clinical Practice

These data provide evidence that zolmitriptan nasal spray can be used as a first line therapy in the acute treatment of CH and in particular, given the safety data for the use of zolmitriptan 15 mg/day (Palmer & Spencer, 1997) although in migraine patients, it seems a possible advantage that patients with CH could probably use three 5 mg doses in 24 h.

Other Recent Advances

In recent years, the neuromodulatory procedures such as deep brain stimulation (Leone, 2006) and occipital nerve stimulation (Burns et al., 2007; Magis et al., 2007) appear to be an effective treatment in medically intractable chronic CH patients.

How Do the Trial Results Fit into the Emerging Treatment and Research Framework?

CH is the most painful form of primary headache known and thus treatments need to work quickly. At present there are relatively few well designed, controlled studies that showed clear evidence of efficacy in CH including sumatriptan 20 mg nasal spray (van Vliet *et al.*, 2003), sumatriptan 6 mg subcutaneous injections (Ekbom & The Sumatriptan Cluster Headache Study Group, 1991) and most recently oxygen (Cohen *et al.*, 2007). There is an ongoing need for more studies to provide a solid evidence base for the treatment of this condition.

Summary of How to Treat the Disorder Incorporating the Results of the New Trial Data

The treatment of CH can be divided into acute therapy aimed at aborting attacks and prophylactic therapy aimed at rapid suppression of attack frequency (Goadsby *et al.*, 2007). Current first line acute treatments include subcutaneous sumatriptan 6 mg, which has a rapid effect and high response rate (Ekbom *et al.*, 1993; Ekbom & The Sumatriptan Cluster Headache Study Group, 1991), and can be used twice daily, on a long-term basis if necessary without risk of tachyphylaxis and rebound (Ekbom *et al.*, 1992). Sumatriptan 20 mg nasal spray (van Vliet *et al.*, 2003) and zolmitriptan 5 mg nasal spray (Rapoport *et al.*, 2007; Cittadini *et al.*, 2006); inhalation of 100% oxygen, at 7–12 l/min for 15–20 min is also safe and effective (Cohen *et al.*, 2007; Fogan, 1985). Second line treatments include: subcutaneous octreotide 100 µg which has recently shown moderate effect in the treatment of acute CH attack (Matharu *et al.*, 2004), and can be useful in patients that are unresponsive or intolerant to triptans. Lidocaine solution 20–60 mg, given as nasal drops (4–6%), or as a spray nasal in the nostril on the painful side has limited efficacy (Robbins, 1995). The preventive treatments can be divided in short and long-term prophylaxis. The short-term preventives include corticosteroids (Couch & Ziegler, 1978), which is used as transitional therapy in conjunction with other approaches until the latter are effective. Methysergide (Curran *et al.*, 1967) is a good option in patients with short bouts that last less than 6 months. However, methysergide is no longer available in the US. Greater occipital nerve (GON) injection is another option as short-term treatment and consists of injection of local anesthetic and corticosteroids around the GON ipsilateral to the affected side (Ambrosini *et al.*, 2005). The long-term preventives include verapamil, which is the drug of choice in both episodic and chronic CH (Leone *et al.*, 2000; Bussone *et al.*, 1990; Gabai & Spierings, 1989) and clinical experience has demonstrated that higher doses are needed in order to treat this condition in contrast to the dose common used in cardiological field. Verapamil can cause heart block by slowing the conduction, therefore checking the PR interval prolongation on ECG can monitor potential development of heart block (Cohen *et al.*, 2007a). Another effective treatment is lithium with the efficacy more evident for chronic compared to episodic CH. Other treatments such as topiramate, valproate, pizotifen and gabapentin are employed without clear evidence of efficacy (Goadsby *et al.*, 2007).

References

Ambrosini, A., Vandenheede, M., Rossi, P., Aloj, F., Sauli, E., Pierelli, F., *et al.* (2005). Suboccipital injection with a mixture of rapid- and long-acting steroids in cluster headache: a double-blind placebo-controlled study. *Pain*, 118, 92–96.

Andersson, P.G., & Jespersen, L.T. (1986). Dihydroergotamine nasal spray in the treatment of attacks of cluster headache. *Cephalalgia*, 6, 51–54.

Bahra, A., Gawel, M.J., Hardebo, J.-E., Millson, D., Brean, S.A., & Goadsby, P.J. (2000). Oral zolmitriptan is effective in the acute treatment of cluster headache. *Neurology*, 54, 1832–1839.

Bahra, A., May, A., & Goadsby, P.J. (2002). Cluster headache: a prospective clinical study in 230 patients with diagnostic implications. *Neurology*, 58, 354–361.

Burns, B., Watkins, L., & Goadsby, P.J. (2007). Successful treatment of medically intractable cluster headache using occipital nerve stimulation (ONS). *The Lancet*, 369, 1099–1106.

Bussone, G., Leone, M., Peccarisi, C., Micieli, G., Granella, F., Magri, M., *et al.* (1990). Double blind comparison of lithium and verapamil in cluster headache prophylaxis. *Headache*, 30, 411–417.

Charlesworth, B.R., Dowson, A.J., Purdy, A., Becker, W.J., Boes-Hansen, S., & Farkkila, M. (2003). Speed of onset and efficacy of zolmitriptan nasal spray in the acute treatment of migraine: a double-blind, placebo-controlled, dose-ranging study versus zolmitriptan tablet. *CNS Drugs*, 17, 653–667.

Cittadini, E., May, A., Straube, A., Evers, S., Bussone, G., & Goadsby, P.J. (2006). Effectiveness of intranasal zolmitriptan in acute cluster headache. A randomized, placebo-controlled, double-blind crossover study. *Archives of Neurology*, 63, 1537–1542.

Cohen, A.S., Matharu, M.S., & Goadsby, P.J. (2007a). Electrocardiographic abnormalities in patients with cluster headache on verapamil therapy. *Neurology*, 69, 668–675.

Cohen, A.S., Matharu, M.S., Burns, B., & Goadsby, P.J. (2007b). Randomized double-blind, placebo-controlled trial of high-flow inhaled oxygen in acute cluster headache. *Cephalalgia*, 27, 1188.

Couch, J.R., & Ziegler, D.K. (1978). Prednisone therapy for cluster headache. *Headache*, 18, 219–221.

Curran, D.A., Hinterberger, H., & Lance, J.W. (1967). Methysergide. *Research and Clinical Studies in Headache*, 1, 74–122.

Ekbom, K., & The Sumatriptan Cluster Headache Study Group (1991). Treatment of acute cluster headache with sumatriptan. *New England Journal of Medicine*, 325, 322–326.

Ekbom, K., Waldenlind, E., Cole, J.A., Pilgrim, A.J., & Kirkham, A. (1992). Sumatriptan in chronic cluster headache: results of continuous treatment for eleven months. *Cephalalgia*, 12, 254–256.

Ekbom, K., Monstad, I., Prusinski, A., Cole, J.A., Pilgrim, A.J., & Noronha, D. (1993). Subcutaneous sumatriptan in the acute treatment of cluster headache: a dose comparison study. *Acta Neurologica Scandinavica*, 88, 63–69.

Fogan, L. (1985). Treatment of cluster headache: a double blind comparison of oxygen vs air inhalation. *Archives of Neurology*, 42, 362–363.

Gabai, I.J., & Spierings, E.L.H. (1989). Prophylactic treatment of cluster headache with verapamil. *Headache*, 29, 167–168.

Goadsby, P.J. (2000). The pharmacology of headache. *Progress in Neurobiology*, 62, 509–525.

Goadsby, P.J., & Edvinsson, L. (1994). Peripheral and central trigeminovascular activation in cat is blocked by the serotonin (5HT)-1D receptor agonist 311C90. *Headache*, 34, 394–399.

Goadsby, P.J., & Yates, R. (2006). Zolmitriptan intranasal: a review of the pharmacokinetics and clinical efficacy. *Headache*, 46, 138–149.

Goadsby, P.J., Cohen, A.S., & Matharu, M.S. (2007). Trigeminal autonomic cephalalgias – diagnosis and treatment. *Current Neurology and Neuroscience Reports*, 7, 117–125.

Headache Classification Committee of The International Headache Society (2004). *The International Classification of Headache Disorders* (2nd ed.). *Cephalalgia*, 24(Suppl. 1), 1–160.

Leone, M. (2006). Deep brain stimulation in headache. *Lancet Neurology*, 5, 873–877.

Leone, M., D'Amico, D., Frediani, F., Moschiano, P., Grazzi, L., Attanasio, A., et al. (2000). Verapamil in the prophylaxis of episodic cluster headache: a double-blind study versus placebo. *Neurology*, 54, 1382–1385.

Magis, D., Allena, M., Bolla, M., De Pasqua, V., Remacle, J.M., & Schoenen, J. (2007). Occipital nerve stimulation for drug-resistant chronic cluster headache: a prospective pilot study. *Lancet Neurology*, 6, 314–321.

Matharu, M.S., Levy, M.J., Meeran, K., & Goadsby, P.J. (2004). Subcutaneous octreotide in cluster headache – randomized placebo-controlled double-blind cross-over study. *Annals of Neurology*, 56, 488–494.

Mathew, N.T., Kailasam, J., & Meadors, L. (2004). Early treatment of migraine with rizatriptan: a placebo-controlled study. *Headache*, 44, 669–673.

Palmer, K.J., & Spencer, C.M. (1997). Zolmitriptan. *CNS Drugs*, 7, 468–478.

Rapoport, A.M., Mathew, N.T., Silberstein, S.D., Dodick, D., Tepper, S.J., Sheftell, F.D., et al. (2007). Zolmitriptan nasal spray in the acute treatment of cluster headache: a double-blind study. *Neurology*, 69, 821–826.

Robbins, L. (1995). Intranasal lidocaine for cluster headache. *Headache*, 35, 83–84.

Snijders, T.A.B., & Bosker, R.J. (1999). *Multilevel Analysis. An Introduction to Basic and Advanced Multilevel Modelling* (1st ed.). London: Sage Publications.

Tfelt-Hansen, P. (1998). Efficacy and adverse events of subcutaneous, oral, and intranasal sumatriptan used for migraine treatment: a systematic review based on number needed to treat. *Cephalalgia*, 18, 532–538.

van Vliet, J.A., Bahra, A., Martin, V., Aurora, S.K., Mathew, N.T., Ferrari, M.D., et al. (2003). Intranasal sumatriptan in cluster headache – randomized placebo-controlled double-blind study. *Neurology*, 60, 630–633.

Yang, M., Goldstein, H., & Heath, A. (2000). Multilevel models for repeated binary outcomes: attitudes and voting over the electoral cycle. *Journal of the Royal Statistical Society (A)*, 163, 49–62.

Zingmark, P.-H., Yates, R., Hedlund, C., & Kagedal, M. (2003). True nasopharyngeal absorption of zolmitriptan following administration of zolmitriptan nasal spray. *European Journal of Neurology*, 10(Suppl. 1), 76.

Progress in Neurotherapeutics and Neuropsychopharmacology, 3:1, 137–151 © 2008 Cambridge University Press
DOI: 10.1017/S1748232107000110   Printed in the United Kingdom

Optimal Dosing of Immunomodulating Drugs: A Dose-Comparison Study of GA in RRMS

Daniel Wynn
Consultants in Neurology, Northbrook, IL, USA; Email: dwynnmd@dwynnmd.interaccess.com

Catherine Meyer
Consultants in Neurology, Northbrook, IL, USA; Email: Research@CINLTD.com

Neil Allen
Consultants in Neurology, Northbrook, IL, USA; Email: Research@CINLTD.com

Dennis O'Brien
Billings Clinic, Billings, MT, USA

ABSTRACT

Background: Though indications of a dose–response for glatiramer acetate (GA) were apparent during early drug development and clinical testing, no formal dose-comparisons of GA had been conducted before the present study. *Design/Methods*: This multicenter, randomized, double-blind study compared the safety and efficacy of two GA doses: 20 mg/day, the currently approved dose, versus 40 mg/day. Relapsing–remitting multiple sclerosis (RRMS) patients with active disease (1–15 gadolinium-enhancing (GdE) lesions on screening magnetic resonance imaging (MRI) and ≥ 1 relapse in the previous year) were eligible. The primary outcome was change from baseline in total number of GdE lesions at 7, 8, and 9 months. Other outcomes included effects on relapse, changes in expanded disability status scale (EDSS) scores, and responder analyses. *Results*: Benefits of the 40 mg GA dose versus the 20 mg dose on GdE lesions were evident by month 3. Additionally, significant advantages of the 40 mg dose were observed for time to first relapse and proportion of relapse-free patients. There was a trend for better outcomes with 40 mg/day GA for the primary efficacy measure, but the difference between doses was not statistically significant. Both GA doses were safe and similarly well tolerated. *Interpretation*: A 40 mg/day GA dosage may be more effective than the 20 mg/day recommended dosage for reducing disease activity, and appears to have an earlier onset of action. A large, phase III study is underway to confirm these findings.

Correspondence should be addressed to: Daniel Wynn, Consultants in Neurology, Northbrook, IL, USA; Email: dwynnmd@dwynnmd.interaccess.com

Key words: dose–response, glatiramer acetate, multiple sclerosis, relapsing–remitting.

Introduction

Glatiramer acetate (GA; Copaxone®) has been shown in three pivotal clinical trials (Comi *et al.*, 2001; Johnson *et al.*, 1995; 1998; Bornstein *et al.*, 1987); in an ongoing long-term (>10 years), open-label follow-up study (Ford *et al.*, 2006); and during postmarketing experience, to be safe and effective for reducing relapse rate, delaying disability, and improving magnetic resonance imaging (MRI) measures of disease burden in patients with relapsing–remitting multiple sclerosis (RRMS). MS is a heterogenous disease and GA, like other immunomodulators used in MS, is not effective in all patients. Dose-comparison studies of the interferon beta (IFNβ) drugs suggest that higher rather than lower doses of these agents are more effective, up to a certain threshold, at which the risk:benefit ratio of the drug becomes unfavorable (Hughes *et al.*, 2001; Ebers *et al.*, 1998; The IFNB Multiple Sclerosis Study Group, 1993). Although optimization of GA dosing could improve therapeutic outcomes, clinical experience with GA doses other than the currently approved dosage, 20 mg/day, is limited.

GA was originally synthesized to induce experimental autoimmune encephalomyelitis (EAE), an animal model of MS. However, instead of inducing disease it was protective in a variety of species, and also showed a therapeutic effect in animals with EAE. This finding prompted small studies in MS patients, the results of which were suggestive of a therapeutic dose–response. In a pilot study that included four patients with very advanced MS (three other study patients had disseminated encephalomyelitis), intramuscular (IM) GA doses of 2–3 mg every 2 or 3 days for 3 weeks, then once weekly for 2–5 additional months were evaluated (Abramsky *et al.*, 1977). This dose had no adverse effects but only slight symptom improvement was noted in two of the four MS patients. Another study with 16 MS patients (4 RRMS and 12 chronic progressive) assessed the safety and efficacy of GA 5 mg IM, administered with regularly reduced frequency over a 6-month period (Bornstein *et al.*, 1982). GA was administered five times per week for 3 weeks, then thrice weekly for 3 weeks, twice weekly for 3 weeks, then once weekly for the remainder of a 6-month period. Several patients initially demonstrated disease improvement, but, as the dosing frequency was reduced, improvements disappeared. Over the course of the next year, the GA dosage was incrementally increased to 20 mg/day in these patients. Fifteen subjects completed the study, with 2 of 3 RRMS patients and 2 of 12 chronic progressive patients described as "improved."

The promising results observed with the 20 mg/day dosage led to the first pivotal study of GA, which included 50 MS patients who received GA 20 mg/day subcutaneously (SC) or placebo for 2 years (Bornstein *et al.*, 1987). Compared with placebo, GA was associated with improvement in relapse rate and decreased disability. Treatment was well tolerated, and 20 mg/day became the established dosage in larger clinical trials and was approved by the FDA for treatment of RRMS.

Until now, no formal dose-comparison studies of GA have been conducted and the optimal dose of GA remains unknown. The excellent safety and tolerability of the currently approved GA dose suggested that although efficacy might be improved at higher doses, patient safety would not be compromised. This review describes the first formal dose-comparison study of GA. (This study has been reported previously (Cohen *et al.*, 2007).)

Clinical Trial Methods

Patients

Male and female patients aged 18–50 with clinically definite MS according to the Poser criteria (Poser *et al.*, 1983) were enrolled between October 2003 and January, 2005. Key inclusion criteria were 1–15 gadolinium-enhancing (GdE) lesions on screening MRI, at least 1 relapse in the previous year, and expanded disability status scale (Kurtzke, 1983) (EDSS) score between 0 and 5.0, inclusive. Key exclusion criteria were relapse occurrence or steroid treatment within 30 days of the screening visit or between the screening and baseline visits, prior use of GA, use of an IFNβ drug within 60 days, immunosuppressant use within 6 months, sensitivity to mannitol, prior use of cladribine or total lymphoid irradiation, and inability to undergo MRI with paramagnetic contrast agents.

All patients provided written informed consent before randomization to treatment.

Study Design

The trial was a multicenter (18 clinical sites), randomized, double-blind, parallel-group, dose-comparison study. Patients were evenly randomized to receive a single daily SC injection of GA 20 mg or GA 40 mg for 9 months. For study purposes, a month was defined as 28 ± 4 days. The baseline visit was conducted within 14 days of screening. At each study site, a treating neurologist supervised overall medical management, including safety monitoring. An examining neurologist performed neurological testing, recorded 25′ walk time, and calculated functional system (FS) scores and EDSS score (Neurostatus, L. Kappos, MD, Department of Neurology, University Hospital, Basel, Switzerland) at scheduled and unscheduled visits. Neurological exams were performed at baseline and every 3 months thereafter.

Brain MRIs were performed at screening (MRIs obtained at screening were used as the pretreatment baseline images) and at months 3, 7, 8, and 9, or at early termination if the patient had been in the study for at least 3 months. Scheduled

MRIs were not delayed if the patient was receiving steroid therapy for a confirmed relapse.

Vital signs, adverse events (AEs), and concomitant medications were assessed at baseline and at months 1, 3, 6, 7, 8, and 9, or early termination. Laboratory assessments (hematology, serum chemistries, and urinalysis) and EKGs were performed at baseline and at months 1, 3, 6, and 9, or early termination. Blood samples were collected at baseline and at 3-month intervals thereafter to assess anti-GA antibodies.

A relapse was defined as the appearance of one or more new neurologic symptoms or reappearance of one or more previous symptoms persisting at least 48 h, not accompanied by fever or infection, and occurring after ≥30 days of stable or improving neurologic function. Patients were examined within 7 days of a suspected relapse. An event was considered a relapse only if the examining neurologist's assessment corresponded to an increase of at least 0.5 EDSS steps, 1 grade in 2 or more FS scores, or 2 grades in a single FS score. On-study relapses could be treated by the treating neurologist with a standard 1000 mg dose of IV methylprednisolone for 3 consecutive days without an oral taper.

The protocol was approved by the institutional review boards of the participating centers. An independent Drug Safety Monitoring Board met five times to review study conduct and blinded safety data. A 6th meeting was held to review unblinded safety results. The Data Safety Monitoring Board (DSMB) could terminate the study early in the event of safety concerns.

MRI Scanning Techniques and Analyses

The MRI Analysis Center in the Neuroimaging Research Unit, San Raffaele Scientific Institute, Milan, Italy, performed MRI analyses. All sites had 1.0-T or 1.5-T scanners. Dual-echo spin echo sequences were used to obtain proton-density and T2-weighted images (repetition time (TR) 2200–3000, echo time (TE) 15 to 50/80 to 100, echo train length 4–6, 3-mm slice thickness, and 44 contiguous axial slices). T1-weighted images (TR 450–660, TE 10–20) with the same scan geometry as above were obtained before and 5 min after administration of Gd 0.1 mmol/kg. Slices ran parallel to a line joining the inferoanterior and inferoposterior parts of the corpus callosum. Patients were carefully repositioned at follow-up visits according to published guidelines (Miller *et al.*, 1991).

Investigators were blinded to MRI results during the study. Image quality was reviewed at the MRI analysis center and unsatisfactory images were rejected but not repeated. Identification of GdE, T2-hyperintense, and T1-hypointense lesions were based on consensus of two experienced examiners, as previously described (Filippi *et al.*, 1998; Barkhof *et al.*, 1997). Lesions were outlined by trained technicians using a semiautomated segmentation technique based on local thresholding (Rovaris *et al.*, 1997). Lesion volumes were calculated automatically. Using the same measurement techniques as those in a previous study (Rovaris *et al.*, 1997), the median intraobserver coefficient of variation for T2 lesion loads was 1.6% (range: 1.8–6.2%) and was 4.0% (range: 2.2–8.4%) for T1 lesion loads.

Outcome Measures

The primary efficacy measure was the total number of GdE MRI lesions at months 7, 8, and 9. Secondary efficacy outcomes included the number of new GdE lesions and total number of new T2-hyperintense lesions at months 8 and 9, change from baseline to termination in T2 lesion volume and relapse rate, and change from baseline to each visit in 25' walk time. Prospective exploratory outcomes were changes from baseline to termination in total GdE and T1-hypointense lesion volumes, MRI metrics at month 3, and change from baseline EDSS scores at each visit.

Post hoc analyses were also performed, including time to first relapse, proportion of relapse-free patients, and "responder" analyses, which were based on occurrence of relapses, EDSS progression, and presence of GdE lesions and/or new T2 lesions at months 7, 8, and 9.

Statistical Analyses

Sample size calculations were based on the European/Canadian MRI study of GA (Comi *et al.*, 2001). It was estimated that 50 evaluable patients per group would provide 90% power to detect a 60% treatment effect between groups in total number of GdE lesions at months 7, 8, and 9, with 2-sided $\alpha = 0.05$. All analyses used intention-to-treat (ITT) principles; however, to be included in the primary efficacy analysis, patients must have had at least one MRI scan at months 7, 8, or 9.

Total number of GdE lesions at months 7, 8, and 9, and other analyses of GdE and T2 lesions used quasi-likelihood (overdispersed) Poisson regression (SAS PROC GENMOD), using DIST = POI and DSCALE in the options of the MODEL statement with an offset based on the log of proportion of available scans (1/3, 2/3, or 3/3). Covariates in the model included baseline GdE count, center effect, and treatment effect. Numbers of patients who withdrew early due to AEs were compared using Fisher's exact test, and time to withdrawal was analyzed by log-rank test.

Relapse rates were analyzed using Poisson regression with relapse rate in the year before entry and baseline EDSS scores as covariates. Comparisons of proportions of relapse-free patients were made using chi-square test. Time to first confirmed relapse was analyzed using Kaplan–Meier technique and compared between treatments by a log-rank test.

In post hoc analyses, patients were considered responders if they: (1) were relapse-free with no GdE lesions at months 7, 8, and 9, or had a reduction in the mean number of GdE lesions of at least 50% versus baseline; or (2) were relapse-free with no EDSS progression; had no GdE lesions at months 7, 8, and 9; and had no new T2-hyperintense lesions at the last assessment. Responder comparisons were performed using logistic regression adjusted for clinical site and number of baseline GdE lesions.

All p values were 2-tailed. Data analysis was performed by Teva Pharmaceutical Industries, Israel, and study investigators were given independent access to data.

Results

Patient Accounting

Of 229 patients screened, 90 patients were randomized (Figure 1). Most excluded patients lacked GdE lesions on screening MRI. Demographic and disease

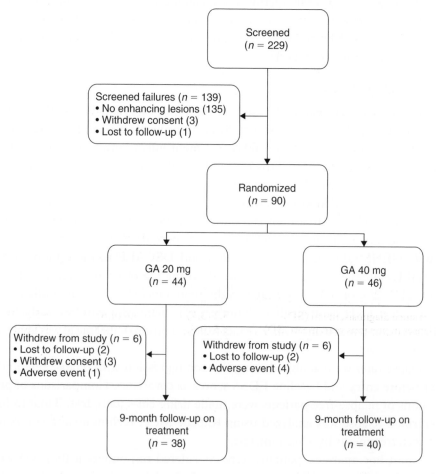

Fig. 1.
Patient disposition. (*Source*: With permission, **Cohen *et al.*** (2007). *Neurology*, 68, 939–944.)

characteristics at baseline were well matched between treatment groups (Table 1). The group of all patients had active disease with a mean of 1.5 relapses in the year before study entry and a mean of 3.4 ± 3.2 GdE lesions at the baseline visit.

Thirty-nine patients in the GA 20 mg/day group and 42 patients in the 40 mg/day group had at least one MRI during months 7, 8, and 9, and are included in the primary efficacy analysis. Overall, 38 patients receiving 20 mg/day and 40 patients receiving 40 mg/day GA completed 9 months of double-blind treatment.

Efficacy

MRI outcomes. A summary of MRI outcomes is shown in Table 2. Decreases from baseline in total number of GdE lesions at months 7, 8, and 9 (the primary endpoint) were apparent in both GA dose groups (65% decrease with GA 20 mg/day and 75% decrease with GA 40 mg/day, $p < 0.0001$ both comparisons). Figure 2 shows mean number of GdE lesions at each study visit. There was a trend favoring 40 mg/day for the primary endpoint (38% reduction versus 20 mg/day, $p = 0.0898$). An advantage of the higher GA dose on GdE lesion count was apparent by month 3 (a 52% reduction, $p = 0.0051$).

Some secondary and prespecified exploratory MRI endpoints also favored the 40 mg/day GA dosage; specifically, change from baseline in GdE lesion volume and numbers of new GdE lesions and new T2-hyperintense lesions at months 8 and 9 (Table 2). There were no differences between treatment groups for change from baseline total T2-hyperintense or T1-hypointense lesion volumes.

Table 1. **Baseline Demographic and Disease Characteristics**

CHARACTERISTIC	GA 20 mg (*n* = 44)	GA 40 mg (*n* = 46)	TOTAL (*n* = 90)
Age, mean (SD), years	37.1 (7.0)	37.4 (6.5)	37.2 (6.7)
Female (%)	31 (71%)	37 (80%)	68 (76%)
Caucasian (%)	38 (86%)	44 (96%)	82 (91%)
Years since symptom onset, mean (SD)	7.4 (6.2)	6.7 (6.4)	7.1 (6.3)
Years since diagnosis, mean (SD)	3.2 (3.7)	3.8 (4.8)	3.5 (4.3)
Relapses in previous year, mean (SD)	1.5 (0.8)	1.5 (0.8)	1.5 (0.8)
Actual EDSS score, mean (SD)	2.0 (1.2)	2.1 (1.0)	2.0 (1.1)
Converted EDSS score, mean (SD)	2.0 (1.2)	2.0 (0.9)	2.0 (1.0)
T25FW, mean (SD), seconds	4.9 (1.3)	5.1 (1.3)	5.0 (1.2)
GdE lesion number, mean (SD)	3.4 (3.3)	3.4 (3.1)	3.4 (3.2)
GdE lesion number, median (range)	2.0 (1–15)	2.0 (1–14)	2.0 (1–15)
GdE lesion volume, mean (SD), ml	0.59 (0.686)	1.17 (3.74)	0.89 (2.73)
T2-hyperintense lesion volume, mean (SD), ml	16.97 (15.83)	18.89 (14.71)	17.96 (15.21)
T1-hypointense lesion volume, mean (SD), ml	3.65 (6.38)	4.39 (4.97)	4.03 (5.67)

T25FW = Timed 25-Foot Walk.
Source: With permission, **Cohen et al.** (2007). *Neurology,* 68, 939–944.

Table 2. **MRI Results**

ENDPOINT	GA 20 mg (n = 44)	GA 40 mg (n = 46)	EFFECT SIZE (95% CI)	p VALUE
Primary endpoints				
Total number of GdE lesions at months 7, 8, 9; mean (SD)*	3.62 (4.06)	2.26 (4.06)	Rate ratio 0.62 (0.36, 1.08)	0.0898
Secondary endpoints				
Total number of new GdE lesions at months 8, 9; mean (SD)	1.41 (1.86)	1.00 (1.91)	Rate ratio 0.73 (0.39, 1.35)	0.311
Total number of new T2-hyperintense lesions at months 8, 9; mean (SD)	1.38 (1.76)	1.00 (2.00)	Rate ratio 0.70 (0.38, 1.30)	0.256
T2-hyperintense lesion volume change LOV versus baseline, mm^3, adjusted mean (SE)	800 (1144)	1516 (1095)	Difference 715 (−3678, 2248)	0.631
Prespecified exploratory endpoints				
GdE lesion volume change LOV versus baseline, mm^3, adjusted mean (SE)	−684 (50.81)	−801 (49.55)	Difference 117 (−16, 251)	0.0841
T1-hypointense lesion volume change LOV versus baseline, mm^3, adjusted mean (SE)	122.29 (115.71)	32.23 (109.72)	Difference 90.16 (−208.10, 388.42)	0.548
Number of GdE lesions at month 3, mean (SD)	2.61 (4.22)	1.33 (1.58)	Rate ratio 0.48 (0.29, 0.82)	0.0051

LOV = last observed value; MSFC = multiple sclerosis functional composite; NNT = number needed to treat.
*39 of 44 patients on 20 mg and 42 of 46 patients on 40 mg had at least one MRI scan at months 7, 8, or 9 and were included in the ITT analysis of the primary efficacy endpoint.
Source: With permission, **Cohen *et al.*** (2007). *Neurology*, 68, 939–944.

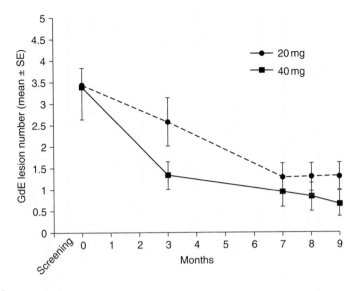

Fig. 2.
Mean number of GdE lesions at each study visit. (*Source*: With permission, **Cohen** *et al.*
(2007). *Neurology*, 68, 939–994.)

Clinical outcomes. Relapse rate in both groups decreased during treatment
compared with the previous year. On-study relapses were less frequent in the
40 mg/day GA group, although the difference between treatment arms was not
statistically significant (relative risk 0.59, 95% CI: 0.31, 1.16) (Table 3). Post hoc
analyses showed a significantly higher proportion of relapse-free patients in the
40 mg/day GA dose group compared with the 20 mg/day group (76.1% versus
52.3%, respectively; $p = 0.0183$) and a significant delay in time to first relapse
(213 days versus 80 days, respectively; $p = 0.0367$).

No significant changes from baseline in 25′ walk times at each visit were
observed in either treatment group (data not shown). Similarly, no significant
changes from baseline EDSS scores at each visit were noted, and there were no
significant differences between GA dosage groups for either measure. The post
hoc responder analyses demonstrated significant benefits of the 40 mg/day GA
dosage (Table 3).

Safety and Tolerability

Safety profiles were similar in both GA treatment groups. There were no deaths
during the study. Early withdrawals due to an AE were infrequent: 1 patient
(2.3%) in the 20 mg/day group and 4 patients (8.7%) in the 40 mg/day group
terminated early ($p = 0.36$). The patient receiving 20 mg/day withdrew after
experiencing severe dyspnea, speech disorder, and panic reaction immediately
after injection, which was considered related to study drug. AEs leading to early

Table 3. **Clinical Efficacy Results**

ENDPOINT	GA 20 mg (n = 44)	GA 40 mg (n = 46)	EFFECT SIZE (95% CI)	*p* VALUE
Secondary endpoints				
Total number of confirmed relapses, mean (SD)	0.52 (0.59)	0.30 (0.59)	Rate ratio 0.59 (0.31, 1.16)	0.121
MSFC change at each visit versus baseline			No change or between-group difference	
Prespecified exploratory and post hoc endpoints				
Relapse-free patients	23/44 (52.3%) NNT = 1.9	35/46 (76.1%) NNT = 1.3	Risk ratio 0.50 (0.27, 0.91)	0.0183
Time to first confirmed relapse (20th percentile), days	80	213		0.0367
EDSS change at each visit versus baseline			No change or between-group difference	
Responders*	15/39 (38.5%) NNT = 2.6	29/42 (69.0%) NNT = 1.5	Odds ratio 3.51 (1.39, 8.88)	0.0078
Responders†	5/37 (13.5%) NNT = 7.4	13/40 (32.5%) NNT = 3.1	Odds ratio 3.12 (1.00, 11.13)	0.0049

LOV = last observed value; MSFC = multiple sclerosis functional composite; NNT = number needed to treat.
*Relapse-free with no GdE lesions at months 7, 8, and 9 or a reduction in the mean number reduced by at least 50% versus baseline.
†Relapse-free; no EDSS progression; no GdE lesions at months 7, 8, and 9; and no new T2-hyperintense lesions at the last assessment.
Source: With permission, **Cohen *et al.*** (2007). *Neurology,* 68, 939–944.

Table 4. **Number and Percentage of Patients Experiencing AEs with Frequency Differing by ⩾5% in the 40 mg Group Compared with the 20 mg Group**

AE	GA 20 mg ($n = 44$)	GA 40 mg ($n = 46$)
Injection-site burning	6 (13.6%)	13 (28.3%)
Injection-site mass	9 (20.5%)	16 (34.8%)
Injection-site pain	9 (20.5%)	14 (30.4%)
Urticaria	1 (2.3%)	5 (10.9%)
Any symptom of IPIR	10 (22.7%)	15 (32.6%)
Palpitations	1 (2.3%)	5 (10.9%)
Flushing	6 (13.6%)	9 (19.6%)
Affect lability	0	6 (13%)
Muscle cramp	0	3 (6.5%)
Pharyngitis	0	3 (6.5%)
Headache	4 (9.1%)	7 (15.2%)
Hypoesthesia	4 (9.1%)	7 (15.2%)
Paresthesia	6 (13.6%)	1 (2.2%)

Source: With permission, **Cohen *et al.*** (2007). *Neurology*, 68, 939–944.

withdrawal in the 40 mg/day group included immediate post-injection reaction (IPIR, $n = 2$), injection-site reaction ($n = 1$), and increased fatigue ($n = 1$). There was no difference between groups in mean time to early withdrawal ($p = 0.95$).

Two serious AEs occurred during the study. A patient in the 40 mg/day dose group experienced an IPIR that required hospitalization and the patient subsequently withdrew from the study. A patient in the 20 mg/day GA group was involved in a motor vehicle accident, which was not considered related to study drug.

Injection-site reactions were the most common AEs, with similar frequency in both dose groups. AEs with at least 5% higher frequency in the 40 mg/day group versus the 20 mg/day group are shown in Table 4. IPIRs occurred more frequently in the higher GA dose group (32.6% versus 22.7% with 20 mg/day); all resolved without sequelae.

Unique Aspects of the Trial

Clinical studies have demonstrated the efficacy of approved dosages of the immunomodulatory drugs, GA, IFNβ, natalizumab, and the neoplastic agent, mitoxantrone, in RRMS patients. However, relatively few studies have been conducted solely to determine the best use or the optimal dose of these agents. At the currently approved dosage, 20 mg/day, long-term GA is safe and well tolerated; patients who continue in the long-term open-label GA extension study (now in its 14th year) continued to do well after more than a decade of continuous therapy (Ford *et al.*, 2006).

This controlled, prospective, comparative study is the first formal dose-optimization trial of GA in RRMS patients.

Conclusions

The 40 mg/day GA dosage was more effective on MRI and clinical measures of disease activity than the 20 mg/day dosage, without compromising safety. GA 40 mg/day had more rapid and greater anti-inflammatory effects than the lower dose, as indicated by the significant difference in number of GdE lesions on MRI at month 3 and the trend for reductions in GdE lesions at months 7, 8, and 9. The higher GA dose also had significant benefits on time to first relapse and proportion of relapse-free patients.

Influence on the Field

Most dose-comparison studies of the various IFNβ drugs show that higher tested doses (SC IFNβ-1b 8 MIU versus 1.6 MIU and SC IFNβ-1a 44 μg versus 22 μg) are more effective than lower doses for reducing disease activity (Hughes *et al.*, 2001; Ebers *et al.*, 1998; The IFNB Multiple Sclerosis Study Group, 1993). However, these studies also suggest there is an efficacy threshold for these agents (Clanet *et al.*, 2002; Jacobs *et al.*, 2000). Whether even higher doses of IFNβ than those tested would improve efficacy is unknown. Importantly, the risk:benefit ratio of these drugs increases at higher doses; for example, neutralizing antibody (NAb) development, the occurrence of certain side effects, and potential for hepatic toxicity are elevated as doses of IFNβ increase (The Once Weekly Interferon for MS Study Group, 1999).

Results of this study indicate that doubling the currently approved GA dose increases therapeutic benefits without increasing safety risks. Whether 40 mg represents a "threshold dose" for GA is unknown. There was a similar frequency of injection-site reactions, the most commonly reported AE, with both GA doses, but IPIRs were more common with the higher dose and injections were somewhat more painful. Tolerability, rather than safety, may ultimately limit the GA dose.

How the Trial Results Fit into the Emerging Treatment and Research Framework

Determining the safety and efficacy of higher doses of immunomodulatory therapies has become particularly relevant since the observation that neuroinflammation need not always be destructive, and, in some cases, is protective. A widely accepted model of MS pathogenesis involves activation of T helper type 1 (Th1) cells by an unknown autoantigen(s). These cells typically express proinflammatory cytokines, which activate macrophages and promote myelin damage. Nevertheless, recent data suggest components of the inflammatory response in the CNS also may promote neuroprotection and/or protective autoimmunity (Kipnis *et al.*, 2004). For example, Th1 cells express brain-derived neurotrophic factor (BDNF), which induces neuronal outgrowth, remyelination, regeneration, and rescue of degenerating neurons at the site of CNS lesions in MS patients (Hohlfeld *et al.*,

2000). Thus, there may be a "too high" dose, at which an immunomodulating agent interferes with protective inflammation. Along these lines, a dramatic example of interference with protective inflammation is the increased risk of progressive multifocal leukoencephalopathy (PML) with natalizumab, which is thought to be due to decreased immune surveillance that in normal circumstances would have prevented the JC virus (the cause of PML) from entering the CNS (Berger & Koralnik, 2005).

Whether the 40 mg/day dosage boosts the purported neuroprotective mechanisms of GA is not as easily determined. GA-reactive T cells are primarily of the Th2 phenotype, which express anti-inflammatory cytokines (e.g. IL-10, TGF-β) as well as BDNF (Aharoni *et al.*, 2003). GA also appears to augment protective autoimmunity (Kipnis & Schwartz, 2002). However, treatment effects on disease progression take longer to discern than effects on inflammation. In this 9-month study, there was no significant improvement or worsening from baseline in EDSS scores in either GA dose group. Further study of this dosage may provide more information regarding its effects toward neuroprotection.

Translation to Clinical Practice

These data suggest 40 mg/day GA confers greater efficacy in RRMS patients without compromising safety. The 40 mg/day dosage was associated with no unexpected AEs, however, it was slightly less well tolerated than the 20 mg/day dosage with respect to IPIRs and injection-site reactions.

More study is needed to establish effects of long-term treatment with a 40 mg GA dose. At this writing, a large (~1000 RRMS patients), phase III study is underway to confirm sustainability of more rapid and beneficial effects of 40 mg/day GA and to confirm the risk:benefit ratio of this dose. Anticipated completion of the study occurs in March 2009 (www.clinicaltrials.gov; identifier: NCT00337779).

Acknowledgments

Co-investigators in the 9006 Dose Comparison Study Group include J.A. Cohen, MD, Mellen Center for MS Treatment and Research, Cleveland Clinic Foundation, Cleveland, OH; M. Rovaris, MD and M. Filippi, MD, Neuroimaging Research Unit, Department of Neurology, San Raffaele Scientific Institute, Milan, Italy; A.D. Goodman, MD, Department of Neurology, University of Rochester, Rochester, NY; and D. Ladkani, PhD, Teva Pharmaceuticals, Petach Tiqva, Israel. Pippa Loupe, PhD, Teva Neuroscience, Kansas City, MO and Sheila Owens, BS, Medical Communication Company, Doylestown, PA provided assistance with manuscript development. The study was funded by Teva Pharmaceuticals Inc., Petach Tiqva, Israel.

References

Abramsky, O., Teitelbaum, D., & Arnon, R. (1977). Effect of a synthetic polypeptide (COP 1) on patients with multiple sclerosis and with acute disseminated encephalomyelitis. *Journal of the Neurological Sciences*, 31, 433–438.

Aharoni, R., Kayhan, B., Eilam, R., Sela, M., & Arnon, R. (2003). Glatiramer acetate-specific T cells in the brain express T helper 2/3 cytokines and brain-derived neurotrophic factor *in situ*. *Proceedings of the National Academy of Sciences of the United States of America*, 100, 14157–14162.

Barkhof, F., Filippi, M., van Waesberghe, J.H., Molyneux, P., Rovaris, M., Lycklama, A., *et al.* (1997). Improving interobserver variation in reporting gadolinium-enhanced MRI lesions in multiple sclerosis. *Neurology*, 49, 1682–1688.

Berger, J.R., & Koralnik, I.J. (2005). Progressive multifocal leukoencephalopathy and natalizumab – unforeseen consequences. *New England Journal of Medicine*, 353, 414–416.

Bornstein, M.B., Miller, A.I., Teitelbaum, D., Arnon, R., & Sela, M. (1982). Multiple sclerosis: trial of a synthetic polypeptide. *Annals of Neurology*, 11, 317–319.

Bornstein, M.B., Miller, A., Slagle, S., Weitzman, M., Crystal, H., Drexler, E., *et al.* (1987). A pilot trial of Cop 1 in exacerbating–remitting multiple sclerosis. *New England Journal of Medicine*, 317, 408–414.

Clanet, M., Radue, E.W., Kappos, L., Hartung, H.P., Hohlfeld, R., Sandberg-Wollheim, M., *et al.* (2002). A randomized, double-blind, dose-comparison study of weekly interferon beta-1a in relapsing MS. *Neurology*, 59, 1507–1517.

Cohen, J.A., Rovaris, M., Goodman, A.D., Ladkani, D., Wynn, D., & Filippi, M. (2007). Randomized, double-blind, dose-comparison study of glatiramer acetate in relapsing–remitting MS. *Neurology*, 68, 939–944.

Comi, G., Filippi, M., Wolinsky, J.S., & European/Canadian Glatiramer Acetate Study Group (2001). European/Canadian multicenter, double-blind, randomized, placebo-controlled study of the effects of glatiramer acetate on magnetic resonance imaging – measured disease activity and burden in patients with relapsing multiple sclerosis. *Annals of Neurology*, 49, 290–297.

Ebers, G., & PRISMS (Prevention of Relapses and Disability by Interferon beta-1a Subcutaneously in Multiple Sclerosis) Study Group (1998). Randomised double-blind placebo-controlled study of interferon beta-1a in relapsing/remitting multiple sclerosis. *Lancet*, 352, 1498–1504.

Filippi, M., Gawne-Cain, M.L., Gasperini, C., van Waesberghe, J.H., Grimaud, J., Barkhof, F., *et al.* (1998). Effect of training and different measurement strategies on the reproducibility of brain MRI lesion load measurements in multiple sclerosis. *Neurology*, 50, 238–244.

Ford, C.C., Johnson, K.P., Lisak, R.P., Panitch, H.S., Shifroni, G., & Wolinsky, J.S. (2006). A prospective open-label study of glatiramer acetate: over a decade of continuous use in MS patients. *Multiple Sclerosis*, 12, 309–320.

Hohlfeld, R., Kerschensteiner, M., Stadelmann, C., Lassmann, H., & Wekerle, H. (2000). The neuroprotective effect of inflammation: implications for the therapy of multiple sclerosis. *Journal of Neuroimmunology*, 107, 161–166.

Hughes, R.A.C., PRISMS (Prevention of Relapses and Disability by Interferon-β-1a Subcutaneously in Multiple Sclerosis) Study Group, & the University of British Columbia MS/MRI Analysis Group (2001). PRISMS-4: long-term efficacy of interferon-β-1a in relapsing MS. *Neurology*, 56, 1628–1636.

Jacobs, L., Rudick, R., & Simon, J. (2000). Extended observations on MS patients treated with IM interferon-beta1a (Avonex): implications for modern MS trials and therapeutics. *Journal of Neuroimmunology*, 107, 167–173.

Johnson, K.P., Brooks, B.R., Cohen, J.A., Ford, C.C., Goldstein, J., Lisak, R.P., *et al.* (1995). Copolymer 1 reduces relapse rate and improves disability in relapsing–remitting multiple sclerosis: results of a phase III multicenter, double-blind placebo-controlled trial. The Copolymer 1 Multiple Sclerosis Study Group. *Neurology*, 45, 1268–1276.

Johnson, K.P., Brooks, B.R., Cohen, J.A., Ford, C.C., Goldstein, J., Lisak, R.P., *et al.* (1998). Extended use of glatiramer acetate (copaxone) is well tolerated and maintains its clinical effect on multiple sclerosis relapse rate and degree of disability. The Copolymer 1 Multiple Sclerosis Study Group. *Neurology*, 50, 701–708.

Kipnis, J., & Schwartz, M. (2002). Dual action of glatiramer acetate (Cop-1) in the treatment of CNS autoimmune and neurodegenerative disorders. *Trends in Molecular Medicine*, 8, 319–323.

Kipnis, J., Aviden, H., Caspi, R.R., & Schwartz, M. (2004). Dual effect of CD4+CD25+ regulatory T cells in neurodegeneration: a dialog with microglia. *Proceedings of the National Academy of Sciences of the United States of America*, 101, 14663–14669.

Kurtzke, J.F. (1983). Rating neurologic impairment in multiple sclerosis: an expanded disability status scale (EDSS). *Neurology*, 33, 1444–1452.

Miller, D.H., Barkhof, F., Berry, I., Kappos, L., Scotti, G., & Thompson, A.J. (1991). Magnetic resonance imaging in monitoring the treatment of multiple sclerosis: concerted action guidelines. *Journal of Neurology Neurosurgery and Psychiatry*, 54, 683–688.

Poser, C.M., Paty, D.W., Scheinberg, L., McDonald, W.I., Davis, F.A., Ebers, G.C., *et al.* (1983). New diagnostic criteria for multiple sclerosis: guidelines for research protocols. *Annals of Neurology*, 13, 227–231.

Rovaris, M., Filippi, M., Calori, G., Rodegher, M., Campi, A., Colombo, B., *et al.* (1997). Intra-observer reproducibility in measuring new putative MR markers of demyelination and axonal loss in multiple sclerosis: a comparison with conventional T2-weighted images. *Journal of Neurology*, 244, 266–270.

The IFNB Multiple Sclerosis Study Group (1993). Interferon beta-1b is effective in relapsing–remitting multiple sclerosis. I. Clinical results of a multicenter, randomized, double-blind, placebo-controlled trial. *Neurology*, 43, 655–661.

The Once Weekly Interferon for MS Study Group (1999). Evidence of interferon beta-1a dose response in relapsing–remitting MS: the OWIMS Study. *Neurology*, 53, 679–686.

Progress in Neurotherapeutics and Neuropsychopharmacology, 3:1, 153–165 © 2008 Cambridge University Press
DOI: 10.1017/S1748232107000043   Printed in the United Kingdom

Tetrathiomolybdate versus Trientine in the Initial Treatment of Neurologic Wilson's Disease

George J. Brewer
Department of Human Genetics, Department of Internal Medicine, University of Michigan, Ann Arbor, MI, USA; Email: brewergj@umich.edu

Fred Askari
Department of Internal Medicine, University of Michigan, Ann Arbor, MI, USA; Email: faskari@med.umich.edu

Matthew T. Lorincz
Department of Neurology, University of Michigan, Ann Arbor, MI, USA; Email: lorincz@umich.edu

Martha Carlson
Department of Pediatrics-Neurology, University of Michigan, Ann Arbor, MI, USA; Email: marthac@umich.edu

Michael Schilsky
Department of Internal Medicine, Cornell University, New York, NY, USA; Email: mls2003@med.cornell.edu

Karen J. Kluin
Department of Neurology, Department of Speech Pathology, University of Michigan, Ann Arbor, MI, USA; Email: niulk@umich.edu

Peter Hedera
Department of Neurology, Vanderbilt University, Nashville, TN, USA; Email: peter.hedera@Vanderbilt.Edu

Paolo Moretti
Departments of Neurology and Molecular and Human Genetics, Baylor College of Medicine, Houston, TX, USA; Email: pmoretti@bcm.tmc.edu

John K. Fink
Department of Neurology, University of Michigan, Ann Arbor, MI, USA; Email: jkfink@umich.edu

Roberta Tankanow
College of Pharmacy, University of Michigan, Ann Arbor, MI, USA; Email: robertat@umich.edu

Robert B. Dick
Department of Human Genetics, University of Michigan, Ann Arbor, MI, USA; Email: bobdick@umich.edu

Julia Sitterly
Department of Human Genetics, University of Michigan, Ann Arbor, MI, USA; Email: sitterly@umich.edu

ABSTRACT

Background: The initial treatment of the neurologic presentation of Wilson's disease is problematic. Penicillamine, used for years on most patients, causes neurologic worsening in up to half of such patients, and half of those who worsen never recover. Zinc, ideal for maintenance therapy, is too slow for these acutely ill patients. We have developed tetrathiomolybdate (TM) for this type of patient, and it has worked well in open label studies. Trientine, another anticopper drug on the market approved for penicillamine intolerant patients, had not been tried in this type of patient. Here, we report on a double blind trial of TM versus trientine in the neurologically presenting Wilson's disease patient. *Design and Methods*: The study was a double blind design in which patients received either TM plus zinc, or trientine plus zinc, for 8 weeks★. Patients were accepted if they presented with neurologic symptoms from Wilson's disease, if they had not been treated longer than 4 weeks with penicillamine or trientine. Patients were followed in the hospital for the 8 weeks of treatment with weekly semiquantitative neurologic and speech examinations, to evaluate possible neurologic worsening. They also had blood and urine studies done weekly. At discharge from hospital theywere continued on zinc maintenance therapy, and returned at yearly intervals for 3 years for further evaluation. *Results*: Twenty-three patients were entered into the trientine arm and 6 reached criteria for neurologic deterioration, while 25 patients were entered into the TM arm and only 1 deteriorated ($p < 0.05$). One patient on trientine had an adverse event while 7 on TM had adverse events. All adverse events were mild. Four patients in the trientine arm died during follow-up, 3 having shown initial neurologic deterioration, 2 patients in the TM arm died. In those patients who did not deteriorate or die, neurologic and speech recovery over 3 years was good. *Interpretation*: TM is a superior choice to trientine for the initial therapy of neurologic Wilson's disease.

Key words: copper toxicity, double blind trial, neurologic damage, tetrathiomolybdate, trientine, Wilson's disease.

Introduction and Overview

Wilson's disease is an autosomal recessive disease of copper accumulation and copper toxicity (Brewer, 2005; 2004; 2001; Brewer & Askari, 2005; Schilsky, 1996; Scheinberg & Sternlieb, 1984). Copper is an essential trace element but most diets contain a little more copper than is needed. Normal people attain a neutral copper balance by excreting excessive copper in the bile. In Wilson's disease, mutations

★This study was originally published in reference 1.

Correspondence should be addressed to: George J. Brewer, MD, Department of Human Genetics and Department of Internal Medicine, University of Michigan Medical School, 5024 Kresge Bldg. II, Ann Arbor, MI 48109-0534, USA; Ph: +1 734 764 5499; Fax: +1 734 615 2048; Email: brewergj@umich.edu

exist in both copies of a gene called ATP7B (Bull *et al.*, 1993; Tanzi *et al.*, 1993; Yamaguchi *et al.*, 1993), which codes for a protein in the liver that is required for biliary copper excretion, and these patients accumulate a little copper every day of their lives. The excess copper is initially stored in the liver. As the storage capacity of the liver is exceeded, the liver is damaged, and about half of the patients present with liver disease. If the liver disease is subclinical, excess copper begins to circulate and accumulate in other organs. The next most sensitive organ is the brain, and the other half of patients present with a neurologic movement disorder, with symptoms such as tremor, dystonia, dysphagia, dysarthria, and incoordination (Brewer *et al.*, 2006; Brewer, 2005; Fink *et al.*, 1999; Brewer & Yuzbasiyan-Gurkan, 1992). In the US and Europe the age of presentation is generally late teenage years or twenties. In India and the Far East, the disease tends to present much earlier. If undiagnosed and untreated, the disease is usually progressive and fatal.

About half of the patients who present neurologically, have behavioral disturbances (Brewer, 2005; Akil *et al.*, 1991). These may predate neurologic symptoms by many years, and consist of personality changes, depression, disinhibition, and sometimes psychosis. The personality changes include temper tantrums, bouts of crying, and mood swings. Patients have difficulty focusing on tasks.

The only practical treatment for many years was an oral copper chelator, D-penicillamine, introduced by Walshe in 1956 (Walshe, 1956). Penicillamine is toxic to many patients, and later Walshe introduced another chelator, trientine, which is approved for use in penicillamine intolerant patients (Walshe, 1982). Zinc acetate, which blocks intestinal copper absorption, was approved for the maintenance therapy of Wilson's disease in the US in 1997, based on our work (Brewer *et al.*, 1998; 1994; 1993; 1983; Yuzbasiyan-Gurkan *et al.*, 1992; Brewer *et al.*, 1987; Hill *et al.*, 1987), and on supporting work carried out in the Netherlands (Hoogenraad *et al.*, 1987; 1979).

Purpose of Our Trial

Penicillamine, as the only drug available, was used for years as the major treatment for Wilson's disease, including patients presenting with neurologic disease. Many of these patients worsened neurologically. A retrospective survey indicated that about half of neurologically presenting, penicillamine treated, patients worsened neurologically, usually within the first few weeks of therapy, and half of those who worsened, never recovered to their prepenicillamine baseline (Brewer, 1987). Many were left permanently severely disabled. The mechanism seems to be that penicillamine mobilizes some of the stored copper from the liver, flushing it through the circulation for excretion in the urine. During this process, brain copper is further elevated, causing more toxicity. Zinc is too slow acting for initial therapy of these acutely ill patients. Trientine had not been evaluated in this type of patient, but since its chelation mechanism was much like penicillamine, it also seemed to have the same risk of inducing neurologic worsening.

Because of the need for an appropriate therapy for this type of patient, we developed tetrathiomolybdate (TM) (Brewer, 2005; Brewer *et al.*, 2006; 2003; 1996; 1994; 1991). It performed well in an open label trial (see next section), so we planned the trial presented here, a double blind comparison of TM and trientine for the initial treatment of neurologically presenting Wilson's disease.

Tetrathiomolybdate

TM is known to work as an anticopper drug by forming a tripartite complex with protein and copper (Mason, 1990; Bremner *et al.*, 1982; Gooneratne, 1981; Mills *et al.*, 1981a, b). It is possible to have two mechanisms of action by giving it with food, where it complexes food and endogenously secreted copper with food protein, and prevents the copper absorption, and by giving it without food, where much of the TM is absorbed and forms a complex with albumin and freely available copper (the potentially toxic copper). This complex is very strong and the bound copper is not available for cellular uptake. This complex builds up in the blood to a plateau, and is slowly broken down by the liver.

A good deal of preclinical work has been done with rats, to study the anticopper mechanisms and toxicity of TM. All of the toxicities could be overcome by copper supplementation, indicating they were due to copper deficiency. The main veterinary use has been to treat copper poisoned sheep, who usually die of acute liver failure (Gooneratne, 1981). The use of TM has been very effective in saving these sheep.

We carried out an open label study of TM in neurologically presenting Wilson's disease patients that ultimately included 55 subjects (Brewer *et al.*, 2003; 1996; 1994; 1991). During this research we carried out dose ranging studies in treatments that lasted 8 weeks, the limit the FDA would allow for a drug that had not had a formal toxicity assessment. We settled on a dose of 20 mg three times/day with food (to block copper absorption) and 20 mg three times/day between meals (to be absorbed and complex "free" copper in the body). These patients were transitioned to maintenance zinc therapy. We found that results were unaffected by adding zinc therapy at the 6 week point, or giving it from the beginning (Brewer, 2003). We used semiquantitative neurologic and speech scoring tests weekly to assess the preservation of neurologic function. Only 2 of the 55 patients (3.6%) reached our criteria for neurologic worsening, while the vast majority (96.4%) were stable during TM therapy, and then recovered during the first 2 years of zinc therapy (Brewer, 2003). We hypothesize that an occasional patient will worsen neurologically due to the natural history of their disease, irrespective of drug treatment, while penicillamine-induced worsening is a drug-catalyzed event. The only toxicity of TM was an occasional patient who had overtreatment anemia, or a mild increase in transaminase enzymes (Brewer, 2003).

Clinical Trial

Subjects

Subjects were patients with neurologically presenting Wilson's disease who had not been treated with penicillamine or trientine for longer than 4 weeks. The diagnosis of Wilson's disease was established by previously published methods, including the presence of Kayser-Fleischer rings, a urine copper over 100 μg/24 h, and a liver biopsy copper value over 200 μg/g dry weight of tissue (Brewer *et al.*, 1998; Hill *et al.*, 1987; Brewer *et al.*, 1983). The presence of one or more neurologic symptoms from Wilson's disease was confirmed by a consulting neurologist. The project was approved by the Institutional Review Board of the University of Michigan Medical School.

Trial Methods

Patients were randomized to one of two arms. In one arm they received TM 20 mg three times/day with meals and 20 mg three times/day between meals for 8 weeks. In the other arm patients received 500 mg of trientine hydrochloride two times between meals for 8 weeks. Trientine and TM were placed in identical type capsules. Patients received placebo as appropriate so that all patients got the same number of pills at the same time. Patients in both arms received 50 mg of zinc two times/day, between meals. All patients were hospitalized for the 8 weeks of the study. Blood was drawn to measure safety variables (blood counts and liver function tests) weekly. These were done in the University of Michigan Health system hematology and biochemistry laboratories. Neurologic and speech function (see next section) were assessed weekly. After the 8 week hospitalization, patients were discharged on maintenance zinc therapy, and returned annually for 3 years for reevaluation which included semiquantitative neurologic and speech examinations.

Two types of adverse events were expected based on prior work, anemia/leukopenia and transaminase elevations (Brewer, 2003). Criteria for anemia/leukopenia were a drop to 80% of baseline of either hemoglobin levels or white blood cell count. Criteria for transaminase elevations were a quadrupling of baseline values of either aspartate aminotransferase (AST) or alanine aminotransferase (ALT), which resulted in discontinuation of the drug (TM or trientine). If anemia or leukopenia reached criteria, the patient was taken off TM or trientine until recovery, then started back at half dose levels. If blood counts then dropped by 20%, the drug was discontinued.

Instruments

The semiquantitative neurologic and speech examinations have been standardized for Wilson's disease and repeatedly evaluated in this disease, with several publications based on these methods (Brewer *et al.*, 2003; 1996; 1994; 1991). In brief, the neurologic examination assesses the various possible neurologic abnormalities in Wilson's disease, with each evaluation resulting in a score of 0 (normal) to 3 (severe). These scores are totaled and the final score ranges from 0 to 38. Since there is mild fluctuation from day to day, a replicable increase of 5 is set as indicating neurologic deterioration. The speech evaluation similarly evaluates various abnormalities of speech, with a final score that varies from 0 (normal) to 7 (anarthric). A replicable increase of 3 points is considered evidence of speech deterioration.

Primary and Secondary Outcomes

The two primary outcomes were deterioration in either the semiquantitative neurologic or speech examinations such that they reached criteria for neurologic worsening. Secondary outcomes included semiquantitative neurologic and speech scores over years of follow-up, the relationship of baseline scores on these tests to neurologic worsening, death, 24 h urine copper and nonceruloplasmin plasma copper over years of follow-up, and adverse events of anemia/leukopenia or transaminase elevations.

Analyses

The rate of neurologic deterioration on TM versus the rate on trientine was tested for statistical significance with the Chi square test. The rate of death in those patients who worsened neurologically versus the rate of death in those who didn't worsen neurologically was also tested for significance using the Chi square test, as was the rate of adverse events in the TM arm versus the trientine arm. The baseline speech scores of patients who worsened neurologically versus the baseline speech scores of those who didn't worsen were compared for statistical significance by t-test.

Results

Efficacy: The primary outcome results, number of deteriorations in semiquantitative neurologic and speech scores, are shown in Tables 1 and 2, respectively. There is a significantly greater rate of neurologic deterioration with trientine than with TM (Table 1). None of the speech scores reached our criteria for deterioration, but it can be noted that all of the speech scores of the patients who deteriorated neurologically were at least mildly worse (Table 2).

Regarding secondary outcomes, Table 3 shows the decline in mean semiquantitative neurologic and speech scores (decline in scores means improvement) over 3 years of maintenance zinc therapy in patients who did not deteriorate or die. In general the scores show a steady decline over the 3 years, and there is no difference between the TM and trientine arms.

Another secondary outcome was whether baseline scores on the neurology and speech tests were predictive of neurologic deterioration. Although the baseline

Table 1. **Patients' Semiquantitative Neurologic Scores**

NUMBER OF PATIENTS	NUMBER DETERIORATED	BASE LINE SCORES OF PATIENTS WHO DETERIORATED	SCORES AT PEAK OF DETERIORATION	WEEK OF TREATMENT IN WHICH PEAK DETERIORATION OCCURRED
TM arm				
25	1[*]	7.5	13	4
Trientine arm				
23	6[*]	7.0	20.0	7
		10.5	22.5	8
		3.5	10.5	4
		15.0	20.5	6
		11.5	17.5	38[**]
		11.0	17.3	7

[*]Significantly different ($p < 0.05$).
[**]This patient was reported by his family to have deteriorated shortly after discharge (at 8 weeks) to his home in Venezuela. On readmission at 38 weeks he was found to have reached criteria for worsening in spite of good evidence of compliance with maintenance therapy.

Table 2. **Patients' Semiquantitative Speech Scores**

NUMBER OF PATIENTS	NUMBER DETERIORATED	BASE LINE SPEECH SCORES OF PATIENTS WHO DETERIORATED ON NEUROLOGIC TEST	SPEECH SCORES AT THEIR PEAK	WEEK OF TREATMENT IN WHICH HIGHEST SPEECH SCORE OCCURRED
TM arm				
25	0	5.0	6.0	4
Trientine arm				
23	0	5.0	6.0	1
		4.5	6.0	3
		4.0	4.5	5
		5.0	6.0	7
		4.0	6.0	38
		5.0	7.0	5

neurology scores were slightly higher in patients who deteriorated, they were not significantly different. The speech scores, however, proved to be more predictive. The baseline speech scores of patients who deteriorated (shown in Table 2), averaged 4.6, while the baseline speech scores of patients who didn't deteriorate averaged 3.3. These two are significantly different ($p < 0.04$). These data suggest that a high baseline speech score may be predictive of neurologic deterioration.

Death was also a secondary outcome. Table 4 summarizes the deaths in study patients, giving the months until death from time of entry into the study, the cause of death to the extent known, and whether the patient deteriorated neurologically on initial treatment. Four patients died on the trientine arm and two on the TM arm. The incidence of death is not significantly different. However, out of seven patients who worsened, four died, while only two out of 41 patients who didn't worsen died. This difference is significant ($p < 0.01$). Neurologic worsening forecasts poor survival.

Two other secondary outcomes were nonceruloplasmin blood copper and 24 h urine copper, during follow-up. The data are given in Table 5. There is a robust reduction in both to what we consider good copper control values after 1 year of zinc therapy, and the reductions are generally equivalent in both the TM and trientine arms.

Tolerability: Both TM and trientine were well-tolerated by the patients.

Safety: The adverse events are shown in Table 6. Four patients reached criteria for transaminase elevations, and they were all in the TM arm. Four patients also reached criteria for anemia and/leukopenia. Three of these were in the TM arm and one in the trientine arm (Table 6). Seven of 25 TM patients with adverse events versus one out of 23 for trientine is significantly different ($p < 0.03$) so it

Table 3. **Decline in Mean Semiquantitative Neurologic and Speech Scores Over Years of Maintenance Therapy**

	TM		TRIENTINE	
	MEAN	SD	MEAN	SD
Neurology scores				
Initial	6.3	3.4	7.1	5.4
Year 1	3.5	5.4	5.5	5.0
Year 2	2.4	1.5	2.9	3.8
Year 3	1.4	1.7	4.4	5.6
Speech scores				
Initial	3.1	1.5	3.5	1.6
Year 1	2.5	2.0	3.1	2.1
Year 2	2.4	1.5	2.4	1.9
Year 3	1.7	1.4	2.1	1.7

Table 4. **Deaths in the 48 Patients**

MONTHS UNTIL DEALTH	CAUSE OF DEATH	DETERIORATED INITIALLY
TM arm		
14	Severe neurologic impairment	No
17.5	Leukemia	Yes
Trientine arm		
22	Severe neurologic impairment and infection	Yes
11.5	Severe neurologic impairment	Yes
12	Severe neurologic impairment	No
6	Severe neurologic impairment and pulmonary congestion	Yes

can be concluded that TM has more side effects than trientine, at least at these dosages, and during an 8 week trial.

Unique Aspects of the Trial

This is the first double blind trial of one anticopper drug against another in any aspects of Wilson's disease. Second, no one has evaluated trientine as an initial treatment for neurologically presenting Wilson's, so this trial provides novel data on that aspect of disease management. Third, this was a head-to-head comparison of a new drug (TM) developed for treating neurologically presenting Wilson's disease, versus trientine in a randomized double blind trial. The results indicate TM is superior in terms of efficacy for the primary outcome, rate of neurologic worsening.

Table 5. **Nonceruloplasmin Blood Copper and 24 h Urine Copper Initially and After 1 Year of Therapy**

	INITIAL		1 YEAR	
	MEAN	SD	MEAN	SD
TM arm				
Nonceruloplasmin blood copper (µg/dl)	17.2	2.3	7.4	1.7
24 h urine copper (µg)	240	20	89	10
Trientine arm				
Nonceruloplasmin blood copper	10.7	2.2	7.3	1.5
24 h urine copper	270	60	116	30

Table 6. **Adverse Events**

TREATMENT	TRANSAMINASE INCREASES			
	AST (U/l)		ALT (U/l)	
	BASELINE	PEAK	BASELINE	PEAK
TM	24	72	28	320[*]
TM	23	96[*]	35	333[*]
TM	55	168	46	504[*]
TM	23	72	27	240[*]

TREATMENT	ANEMIA/LEUKOPENIA			
	HEMOGLOBIN (g/dl)		WBC COUNTS ($10^3/\mu l$)	
	BASELINE	AT NADIR	BASELINE	AT NADIR
Trientine	13.1	11.1	3.9	2.8[*]
TM	12.6	8.9[*]	3.0	1.5[*]
TM	13.7	11.2	3.9	1.9[*]
TM	13.4	10.8[*]	2.2	2.1

*Indicates reached criteria for adverse event.

The results also suggest that the secondary outcome of whether baseline speech score is predictive of neurologic worsening was positive, in that patients with higher speech scores at baseline deteriorated significantly more often than patients with lower speech scores.

Another secondary outcome was death, which occurred more often in the trientine arm, but not significantly so. However, neurologic worsening is a grave prognostic sign, in that four out of the seven patients who worsened died, while only three of the 41 who didn't worsen died, a significant difference.

In terms of adverse events, TM had significantly more total events than did trientine.

Translation to Clinical Practice

Table 7 summarizes our recommendations for anticopper therapy of various stages or types of patients with Wilson's disease. It can be seen that zinc fulfills most of the needs for maintenance therapy. For the liver failure presentations we have recently shown that a combination of trientine and zinc for initial therapy works very well (Askari, 2003). However, the question that has remained is how to treat the neurologically presenting patient. Penicillamine is contraindicated because of its high rate of catalyzing neurologic worsening, and zinc is too slow acting. As a result of this trial we now know that trientine too has an unacceptably high rate of inducing neurological worsening, and we have confirmed our open label study that TM has a very low rate of associated neurologic worsening (3–4%). An occasional patient will worsen neurologically because of the natural history of the disease, and that may be seen with TM, while penicillamine and trientine cause a drug-catalyzed worsening. Thus, TM is a promising therapeutic. TM is not yet commercially available but is expected to be available by the end of 2007.

Lowering the frequency of side effects during TM therapy is desirable, although even though both side effects observed are benign and respond quickly to a drug holiday followed by a lower dose. At present we are studying whether a

Table 7. **Recommendations for Wilson's Disease Anticopper Treatments**

DISEASE STAGE OR TYPE OF PATIENT	RECOMMEND THERAPY
Initial therapy of neurologic presentation	? (TM proposed)
Initial therapy of liver failure presentation	Trientine plus zinc
Maintenance therapy	Zinc
Presymptomatic diagnosis	Zinc
Pediatric patients	
Symptomatic	As above for neurologic or liver failure
Asymptomatic or previously treated	Zinc, in reduced doses
Pregnant patients	Zinc

lower dose of TM given for a longer period of time will maintain efficacy, while lreducing side effects.

Acknowledgements

This work has been supported by grant FD-U-000505 from the US Food and Drug Administration's Orphan Products Office, and by the General Clinical Research Center of the University of Michigan Hospitals, supported by the National Institutes of Health (grant number MO1-RR00042).

Pipex Therapeutics Inc. has plans to pursue a New Drug Application for tetrathiomolybdate for the initial treatment of neurologically presenting Wilson's disease. Dr. Brewer has an equity interest in Pipex and is a paid consultant to the company.

References

Akil, M., Schwartz, J.A., Dutchak, D., Yuzbasiyan-Gurkan, V., & Brewer, G.J. (1991). The psychiatric presentations of Wilson's disease. *The Journal of Neuropsychiatry and Clinical Neurosciences*, 3, 377–382.

Askari, F.K., Greenson, J., Dick, R.D., Johnson, V.D., & Brewer, G.J. (2003). Treatment of Wilson's disease with zinc. XVIII. Initial treatment of the hepatic decompensation presentation with trientine and zinc. *The Journal of Laboratory and Clinical Medicine*, 142, 385–390.

Bremner, I., Mills, C.F., & Young, B.W. (1982). Copper metabolism in rats given di- or trithiomolybdates. *Journal of Inorganic Biochemistry*, 16, 109–119.

Brewer, G.J. (2001). *Wilson's Disease: A Clinician's Guide to Recognition, Diagnosis, and Management*. Boston, MA: Kluwer Academic Publishers.

Brewer, G.J. (2004). Wilson's disease. In: Kasper, D.L., Braunward, E., Fauci, A.S., Hauser, S.L., Longo, D.L., & Jameson, J.L. (eds.), *Harrison's Principles of Internal Medicine*. New York, NY: McGraw-Hill Companies, Inc, pp. 2313–2315.

Brewer, G.J. (2005a). Neurologically presenting Wilson's disease: epidemiology, pathophysiology and treatment. *CNS Drugs*, 19, 185–192.

Brewer, G.J. (2005b). Behavioral abnormalities in Wilson's disease. In: Weiner, W.J., Lang, A.E., & Anderson, K.E. (eds.), *Behavioral Neurology of Movement Disorders*. Philadelphia: Lippincott, Williams & Wilkins, pp. 262–274.

Brewer, G.J. (2006). Novel therapeutic approaches to the treatment of Wilson's disease. *Expert Opinion on Pharmacotherapy*, 7, 317–324.

Brewer, G.J., & Askari, F.K. (2005). Wilson's disease: clinical management and therapy. *Journal of Hepatology*, 42, S13–S21.

Brewer, G.J., &Yuzbasiyan-Gurkan, V. (1992). Wilson disease. *Medicine*, 71, 139–164.

Brewer, G.J., Hill, G.M., Prasad, A.S., Cossack, Z.T., & Rabbani, P. (1983). Oral zinc therapy for Wilson's disease. *Annals of Internal Medicine*, 99, 314–319.

Brewer, G.J., Hill, G., Prasad, A., & Dick, R. (1987a). The treatment of Wilson's disease with zinc. IV. Efficacy monitoring using urine and plasma copper. *Proceedings of the Society for Experimental Biology and Medicine*, 184, 446–455.

Brewer, G.J., Terry, C.A., Aisen, A.M., & Hill, G.M. (1987b). Worsening of neurologic syndrome in patients with Wilson's disease with initial penicillamine therapy. *Archives of Neurology*, 44, 490–493.

Brewer, G.J., Dick, R.D., Yuzbasiyan-Gurkan, V., Tankanow, R., Young, A.B., & Kluin, K.J. (1991). Initial therapy of patients with Wilson's disease with tetrathiomolybdate. *Archives of Neurology*, 48, 42–47.

Brewer, G.J., Yuzbasiyan-Gurkan, V., Johnson, V., Dick, R.D., & Wang, Y. (1993). Treatment of Wilson's disease with zinc XII: dose regimen requirements. *The American Journal of the Medical Sciences*, 305, 199–202.

Brewer, G.J., Dick, R.D., Johnson, V., Wang, Y., Yuzbasiyan-Gurkan, V., Kluin, K., *et al.* (1994a). Treatment of Wilson's disease with ammonium tetrathiomolybdate. I. Initial therapy in 17 neurologically affected patients. *Archives of Neurology*, 51, 545–554.

Brewer, G.J., Dick, R.D., Yuzbasiyan-Gurkan, V., Johnson, V., & Wang, Y. (1994b). Treatment of Wilson's disease with zinc. XIII: therapy with zinc in presymptomatic patients from the time of diagnosis. *The Journal of Laboratory and Clinical Medicine*, 123, 849–858.

Brewer, G.J., Johnson, V., Dick, R.D., Kluin, K.J., Fink, J.K., & Brunberg, J.A. (1996). Treatment of Wilson disease with ammonium tetrathiomolybdate. II. Initial therapy in 33 neurologically affected patients and follow-up with zinc therapy. *Archives of Neurology*, 53, 1017–1025.

Brewer, G.J., Dick, R.D., Johnson, V.D., Brunberg, J.A., Kluin, K.J., & Fink, J.K. (1998). Treatment of Wilson's disease with zinc: XV long-term follow-up studies. *The Journal of Laboratory and Clinical Medicine*, 132, 264–278.

Brewer, G.J., Hedera, P., Kluin, K.J., Carlson, M., Askari, F., Dick, R.B., *et al.* (2003). Treatment of Wilson disease with ammonium tetrathiomolybdate: III. Initial therapy in a total of 55 neurologically affected patients and follow-up with zinc therapy. *Archives of Neurology*, 60, 379–385.

Brewer, G.J., Askari, F., Lorincz, M.T., Carlson, M., Schilsky, M., Kluin, K.J., *et al.* (2006). Treatment of Wilson disease with ammonium tetrathiomolybdate: IV. Comparison of tetrathiomolybdate and trientine in a double-blind study of treatment of the neurologic presentation of Wilson disease. *Archives of Neurology*, 63, 521–527.

Bull, P.C., Thomas, G.R., Rommens, J.M., Forbes, J.R., & Cox, D.W. (1993). The Wilson disease gene is a putative copper transporting P-type ATPase similar to the Menkes gene. *Nature Genetics*, 5, 327–337.

Fink, J.K., Hedera, P., & Brewer, G.J. (1999). Hepatolenticular degeneration (Wilson's disease). *The Neurologist*, 5, 171–185.

Gooneratne, S.R., Howell, J.M., & Gawthorne, J.M. (1981). An investigation of the effects of intravenous administration of thiomolybdate on copper metabolism in chronic Cu-poisoned sheep. *The British Journal of Nutrition*, 46, 469–480.

Hill, G.M., Brewer, G.J., Prasad, A.S., Hydrick, C.R., & Hartmann, D.E. (1987). Treatment of Wilson's disease with zinc. I. Oral zinc therapy regimens. *Hepatology*, 7, 522–528.

Hoogenraad, T.U., Koevoet, R., & de Ruyter Korver, E.G. (1979). Oral zinc sulphate as long-term treatment in Wilson's disease (hepatolenticular degeneration). *European Neurology*, 18, 205–211.

Hoogenraad, T.U., Van Hattum, J., & Van den Hamer, C.J.A. (1987). Management of Wilson's disease with zinc sulfate. Experience in a series of 27 patients. *Journal of the Neurological Sciences*, 77, 137–146.

Mason, J. (1990). The biochemical pathogenesis of molybdenum-induced copper deficiency syndromes in ruminants: towards the final chapter. *Irish Veterinary Journal*, 43, 18–21.

Mills, C.F., El-Gallad, T.T., & Bremner, I. (1981a). Effects of molybdate, sulfide, and tetrathiomolybdate on copper metabolism in rats. *Journal of Inorganic Biochemistry*, 14, 189–207.

Mills, C.F., El-Gallad, T.T., Bremner, I., & Weham, G. (1981b). Copper and molybdenum absorption by rats given ammonium tetrathiomolybdate. *Journal of Inorganic Biochemistry*, 14, 163–175.

Scheinberg, I.H., & Sternlieb, I. (1998). Wilson's disease. In: Smith, L.H.J. (ed.), *Major Problems in Internal Medicine*. Philadelphia: W.B. Saunders Company, pp. 1–171.

Schilsky, M.L. (1996). Wilson disease: genetic basis of copper toxicity and natural history. *Seminars in Liver Disease*, 16, 83–95.

Tanzi, R.E., Petrukhin, K., Chernov, I., Pellequer, J.L., Wasco, W., Ross, B., et al. (1993). The Wilson disease gene is a copper transporting ATPase with homology to the Menkes disease gene. *Nature Genetics*, 5, 344–350.

Walshe, J.M. (1956). Penicillamine, a new oral therapy for Wilson's disease. *American Journal of Medicine*, 21, 487–495.

Walshe, J.M. (1982). Treatment of Wilson's disease with trientine (triethylene tetramine) dihydrochloride. *Lancet*, 1, 643–647.

Yamaguchi, Y., Heiny, M.E., & Gitlin, J.D. (1993). Isolation and characterization of a human liver cDNA as a candidate gene for Wilson disease. *Biochemical and Biophysical Research Communications*, 197, 271–277.

Yuzbasiyan-Gurkan, V., Grider, A., Nostrant, T., Cousins, R.J., & Brewer, G.J. (1992). Treatment of Wilson's disease with zinc: X. Intestinal metallothionein induction. *The Journal of Laboratory and Clinical Medicine*, 120, 380–386.

Progress in Neurotherapeutics and Neuropsychopharmacology, 3:1, 167–187 © 2008 Cambridge University Press
DOI: 10.1017/S1748232107000080   Printed in the United Kingdom

Randomized Clinical Trials of Pregabalin for Neuropathic Pain: Methods, Results, and Implications

Robert H. Dworkin

Departments of Anesthesiology and Neurology, University of Rochester School of Medicine and Dentistry, Rochester, NY, USA; Email: robert_dworkin@urmc.rochester.edu

Rajbala Thakur

Department of Anesthesiology, University of Rochester School of Medicine and Dentistry, Rochester, NY, USA; Email: rajbala_thakur@urmc.rochester.edu

Teresa Griesing

Pfizer, Inc., New York, NY, USA; Email: Teresa.Griesing@pfizer.com

Uma Sharma

Pfizer, Inc., Ann Arbor, MI, USA; Email: usharma@mmsholdings.com

James P. Young

Pfizer, Inc., Ann Arbor, MI, USA; Email: Young410@sbcglobal.net

Key words: diabetic peripheral neuropathy, neuropathic pain, postherpetic neuralgia, pregabalin, randomized clinical trials, spinal cord injury.

Introduction and Overview

Neuropathic pain is caused by lesions or diseases affecting somatosensory pathways within the peripheral or central nervous system (IASP Special Interest Group on Neuropathic Pain, 2006; Merskey & Bogduk, 1994). Chronic neuropathic pain is common in clinical practice, and patients with conditions such as diabetic peripheral neuropathy (DPN), HIV sensory neuropathy, and spinal cord injury suffer from neuropathic pain that impairs their health-related quality of life, causing physical disability and emotional distress (Jensen *et al.*, 2007). The distinction between neuropathic pain and non-neuropathic inflammatory or musculoskeletal pain is important because it reflects at least partially distinct pathophysiologic mechanisms and somewhat different patterns of treatment efficacy. Neuropathic

Correspondence should be addressed to: Robert H. Dworkin, PhD, Department of Anesthesiology, University of Rochester School of Medicine and Dentistry, 601 Elmwood Avenue, Box 604, Rochester, NY 14642, USA; Fax: +1 585 473 5007; Email: robert_dworkin@urmc.rochester.edu

pain can be diagnosed based on a medical history of a nervous system lesion or disease consistent with the patient's report of pain and neurological examination findings of negative and positive sensory phenomena in the same area innervated by damaged nervous system pathways (Dworkin *et al.*, 2003a).

Chronic neuropathic pain is more common than generally appreciated, with as many as three million patients with painful DPN (Schmader, 2002) and one million patients with postherpetic neuralgia (PHN) (Bowsher, 1999) in the United States. Until relatively recently, there were few treatments available with established efficacy for patients with chronic neuropathic pain. On the basis of results from randomized placebo-controlled trials published within the past several years (Dworkin *et al.*, in press; Finnerup *et al.*, 2005), an evidence-based treatment approach for patients with chronic neuropathic pain is now possible. In this chapter, we provide an overview of the results of randomized placebo-controlled clinical trials of pregabalin in patients with peripheral and central neuropathic pain, emphasizing research methods, results, and implications for clinical practice.

Objective of the Clinical Trials

The purpose of the randomized trials of pregabalin in patients with painful DPN, PHN, and spinal cord injury was to evaluate efficacy and safety and provide the basis for regulatory approval throughout the world. Although a number of pharmacologic treatments are used for neuropathic pain, many patients fail to obtain adequate relief or cannot tolerate the side effects of existing medications. Because of this, there continues to be a need for additional therapeutic options that provide greater efficacy, improved safety and tolerability, and other clinical benefits, such as greater ease of use and improved patient compliance.

Pregabalin

Pregabalin is a structural derivative of the neurotransmitter gamma-aminobutyric acid (GABA) that does not interact with either GABA-A or GABA-B receptors as shown by radioligand binding and functional electrophysiology *in vitro*. Pregabalin binds potently and with high selectivity to the α_2–δ subunit of voltage-gated calcium channels, as does gabapentin. This binding activity correlates with decreased calcium channel function and decreased release of several neurotransmitters, including glutamate, noradrenaline, and substance P (Dooley *et al.*, 2007; Taylor *et al.*, 2007). This decreased neurotransmitter release is associated with reduced hyperexcitability in animal models of nociceptive and neuropathic pain and occurs preferentially when there is abnormal neuronal activation. Pregabalin has been shown to reduce pain-related behaviors in the formalin footpad model, the carrageenan thermal hyperalgesia model, and rodent models of neuropathic and post-surgical pain. Importantly, pregabalin activity was selectively lost in genetically modified mice deficient in drug binding to the α_2–δ type 1 protein (Field *et al.*, 2006). Furthermore, structure–activity studies with compounds chemically similar to pregabalin suggest that high-affinity binding to the α_2–δ site is required for analgesic action (Belliotti *et al.*, 2005). Pregabalin was found active in several pain-related animal models after intrathecal administration, suggesting that the spinal cord is a site of drug action. In addition, results with genetically modified mice indicate that binding at the α_2–δ site is required for pregabalin actions on neurotransmitter release and activity against seizures and anxiety-related behaviors in mice. Thus, binding at the α_2–δ protein appears to be both necessary and sufficient for pregabalin drug actions (Taylor *et al.*, 2007).

In Phase 1 studies, healthy subjects generally tolerated pregabalin dosages from 75 to 900 mg/day. The results of these studies supported further investigation in patients at dosages up to 600 mg/day. The most frequently reported adverse events in clinical pharmacology studies (occurring in $\geqslant 5\%$ of patients) were dizziness, somnolence, headache, stupor, thinking abnormalities (mostly recall memory difficulties), asthenia, peripheral edema, nausea, euphoria, blurred vision, abnormal gait, constipation, dry mouth, incoordination, and infection. Clinical laboratory test abnormalities were generally sporadic, transient, and considered to be unrelated to pregabalin administration. Overall, there were no clinically important changes in blood pressure or heart rate, and no clinically significant ECG abnormalities were observed. In addition, no clinically significant drug interactions with pregabalin have been found. Pregabalin is not protein bound and elimination is primarily by renal excretion and proportional to creatinine clearance. Unlike several agents commonly used in the treatment of neuropathic pain (tricyclic antidepressants and opioid analgesics), the risk of death associated with intentional or unintentional overdose is low.

Clinical Trials

Pregabalin has been assessed in over 2500 patients for the treatment of neuropathic pain in patients with painful DPN, PHN, and spinal cord injury. The initial clinical program consisted of nine fixed-dosage placebo-controlled randomized trials in two peripheral neuropathic pain conditions (an additional two studies were terminated prematurely): five studies in painful DPN (Richter *et al.*, 2005; Lesser *et al.*, 2004; Rosenstock *et al.*, 2004) and four studies in PHN (Van Seventer *et al.*, 2006; Sabatowski *et al.*, 2004; Dworkin *et al.*, 2003b). Patients from these double-blind trials could subsequently enroll in long-term open-label safety studies. In addition to these nine trials, two additional studies have been completed in patients with neuropathic pain: a flexible- and fixed-dosage randomized trial in patients with either painful DPN or PHN (Freynhagen *et al.*, 2005) and a flexible-dosage randomized trial in patients with spinal cord injury pain (Siddall *et al.*, 2006). It should be noted that there have been randomized trials of pregabalin in other chronic pain conditions, including fibromyalgia (Crofford *et al.*, 2005). Although consideration has been given to whether this chronic pain syndrome has a neuropathic component (Dworkin *et al.*, 2005a), discussion of the methods and results of this trial is beyond the scope of this chapter.

Subjects

The major inclusion criteria in the pregabalin randomized trials for DPN consisted of a diagnosis of painful, diabetic, distal, symmetrical, and sensorimotor polyneuropathy of 1–5 years' duration with hemoglobin A1c ⩽11%. For PHN, patients were required to have pain for more than 3 months but not more than 5 years after the herpes zoster rash had healed before protocol amendments removed the upper limit. For the spinal cord injury trial, patients were required to have a complete or incomplete spinal cord injury (paraplegia or tetraplegia) that had occurred at least 1 year previously and had been non-progressive for at least 6 months, pain beginning after the lesion and persisting for at least 3 months (or 6 months if relapsing/remitting pain), and a diagnosis of central pain that was generally made on the basis that pain was below the level of the lesion. Other inclusion and exclusion criteria were generally the same for all the neuropathic pain randomized trials. At study baseline, patients were required to have a score ⩾40 mm on the visual analog scale (VAS) of the Short-form McGill Pain Questionnaire (SF-MPQ) (Melzack, 1987). At randomization, patients were also required to have an average daily pain score ⩾4 for a baseline week of daily diary numerical pain intensity ratings (see below). Although the initial randomized trials excluded patients who had not responded to previous gabapentin treatment at dosages ⩾1200 mg/day, later studies allowed such patients to be enrolled. Patients were excluded if they had severe non-neuropathic pain or clinically significant or unstable medical or psychological conditions that could confound the interpretation of response to pregabalin.

Patients in the DPN studies and the flexible-dosage DPN or PHN trial were required to discontinue all analgesic medications prior to baseline and antidepressants were prohibited (except for selective serotonin reuptake inhibitors). In the PHN and spinal cord injury trials, patients were allowed to continue stable dosages of certain analgesic, anti-inflammatory, and/or antidepressant medications; however, these medications could not be initiated during the trials. Prohibited medications were subject to appropriate washout periods.

The majority of patients in these trial were white, and the median age was 60 years for the DPN patients, 73 years for the PHN patients, and 50 years for the spinal cord injury patients. Within the DPN patients, treatment groups were well balanced with respect to duration of diabetes, hemoglobin A1c levels, and baseline mean pain score. The majority of patients had type II diabetes, with an average duration of 9 years. Within the PHN patients, duration of disease and baseline mean pain scores were comparable between the placebo and all of the pregabalin groups. Creatinine clearance values were similar within each pain condition but, not unexpectedly, mean clearance was lower in the PHN patients, of whom 43% were at least 75 years of age.

Trial Methods

Each study consisted of two phases (see Figure 1). The baseline phase consisted of a 1-week period during which patients were screened for eligibility to enter the double-blind phase. The subsequent double-blind phase encompassed a titration period that varied among trials from 0 to 2 weeks, followed by a fixed- or flexible-dosage period that varied among trials from 4 to 12 weeks, and a 1-week withdrawal or follow-up phase for patients who did not continue in the extension studies. Patients who completed or discontinued from the double-blind phase could elect to continue in optional open-label extension studies.

In five of the fixed-dosage studies, all patients within each pregabalin treatment group were administered the same dosage of pregabalin. In the remaining four fixed-dosage studies, patients randomized to the 300/600 mg/day pregabalin arm received 300 mg/day if their estimated creatinine clearance (CLcr) was 30–60 ml/min and 600 mg/day if their CLcr was >60 ml/min; within this chapter, presentations of these studies will display the randomized treatment designation (i.e. 300/600 mg/day) whereas pooled analyses will be reported by dosage received (i.e. 300 or 600 mg/day).

In the flexible-dosage randomized trials, dosages of pregabalin were escalated at weekly intervals. In the flexible-dosage study in patients with DPN or PHN (Freynhagen *et al.*, 2005), pregabalin was increased from 150 to 300, 450, and 600 mg/day. A single downward dosage adjustment after weeks 1, 2, 3, or 4 was allowed, at which time the patient remained on this dosage for the remainder of the trial. In the spinal cord injury trial (Siddall *et al.*, 2006), pregabalin was initiated at 150 mg/day, and could then be escalated to 300 mg/day after 1 week based on effectiveness and tolerability, and to 600 mg/day after another week if needed

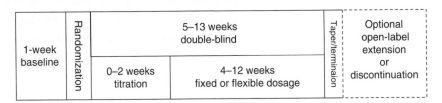

Fig. 1.
Overall study design for clinical trials of pregabalin in neuropathic pain.

for effectiveness. A single dosage reduction for intolerability was permitted after the patient reached 300 or 600 mg/day.

Pregabalin was administered three times daily in the initial neuropathic pain randomized trials, whereas it has been administered twice daily in the more recent trials.

Primary and Secondary Outcomes

The primary efficacy outcome for all of the pregabalin neuropathic pain randomized trials was the endpoint mean pain score, derived from a daily diary pain rating recorded by the patient using an 11-point numerical rating scale ranging from 0 (no pain) to 10 (worst possible pain). Upon awakening, the patient evaluated pain for the previous 24 h by circling the number on the scale that best described his or her pain. Supplemental analyses of the primary endpoint included the proportion of responders (patients who had a $\geqslant 50\%$ reduction from baseline in mean pain score at endpoint) and weekly analysis of pain scores. Because pain reductions of $\geqslant 30\%$ are also considered clinically important by patients (Farrar *et al.*, 2001), analyses were also performed using this additional approach to defining a responder.

The majority of secondary outcomes were assessed using patient self-report questionnaires. Protocol-defined secondary endpoints included: (1) pain ratings using the SF-MPQ present pain intensity, VAS, and pain descriptor scales (Melzack, 1987); (2) sleep interference assessed with an 11-point daily diary numeric rating scale similar to that used for the primary endpoint; (3) Patient Global Impression of Change (PGIC) and Clinical Global Impression of Change (CGIC) rated by the patient and by the clinician on 7-point scales ranging from 1 (very much improved) to 7 (very much worse) (Guy, 1976); and (4) one or more of several health-related quality of life measures, including the SF-36 Health Survey (Ware *et al.*, 1992), Profile of Mood States, Zung Self-Rating Depression Scale, Hospital Anxiety and Depression Scale, Medical Outcomes Study sleep scale, and Euro QOL Health State Profile; detailed discussion of the results of these assessments is beyond the scope of this chapter.

Analysis

All primary and secondary analyses were performed using data from the intention-to-treat (ITT) population. The ITT population consisted of all randomized patients who took at least one dose of study medication. For outcome measures collected using the daily diaries of pain and sleep interference, the following conventions were used:

1. Baseline mean score was calculated as the mean of the last 7 diary entries before taking study medication. Scores did not need to be recorded on consecutive days, and if fewer than 7 scores were recorded

during baseline, the available scores were used to determine the patient's baseline mean.

2. Endpoint mean score was calculated as the mean of the last 7 diary entries while on study medication. Scores did not need to be recorded on consecutive days, and if fewer than 7 scores were recorded by endpoint, available scores were used to determine the mean for all studies except for one of the DPN trials; for this study (040, Table 1), if fewer than 7 post-baseline scores (x) were available, the last 7-x scores from baseline were also used in the calculation of endpoint.

3. Weekly mean score was calculated as the mean of the diary entries for each week in the study. Since each diary entry reflected the previous 24-h period, the week 1 mean was computed using all available entries from days 2 through 8, week 2 from days 9 through 15, and so on.

4. Change from baseline was calculated as the endpoint mean (or weekly mean) score minus the baseline mean score.

5. Responders were defined as patients with 50% or greater and 30% or greater reductions from baseline to endpoint mean pain scores.

Hochberg's multiple comparison procedure was used to protect the type I error rate at the 0.05 level in studies with more than one primary comparison. For all studies, mean pain scores, SF-MPQ scores, mean sleep interference scores, and health-related quality of life assessments were analyzed using an analysis of covariance (ANCOVA) main effects model, including treatment and center as factors and the corresponding baseline score as a covariate. In each case, adjusted least squares means were obtained from the model and 95% confidence intervals (CIs) for the difference in least squares means between each pregabalin and placebo group were constructed.

PGIC and CGIC data were analyzed using the Cochran–Mantel–Haenszel (CMH) test with modified ridit scores, adjusting for center. The proportion of responders was analyzed using the CMH test with table scores, adjusting for center.

Results

The majority of patients completed the studies: 84% in the DPN trials, 77% in the PHN trials, 62% in the trial that enrolled patients with either DPN or PHN, and 63% in the spinal cord injury trial. For pregabalin-treated patients, the most common reason for discontinuation involved adverse events. Discontinuation rates due to adverse events were 9% of pregabalin patients and 4% of placebo patients for the DPN trials, 14% of pregabalin patients and 7% of placebo patients for the PHN trials, and 21% of pregabalin patients and 13% of placebo patients for the spinal cord injury trial.

Table 1. **Endpoint Mean Pain Scores in ITT Analyses of 11 Completed Neuropathic Pain Trials**

STUDY/TREATMENT GROUP	LEAST SQUARES			DIFFERENCE	TREATMENT COMPARISONS FOR PGB VERSUS PLACEBO		
	N	MEAN	SE		95% CI	UNADJUSTED p VALUE	ADJUSTED[A] p VALUE
Painful DPN							
Study 014 [tid] (Richter *et al.*, 2005)							
Placebo	82	5.55	0.23				
PGB 150 mg/day	79	5.11	0.24	−0.44	(−1.08, 0.20)	0.1763	0.1763
PGB 600 mg/day	82	4.29	0.23	−1.26	(−1.89, −0.64)	0.0001	0.0002
Study 029 [tid] (Lesser *et al.*, 2004)							
Placebo	97	5.06	0.21				
PGB 75 mg/day	77	4.91	0.24	−0.15	(−0.76, 0.46)	0.6267	—
PGB 300 mg/day	81	3.80	0.23	−1.26	(−1.86, −0.65)	0.0001	0.0001
PGB 600 mg/day	81	3.60	0.23	−1.45	(−2.06, −0.85)	0.0001	0.0001
Study 040 [tid] (Sharma *et al.*, 2005)							
Placebo	80	4.60	0.26				
PGB 600 mg/day	86	3.96	0.26	−0.64	(−1.37, 0.08)	0.0822	—
AMT 75 mg/day	87	3.67	0.25	−0.93	(−1.65, −0.22)	0.011	—
Study 131 [tid] (Rosenstock *et al.*, 2004)							
Placebo	69	5.46	0.28				
PGB 300 mg/day	75	3.99	0.26	−1.47	(−2.19, −0.75)	0.0001	—
Study 149 [bid] (Sharma *et al.*, 2005)							
Placebo	93	4.66	0.26				
PGB 150 mg/day	96	4.33	0.26	−0.33	(−0.94, 0.28)	0.2849	0.5580
PGB 300 mg/day	96	4.48	0.26	−0.18	(−0.79, 0.43)	0.558	0.5580
PGB 300/600 mg/day[b]	98	3.69	0.25	−0.97	(−1.58, −0.36)	0.0018	0.0054
Postherpetic neuralgia							
Study 030 [tid] (Sharma *et al.*, 2005)							
Placebo	87	5.59	0.21				
PGB 75 mg/day	83	5.46	0.21	−0.14	(−0.71, 0.43)	0.6361	0.7999
PGB 150 mg/day	82	5.52	0.22	−0.07	(−0.64, 0.50)	0.7999	0.7999

	N		SE		CI		
Study 045 [tid] (Sabatowski *et al.*, 2004)							
Placebo	81	6.33	0.22				
PGB 150 mg/day	81	5.14	0.22	−1.20	(−1.81, −0.58)	0.0002	0.0002
PGB 300 mg/day	76	4.76	0.23	−1.57	(−2.20, −0.95)	0.0001	0.0002
Study 127 [tid] (Dworkin *et al.*, 2003b)							
Placebo	84	5.29	0.24				
PGB 300/600 mg/day[b]	88	3.60	0.24	−1.69	(−2.33, −1.05)	0.0001	—
Study 196 [bid] (Van Seventer *et al.*, 2006)							
Placebo	93	6.14	0.23				
PGB 150 mg/day	87	5.26	0.24	−0.88	(−1.53, −0.23)	0.0077	0.0077
PGB 300 mg/day	98	5.07	0.23	−1.07	(−1.70, −0.45)	0.0008	0.0016
PGB 300/600 mg/day[b]	88	4.35	0.24	−1.79	(−2.43, −1.15)	0.0001	0.0003
Painful DPN and PHN							
Study 155 [bid] (Freynhagen *et al.*, 2005)							
Placebo	62	4.98	0.32				
PGB 600 mg/day	128	3.60	0.24	−1.38	(−2.11, −0.65)	<0.001	<0.001
PGB flexible dosage	139	3.81	0.23	−1.17	(−1.90, −0.45)	0.002	0.002
Spinal cord injury							
Study 125 [bid] (Siddall *et al.*, 2006)							
Placebo	67	6.20	0.24				
PGB flexible dosage	69	4.67	0.23	−1.533	(−0.92, −2.15)	<0.001	—

SE = standard error; CI = confidence interval; PGB = pregabalin; AMT = amitriptyline.

[a]Adjustment is based on Hochberg's procedure and applies to all treatment comparisons except PGB 75 mg/day in study 029 (as stated in protocol), and protocols with only 1 PGB treatment group (studies 040, 127, 131, 125).

[b]In studies 127, 149, and 196, patients randomized to the 300/600 mg/day PGB group received either 300 or 600 mg/day based on their CLcr.

EFFICACY

Pregabalin reduced neuropathic pain as measured by endpoint mean pain scores in four of the five completed DPN trials (Table 1, Figure 2). Efficacy was demonstrated for 300 mg/day of pregabalin in two of the three randomized trials and for 600 mg/day in three of the four randomized trials in which these dosages were evaluated. Neither 75 mg/day (evaluated in one study) nor 150 mg/day (evaluated in two studies) significantly reduced pain scores compared with placebo in patients with painful DPN. In one DPN trial that used amitriptyline as a positive control, amitriptyline was significantly more efficacious than placebo in reducing endpoint mean pain scores.

Across the four completed PHN randomized trials, efficacy was demonstrated for 150 mg/day of pregabalin in two of the three trials in which this dosage was evaluated, and for 300 mg/day and 300/600 mg/day in the three trials in which these dosages were evaluated (Table 1, Figure 2). As in the DPN studies, 75 mg/day was not an efficacious dosage.

In the flexible-dosage trial in patients with either painful DPN or PHN, pregabalin dosed flexibly from 150 to 600 mg/day (with an average dosage after escalation of 457 mg/day) and pregabalin at a fixed-dosage of 600 mg/day were

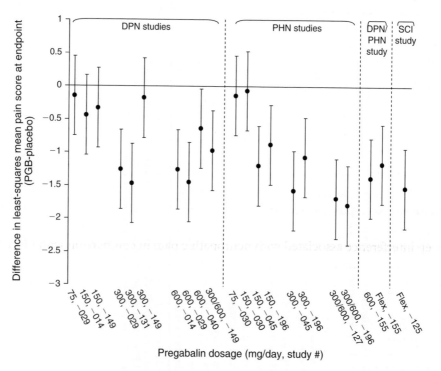

Fig. 2.

Differences (with 95% CIs) in endpoint least squares mean pain scores between pregabalin and placebo for the 5 DPN trials, 4 PHN trials, 1 DPN/PHN trial, and 1 spinal cord injury trial.

both significantly better than placebo and comparable reductions in pain occurred for these dosages. In the spinal cord injury trial, the efficacy of pregabalin dosed flexibly from 150 to 600 mg/day was significant versus placebo, with an average pregabalin dosage after stabilization of 450 mg/day.

Overall, pregabalin treatment was associated with statistically significant reductions in neuropathic pain in patients with painful DPN, PHN, and spinal cord injury pain at dosages from 150 to 600 mg/day (Table 1). Across the seven of nine fixed-dosage trials in DPN and PHN that demonstrated efficacy as well as the flexible-dosage trials in DPN or PHN and spinal cord injury pain, the placebo-corrected treatment differences in pain scores (0–10 scale) for efficacious pregabalin dosages ranged from -0.88 to -1.79; the comparisons with placebo were highly significant ($p < 0.008$) in each case.

In the DPN and PHN trials, the overall proportion of $\geqslant 50\%$ responders was significantly greater in patients treated with 150, 300, or 600 mg/day of pregabalin versus placebo (Figure 3). Using this definition of responder, the proportion of responders in efficacious pregabalin-dosage groups ranged from 39% to 48% (versus from 15% to 30% with placebo) in the DPN studies. Similarly, the proportion of responders in efficacious pregabalin-dosage groups in the PHN studies ranged from 26% to 50% (versus from 8% to 20% with placebo). In the flexible- and fixed-dosage study that enrolled patients with either DPN or PHN, 48% of patients treated with pregabalin dosed flexibly, 52% of patients treated with 600 mg/day of pregabalin, and 24% of patients administered placebo were responders. In the flexible-dosage study in patients with spinal cord injury pain, 22% of pregabalin and 8% of placebo-treated patients were responders. Across the 10 RCTs in patients with DPN or PHN (Figure 3), approximately 2.5 times as many patients treated with 600 mg/day of pregabalin obtained $\geqslant 50\%$ reductions in pain from baseline to endpoint compared to those treated with placebo.

Considering the secondary efficacy outcomes as a group, the pattern of results generally followed that shown for the primary efficacy outcome, supporting a multifaceted response to treatment with pregabalin. Beginning as early as week 1 and throughout the trials, pregabalin in efficacious dosages consistently reduced sleep interference associated with neuropathic pain in comparison with placebo. Across the 10 randomized trials in patients with painful DPN or PHN, patient-assessed global improvement scores demonstrated that the majority of patients who were treated with pregabalin at dosages of 150 mg/day or greater considered themselves improved (Figure 4), with similar findings for clinician-assessed global improvement scores.

TOLERABILITY AND SAFETY

In the randomized trials examining pregabalin in patients with DPN or PHN, 55.9% of placebo- and 71.1% of pregabalin-treated patients had adverse events.

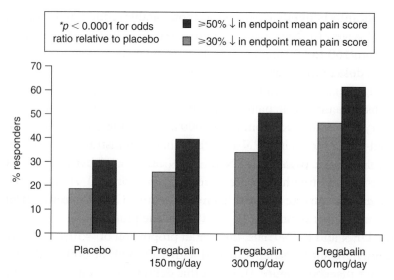

Fig. 3.

Proportions of patients with ⩾50% and ⩾30% pain reductions from baseline to endpoint in the pregabalin DPN and PHN trials (including patients in the fixed-dosage arm of the trial that enrolled patients with either condition).

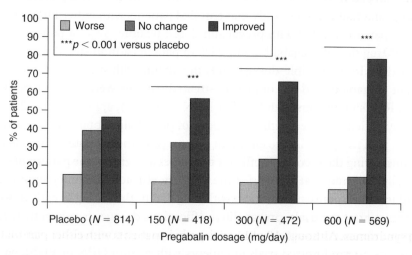

Fig. 4.

Proportions of patients reporting improvement, no change, and worsening on the PGIC scale (condensed from seven to three categories) in the pregabalin DPN and PHN trials (including patients in the fixed-dosage arm of the trial that enrolled patients with either condition).

Adverse events led to discontinuation in 11.4% of patients in these studies. Central nervous system effects (dizziness and somnolence) were the most common reasons pregabalin treatment was interrupted or reduced. Dizziness (23.2%) and somnolence (14.0%) were the most common adverse events; other common adverse events included peripheral edema, dry mouth, asthenia, and blurred vision. The incidence of dizziness, somnolence, and peripheral edema was generally higher at the 300 and 600 mg/day dosages than at the lower dosages. Pregabalin-treated patients gained a mean of 1.6 kg during the pivotal DPN trials, compared with 0.3 kg in placebo-treated patients. Overall, 5.9% of pregabalin-treated and 1.6% of placebo-treated patients in the neuropathic pain randomized trials experienced at least a 7% increase in body weight from baseline to termination.

Dizziness and somnolence, the two most common adverse events in the pregabalin neuropathic pain randomized trials, generally started within 1–2 days of treatment initiation with pregabalin and within 3–5 days with placebo. Many other common adverse events, including other CNS adverse events, had median times to onset within the 1st week in the pregabalin groups. Peripheral edema and weight gain generally had longer median times to onset – 15–22 days for peripheral edema and 11–20 days for weight gain. Because the durations of the trials varied by pain condition, data for the duration of adverse events are difficult to interpret when all studies are combined. Among pregabalin-treated patients who reported dizziness or somnolence but did not discontinue because of these adverse events, dizziness and somnolence resolved in approximately half of the patients.

Although some patients had weight gain and edema concurrently, edema alone did not account for the weight gain observed in pregabalin-treated patients. Neither weight gain nor peripheral edema was associated with cardiovascular complications, systemic changes in laboratory parameters, or clinically important changes in blood pressure. Despite the incidence of weight gain, there were very few discontinuations due to weight gain in patients treated with pregabalin.

Unique Aspects of the Pregabalin Clinical Trials

There are a number of noteworthy aspects of the randomized trials of pregabalin in the treatment of patients with neuropathic pain. One is the large number of multicenter Phase III trials, which were conducted in three different neuropathic pain syndromes. Although 10 of 11 trials were in patients with either painful DPN or PHN, which are both peripheral neuropathic pain conditions, a trial was also conducted in patients with spinal cord injury pain, a central neuropathic pain condition for which few efficacious treatments have been identified.

Also important to note is that the pregabalin trials included two studies that examined flexible dosing (Siddall *et al.*, 2006; Freynhagen *et al.*, 2005). Regulatory agencies generally prefer fixed-dosage studies because they make it possible to determine whether or not specific dosages are efficacious. However, flexible dosing reflects clinical practice much more closely than use of a fixed-dosage because the dosage a patient receives is adjusted on the basis of both effectiveness and tolerability. Interestingly, in the trial with a flexible-dosage arm in patients with either DPN or PHN, the magnitude of benefit was comparable in patients who received flexible dosing of pregabalin between 150 and 600 mg/day (with an average dosage after stabilization of 457 mg/day) and those who were administered a fixed-dosage of 600 mg/day. This suggests that when dosing is individualized, some patients do not require titration to maximum dosages to obtain optimal pain relief and that discontinuation rates may be reduced.

Another noteworthy aspect of the pregabalin trials in neuropathic pain is that concomitant analgesics were permitted in the trials of patients with PHN and spinal cord injury pain. The issue of whether patients should be permitted to remain on stable dosages of concomitant analgesics in clinical trials of new agents for the treatment of neuropathic pain has received a great deal of attention in recent years. On one hand, it is argued that evaluations of a novel treatment in patients who are already being treated with effective treatments will be less likely to demonstrate efficacy (and may lead to regulatory approvals for "add-on" therapy). On the other hand, there are now several medications for neuropathic pain that can be considered first-line (Dworkin *et al.*, in press; Finnerup *et al.*, 2005). It seems likely that patients who are not taking any of these medications or who can be withdrawn from such treatments may not only be relatively unresponsive to existing therapy but may also be less likely to respond to new treatments. Enrolling such patients in clinical trials may therefore make it less likely that new treatments will demonstrate efficacy. Moreover, prohibiting concurrent use of other analgesics in a chronic pain trial may make the results less generalizable to clinical practice, in which combination therapy is very common.

Because the four pregabalin PHN trials enrolled patients who were receiving concomitant analgesics and those who were not, it is possible to compare these two groups with respect to the magnitude of benefit associated with treatment (Dworkin *et al.*, 2005c). For each of the efficacious dosages of pregabalin, the least square differences in endpoint mean pain score between pregabalin and placebo in patients who were and were not receiving concomitant analgesics were minimal and not statistically significant (Figure 5). Importantly, these two groups of patients had equivalent baseline pain, with patients receiving concomitant analgesics having a baseline mean pain score of 6.7 (SD = 1.5) and those not receiving concomitant analgesics having a baseline mean pain score of 6.6 (SD = 1.6). Presumably, one reason for the comparable efficacy of pregabalin in both of these patient groups is their comparable levels of baseline pain, which were in the moderate-to-severe range and allowed pregabalin to show a treatment benefit even in patients receiving other analgesic medications. It is also possible that the mechanism of action of pregabalin targeted underlying pain mechanisms (Woolf, 2004) that did not respond adequately to the analgesic medications that patients in these trials were permitted to continue (e.g. opioid and non-opioid analgesic, anti-inflammatory, and/or antidepressant medications).

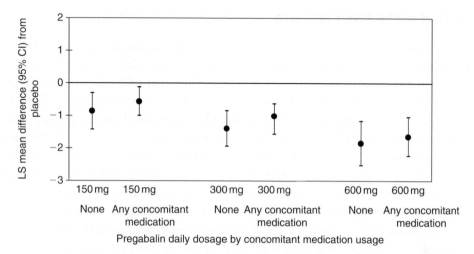

Fig. 5.
Differences in endpoint least squares mean pain scores between pregabalin and placebo in patients receiving any concomitant analgesic medication versus those not receiving such medications in the four PHN trials.

A common concern in clinical trials is whether side effects – for example, sedation or dizziness – can cause patients (or investigators) to become aware of their treatment condition. Although patients in placebo groups often have similar side effects, it is possible that the greater incidence of side effects associated with active treatment could lead to some degree of unblinding. Such compromise of the integrity of the double-blind in a clinical trial could lead to spurious results or an exaggeration of the treatment effect. Of course, it is also possible that patients (and investigators) become aware of patients' treatment conditions because of beneficial effects of the treatment, not its side effects. Several approaches have been suggested for evaluating the role of such unblinding in clinical trials, including asking patients and clinicians at the end of a trial to guess treatment assignment and provide the reasons for these guesses (Moscucci *et al.*, 1987). Although such assessments were not conducted in the pregabalin trials, a strategy used for addressing unblinding was to evaluate treatment efficacy in patients who reported no or few side effects. For example, in one of the PHN trials (Dworkin *et al.*, 2003b), the primary analysis of endpoint mean pain scores was repeated twice – after removing all patients who had one or more of the five side effects reported by more than 10% of pregabalin-treated patients (dizziness, somnolence, peripheral edema, amblyopia, and dry mouth), and after removing all patients who had any of the 11 side effects reported by at least 5% of patients in the pregabalin treatment group. In both of these analyses, there was still significantly greater improvement in the endpoint mean pain scores in patients treated with pregabalin compared with those treated with placebo.

Implications for Future Research

The research design and outcome assessments used in the randomized trials of pregabalin for the treatment of neuropathic pain reflect what is currently state of the art for evaluating treatments for neuropathic pain and other chronic pain conditions (Turk *et al.*, 2006; Dworkin *et al.*, 2005d; Turk *et al.*, 2003). Similar approaches have been used in establishing safety and efficacy in the pivotal trials of gabapentin for PHN (Rice & Maton, 2001; Rowbotham *et al.*, 1998) and duloxetine for painful DPN (Wernicke *et al.*, 2006; Goldstein *et al.*, 2005; Raskin *et al.*, 2005). An increasing number of recent clinical trials, however, have failed to demonstrate efficacy of various other treatments for neuropathic pain. It is unclear whether this reflects medications with limited efficacy or other factors, such as inadequate power to detect modest treatment benefits or increased response rates in placebo groups that make it more difficult to show superiority of the medications (Dworkin *et al.*, 2005b). Until research is conducted that determines whether there are modifiable factors that account for negative trials of efficacious medications for neuropathic pain, the research design and types of outcome assessments used in the randomized trials of pregabalin continue to be preferred by academic investigators, industry, and regulatory agencies for pivotal trials to evaluate the safety and efficacy of medications for neuropathic pain.

One aspect of this approach to neuropathic pain trials is the use of average pain intensity as the primary endpoint. Although primary efficacy analyses have typically examined group differences in mean pain ratings, there has been an increasing emphasis on the use of responder analyses in analgesic clinical trials. One of the primary reasons for this is the presumed greater clinical relevance of these endpoints. In chronic pain clinical trials, it has become common to report the percentages of patients who achieve either $\geqslant 30\%$ or $\geqslant 50\%$ pain reductions from baseline to endpoint (as presented in Figure 3). Although these cut-points identify clinically meaningful levels of improvement (Farrar *et al.*, 2001), the percentages of patients who achieve higher (or lower) levels of relief remain unknown when just one or two definitions of a responder are used. For this reason, it has been argued that a cumulative proportion of responders analysis is preferable (Farrar *et al.*, 2006), which presents the proportions of patients with pain reductions ranging from 0% to 100%, and thereby makes it possible to determine the differences between treatment groups for any level of pain relief within this range. Because this analysis provides considerably more information than analyses examining just one or two definitions of a responder, this approach has been used to present data in the product information for medications recently approved by the United States Food and Drug Administration (FDA) for chronic pain, including DPN and PHN. To date, however, the optimal method for evaluating the statistical significance of group differences in a cumulative proportion of responders analysis has not been determined.

There has been increasing attention to the analysis of missing data in chronic pain clinical trials. In publications of the pregabalin randomized trials, ITT analyses were reported with last observations carried forward for missing data. The FDA has recently suggested that analysis and presentation of pivotal randomized trials of all chronic pain conditions should consider patients who have dropped out of a trial as non-responders (e.g. with ITT analyses using baseline observations carried forward for missing data). Such analyses appear in the FDA-approved pregabalin product information, which therefore presents somewhat different data than the published reports of these pivotal trials.

Relevant Regulatory Issues

The most prominent regulatory issue raised by the clinical trials of pregabalin in patients with neuropathic pain involves the specific indications approved by different regulatory agencies. In the United States, the pregabalin randomized trials in patients with painful DPN and PHN resulted in separate approvals for these two conditions. However, the same trials resulted in approval for the treatment of peripheral neuropathic pain in Europe, where pregabalin was also recently approved for the treatment of central neuropathic pain on the basis of the spinal cord injury trial. These different indications for separate neuropathic pain conditions versus general indications for peripheral or central neuropathic pain reflect different thresholds of comfort regarding the extent to which clinical trial results can be extrapolated from one neuropathic pain condition to another. For example, amitriptyline has well-established efficacy in patients with painful DPN and PHN (Finnerup *et al.*, 2005), but the results of two randomized trials in patients with HIV sensory neuropathy in which it did not differ from placebo (Kieburtz *et al.*, 1998; Shlay *et al.*, 1998) provide the basis for caution regarding the extrapolation of efficacy between different neuropathic pain conditions. Nevertheless, comfort with the validity of such extrapolation may increase as more data become available demonstrating efficacy of pregabalin or other agents for the treatment of diverse types of neuropathic pain.

Implications for Clinical Practice

In recent systematic reviews and treatment guidelines, pregabalin has been considered first-line for the treatment of neuropathic pain (Finnerup *et al.*, 2005), including PHN (Hempenstall *et al.*, 2005; Dubinsky *et al.*, 2004) and painful DPN (Argoff *et al.*, 2006). Other agents that have been considered first-line in the treatment of neuropathic pain include antidepressants (both tricyclic antidepressants and selective serotonin and norepinephrine reuptake inhibitors), gabapentin, opioid analgesics, topical lidocaine, and tramadol (Dworkin *et al.*, in press; Finnerup *et al.*, 2005).

The use of most of these medications for patients with neuropathic pain has long been guided by the rule-of-thumb to "start low and go slow." This approach to titration increases the tolerability of medications with side effects that often cause patients to discontinue treatment. However, slow titration to reach an effective dosage has its own drawbacks, including patients discontinuing treatment during the often lengthy period before an effective dosage is reached. A major advantage of pregabalin in comparison to such treatments is that it can provide pain relief without the necessity of slow titration to reach an effective dosage (Dworkin *et al.*, 2003b; Rowbotham *et al.*, 2003). The results of the pregabalin trials suggest that treatment can be initiated at a dosage of 150 mg/day (75 mg twice daily), which will be effective in some patients, and that titration to 300 mg/day (150 mg twice daily) can occur within a week. Titration in this manner is generally well tolerated, but for patients who are frail, elderly, or overly sensitive to medication side effects, clinicians have anecdotally described initiating treatment with a dosage of 75 mg at bedtime for a week before titrating to 150 mg/day in divided doses.

The analgesic benefits of pregabalin at its starting dosage and the first step of dosage titration suggest that pregabalin is likely to be more effective in the community than medications such as gabapentin or tricyclic antidepressants. This is because in community practice, treatment with these medications is often initiated at low dosages but then not titrated adequately, with patients remaining on subtherapeutic dosages (Oster *et al.*, 2005). This is less likely to occur with pregabalin because treatment can be initiated at an efficacious dosage, and further benefits can occur with titration of the dosage after 1 week.

Summary

The results of the randomized clinical trials discussed in this chapter have demonstrated that pregabalin is safe and efficacious in the treatment of painful DPN, PHN, and spinal cord injury pain. The results of ongoing and planned studies will provide considerable additional data regarding its efficacy in these and other neuropathic pain conditions.

Disclosures

The trials described in this chapter were sponsored by Pfizer, Inc. Dr. Dworkin has received research support, consulting fees, or honoraria in the past year Allergan, CombinatoRx, Dara, Dov, Eli Lilly, Endo, EpiCept, Fralex, Glaxo-SmithKline, GW Pharmaceuticals, Johnson & Johnson, Merck, NeurogesX (also stock options), Novartis, Pfizer, Schwarz Pharma, Supernus, US FDA, US National Institute of Health, US Veterans Administration, Wyeth, and XTL

Biopharmaceuticals. Dr. Thakur has received research support in the past year from Celgene, Cephalon, GlaxoSmithKline, and Pfizer. Drs. Griesing and Mr. Young are currently employed by Pfizer, Inc. and Dr. Sharma was employed by Pfizer, Inc. at the time the studies described in this chapter were conducted.

References

Argoff, C.E., Backonja, M.-M., Belgrade, M.J., Bennett, G.J., Clark, M.R., Cole, B.E., *et al.* (2006). Consensus guidelines: treatment planning and options. *Mayo Clinic Proceedings*, 81(Suppl.), S12–S25.

Belliotti, T., Ekhato, I.V., Capiris, T., Kinsora, J., Vartanian, M.G., Field, M., *et al.* (2005). Structure–activity relationships of pregabalin and analogs that target the α_2-δ protein. *Journal of Medicinal Chemistry*, 48, 2294–2307.

Bowsher, D. (1999). The lifetime occurrence of herpes zoster and prevalence of postherpetic neuralgia: a retrospective survey in an elderly population. *European Journal of Pain*, 3, 335–342.

Crofford, L.J., Rowbotham, M.C., Mease, P.J., Russell, I.J., Dworkin, R.H., Corbin, A.E., *et al.* (2005). Pregabalin for the treatment of fibromyalgia syndrome: results of a randomized, double-blind, placebo-controlled trial. *Arthritis and Rheumatism*, 52, 1264–1273.

Dooley, D.J., Taylor, C.P., Donevan, S., & Feltner, D. (2007). Ca^{2+} channel $\alpha_2\delta$ ligands: novel modulators of neurotransmission. *Trends in Pharmacological Sciences*, 28, 75–82.

Dubinsky, R.M., Kabbani, H., El-Chami, Z., Boutwell, C., & Ali, H. (2004). Practice parameter: treatment of postherpetic neuralgia: an evidence-based report of the Quality Standards Subcommittee of the American Academy of Neurology. *Neurology*, 63, 959–965.

Dworkin, R.H., Backonja, M., Rowbotham, M.C., Allen, R.R., Argoff, C.R., Bennett, G.J., *et al.* (2003a). Advances in neuropathic pain: diagnosis, mechanisms, and treatment recommendations. *Archives of Neurology*, 60, 1524–1534.

Dworkin, R.H., Corbin, A.E., Young, Jr., J.P., Sharma, U., LaMoreaux, L., Bockbrader, H., *et al.* (2003b). Pregabalin for the treatment of postherpetic neuralgia: a randomized, placebo-controlled trial. *Neurology*, 60, 1274–1283.

Dworkin, R.H., Fields, H.L., & Levine, J.D. (eds.) (2005a). Is fibromyalgia a neuropathic pain syndrome? *Journal of Rheumatology*, 32(Suppl. 75), 1–45.

Dworkin, R.H., Katz, J., & Gitlin, M.J. (2005b). Placebo response in clinical trials of depression and its implications for research on chronic neuropathic pain. *Neurology*, 65(Suppl. 4), S7–S19.

Dworkin, R.H., Sharma, U., Young, J., & LaMoreaux, L. (2005c). Pain relief with pregabalin in postherpetic neuralgia (PHN) is not influenced by concomitant medications. *Journal of Pain*, 6(Suppl. 1), S32.

Dworkin, R.H., Turk, D.C., Farrar, J.T., Haythornthwaite, J.A., Jensen, M.P., Katz, N.P., *et al.* (2005d). Core outcome measures for chronic pain clinical trials: IMMPACT recommendations. *Pain*, 113, 9–19.

Dworkin, R.H., O'Connor, A.B., Backonja, M., Farrar, J.T., Jensen, T.S., Kalso, E.A., *et al.* (in press). Pharmacologic management of neuropathic pain: evidence-based clinical recommendations. *Pain*.

Farrar, J.T., Young, J.P., LaMoreaux, L., Werth, J.L., & Poole, M. (2001). Clinical importance of changes in chronic pain intensity on an 11-point numerical pain rating scale. *Pain*, 94, 149–158.

Farrar, J.T., Dworkin, R.H., & Max, M.B. (2006). Use of the cumulative proportion of responders analysis graph to present pain data over a range of cut-off points: making clinical trial data more understandable. *Journal of Pain and Symptom Management*, 31, 369–377.

Field, M.J., Cox, P.J., Stott, E., Melrose, H., Offord, J., Su, T., *et al.* (2006). Identification of the α_2-δ-1 subunit of voltage dependent calcium channels as a novel molecular target for pain mediating the analgesic actions of pregabalin. *Proceedings of the National Academy of Sciences USA,* 103, 17537–17542.

Finnerup, N.B., Otto, M., Jensen, T.S., & Sindrup, S.H. (2005). Algorithm for neuropathic pain treatment: an evidence based proposal. *Pain,* 118, 289–305.

Freynhagen, R., Strojek, K., Griesing, T., Whalen, E., & Balkenohl, M. (2005). Efficacy of pregabalin in neuropathic pain evaluated in a 12-week, randomised, double-blind, multicentre, placebo-controlled trial of flexible- and fixed-dose regimens. *Pain,* 115, 254–263.

Goldstein, D.J., Lu, Y., Detke, M.J., Lee, T.C., & Iyengar, S. (2005). Duloxetine vs. placebo in patients with painful diabetic neuropathy. *Pain,* 116, 109–118.

Guy, W. (1976). *ECDEU Assessment Manual for Psychopharmacology (DHEW Publication No. ADM 76-338).* Washington, DC: U.S. Government Printing Office.

Hempenstall, K., Nurmikko, T.J., Johnson, R.W., A'Hern, R.P., & Rice, A.S.C. (2005). Analgesic therapy in postherpetic neuralgia: a quantitative systematic review. *PLOS Medicine,* 2, 628–644.

IASP Special Interest Group on Neuropathic Pain (2006). Classification and taxonomy. *Neuropathic Pain: Newsletter of the IASP Special Interest Group on Neuropathic Pain,* Issue 7.

Jensen, M.P., Chodroff, M.J., & Dworkin, R.H. (2007). The impact of neuropathic pain on health-related quality of life: review and implications. *Neurology,* 68, 1178–1182.

Kieburtz, K., Simpson, D., Yiannoutsos, C., Max, M.B., Hall, C.D., Ellis, R.J., *et al.* (1998). A randomized trial of amitriptyline and mexiletine for painful neuropathy in HIV infection. *Neurology,* 51, 1682–1688.

Lesser, H., Sharma, U., LaMoreaux, L., & Poole, R.M. (2004). Pregabalin relieves symptoms of painful diabetic neuropathy. *Neurology,* 63, 2104–2110.

Melzack, R. (1987). The short-form McGill Pain Questionnaire. *Pain,* 30, 191–197.

Merskey, H., & Bogduk, N. (eds.) (1994). *Classification of Chronic Pain: Descriptions of Chronic Pain Syndromes and Definitions of Pain Terms* (2nd ed.). Seattle, WA: IASP Press, p. 212.

Moscucci, M., Byrne, L., Weintraub, M., & Cox, C. (1987). Blinding, unblinding, and the placebo effect: an analysis of patients' guesses of treatment assignment in a double-blind clinical trial. *Clinical Pharmacology and Therapeutics,* 41, 259–265.

Oster, G., Harding, G., Dukes, E., Edelsberg, J., & Cleary, P.D. (2005). Pain, medication use and health-related quality of life in older persons with post-herpetic neuralgia: results from a population-based survey. *Journal of Pain,* 6, 356–363.

Raskin, J., Pritchett, Y.L., Wang, F., D'Souza, D.N., Waninger, A.L., Iyengar, S., *et al.* (2005). A double-blind, randomized multicenter trial comparing duloxetine with placebo in the management of diabetic peripheral neuropathic pain. *Pain Medicine,* 6, 346–356.

Rice, A.S.C., & Maton, S. (2001). Gabapentin in postherpetic neuralgia: a randomised, double blind, placebo controlled study. *Pain,* 94, 215–224.

Richter, R.W., Portenoy, R., Sharma, U., Lamoreaux, L., Bockbrader, H., & Knapp, L.E. (2005). Relief of painful diabetic peripheral neuropathy with pregabalin: a randomized, placebo-controlled trial. *Journal of Pain,* 6, 253–260.

Rosenstock, J., Tuchman, M., LaMoreaux, L., & Sharma, U. (2004). Pregabalin for the treatment of painful diabetic peripheral neuropathy: a double-blind, placebo-controlled trial. *Pain,* 110, 628–638.

Rowbotham, M., Young, J.R., Sharma, U., & Knapp, L.K. (2003). Pregabalin shows reduction in pain by day 3 of treatment. *European Journal of Neurology,* 10(Suppl. 1), 73.

Rowbotham, M.C., Harden, N., Stacey, B., Bernstein, P., & Magnus-Miller, L. (1998). Gabapentin for the treatment postherpetic neuralgia: a randomized controlled trial. *JAMA,* 280, 1837–1842.

Sabatowski, R., Galvez, R., Cherry, D.A., Jacquot, F., Vincent, E., Maisonobe, M., *et al.* (2004). Pregabalin reduces pain and improved sleep and mood disturbances in patients with postherpetic neuralgia: results of a randomised, placebo-controlled clinical trial. *Pain*, 109, 26–35.

Schmader, K.E. (2002). The epidemiology and impact on quality of life of postherpetic neuralgia and painful diabetic neuropathy. *Clinical Journal of Pain*, 18, 350–354.

Sharma, U., Young, J., LaMoreaux, L., Emir, B., Fukui, A., Murphy, T.K., & Siffert, J. (2005). Efficacy, safety, and tolerability of pregabalin treatment for neuropathic pain: findings from the analysis of 10 randomized clinical trials. *Presented at the meeting of the American Academy of Physical Medicine and Rehabilitation*, 27–30 October 2005, Philadelphia, Pennsylvania.

Shlay, J.C., Chaloner, K., Max, M.B., Flaws, B., Reichelderfer, P., Wentworth, D., *et al.* (1998). Acupuncture and amitriptyline for pain due to HIV-related peripheral neuropathy: a randomized controlled trial. *JAMA*, 280, 1590–1595.

Siddall, P.J., Cousins, M.J., Otte, A., Griesing, T., Chambers, R., & Murphy, T.K. (2006). Pregabalin in central neuropathic pain associated with spinal cord injury: a placebo-controlled trial. *Neurology*, 67, 1792–1800.

Taylor, C.P., Angelotti, T., & Fauman, E. (2007). Pharmacology and mechanism of action of pregabalin: the calcium channel α_2–δ (alpha$_2$–delta) subunit as a target for antiepileptic drug discovery. *Epilepsy Research*, 73, 137–150.

Turk, D.C., Dworkin, R.H., Allen, R.R., Bellamy, N., Brandenburg, N., Carr, D.B., *et al.* (2003). Core outcome domains for chronic pain clinical trials: IMMPACT recommendations. *Pain*, 106, 337–345.

Turk, D.C., Dworkin, R.H., Burke, L.B., Gershon, R., Rothman, M., Scott, J., *et al.* (2006). Developing outcome measures for pain clinical trials: IMMPACT recommendations. *Pain*, 125, 208–215.

Van Seventer, R., Feister, H.A., Young, Jr., J.P., Stoker, M., Versavel, M., & Rigaudy, L. (2006). Efficacy and tolerability of twice-daily pregabalin for treating pain and related sleep interference in postherpetic neuralgia: a 13-week, randomized trial. *Current Medical Research and Opinion*, 22, 375–384.

Ware, Jr., J.E., Snow, K.K., Kosinski, M., & Gandek, B. (1992). SF-36-item Short Form Health Survey (SF-36): I. conceptual framework and item selection. *Medical Care*, 30, 473–483.

Wernicke, J.F., Pritchett, Y.L., D'Souza, D.N., Waninger, A., Tran, P., Iyengar, S., *et al.* (2006). A randomized controlled trial of duloxetine in diabetic peripheral neuropathic pain. *Neurology*, 67, 1411–1420.

Woolf, C.J. (2004). Pain: moving from symptom control toward mechanism-specific pharmacologic management. *Annals of Internal Medicine*, 140, 441–451.

Progress in Neurotherapeutics and Neuropsychopharmacology, 3:1, 189–197 © 2008 Cambridge University Press
DOI: 10.1017/S1748232107000079   Printed in the United Kingdom

Effect of Methylphenidate in Patients with Acute Traumatic Brain Injury; a Randomized Clinical Trial

Hossein A. Khalili

Department of Neurosurgery, Amiralmomenin Hospital, Shiraz University of Medical Sciences, Grash, Iran;
Email: khalilih@yahoo.com

Kamyar Keramatian

Neuroscience Program, University of British Columbia, Vancouver, Canada; Email: keramatian@gmail.com

ABSTRACT

Background: Traumatic brain injury (TBI) is one of the major causes of death and disability among young people. Methylphenidate is a neural stimulant with possible brain protection properties and has been mainly used in clinic for childhood attention deficit/hyperactivity disorder. TBI patients with late psychosocial problems could benefit from methylphenidate because of the effect on arousal and consciousness level in the sub-acute phase. We studied this effect during the acute phase of moderate and severe TBI. *Design and Methods*: Forty patients with severe TBI (GCS = 5–8) and 40 moderate TBI patients (GCS = 9–12) were randomly divided into treatment and placebo groups on the day of admission. Treatment group received methylphenidate 0.3 mg/kg two times a day orally, beginning on the second day of admission and continuing until being discharged. Admission information and daily Glasgow Coma Scale (GCS) were recorded. Medical, surgical, and discharge plans for patients were decided by attending physicians, who were kept blinded during the course of treatment. *Results*: In the severe TBI patients, both hospital and ICU length of stay, on average, were shorter in the treatment group compared with the control group. In the moderate TBI patients, ICU stay was shorter in the treatment group, there was no significant reduction of the period of hospitalization. *Interpretation*: There were no significant differences between the treatment and control groups in terms of age, sex, post-resuscitation GCS, or brain scan findings, in either severely or moderately impaired TBI patients. Methylphenidate was associated with reductions in ICU and hospital length of stay by 23% in

Correspondence should be addressed to: Hossein A. Khalili, MD, Amiralmomenin Hospital, Grash-Larestan, Fars, Iran;
Ph: +98-9173174156; Email: khalilih@yahoo.com

severe TBI patients ($p = 0.06$ for ICU and $p = 0.029$ for hospital stay time), in the moderately TBI patients who received methylphenidate, there was 26% fall ($p = 0.05$) in ICU length of stay.

Key words: clinical trial, hospitalization length, ICU, methylphenidate, traumatic brain injury.

Introduction and Overview

The prevalence and intensity of traumatic brain injury (TBI) are rising amongst Iranians. Typically, there is a long waiting list of patients with TBI for ICU admission. TBI imposes a heavy financial burden on society. Over the years, a variety of therapeutic modalities have been used in an attempt to improve short- and long-term outcomes of TBI.

Methylphenidate (Ritalin) which has both dopaminergic and slight noradrenergic effects is a central nervous system stimulant with possible neuroprotective properties (Husson *et al.*, 2004; Kajs-Wyllie, 2002). Clinical efficacy of methylphenidate in improving the outcome of TBI has been shown by previous studies. However, to our knowledge, the study presented here provides the first empirical evidence for the efficacy of methylphenidate use in the very acute phase of TBI (Moein *et al.*, 2006).

Purpose of the Trial

Although some studies have shown the effectiveness of methylphenidate on patients' consciousness in the sub-acute and chronic stages of brain injury, the impact of this drug on the acute phase of injury is still unclear. In the study described here, we evaluated the effect of methylphenidate on the most acute stage of TBI.

Agent: Methylphenidate

Methylphenidate (Ritalin) is a central nervous system stimulant with dopaminergic and slight noradrenergic activities (Husson *et al.*, 2004; Kajs-Wyllie, 2002). This drug has been approved by the United States Food and Drug Administration for treatment of children's attention deficit/hyperactivity disorder, narcolepsy, and refractory depression (Kajs-Wyllie, 2002; Challman & Lipsky, 2000). Moreover, neuroprotective effects have been attributed to methylphenidate (Husson *et al.*, 2004).

Several studies have shown that methylphenidate can improve cognitive function and behavior in adults (Jin & Schachar, 2004; Rosati, 2002; Challman & Lipsky, 2000; Whyte *et al.*, 1997; 2004; Speech *et al.*, 1993) and children (Mahalick *et al.*, 1998; Hornyak *et al.*, 1997) with TBI. Methylphenidate also has been reported to enhance arousal and function in the sub-acute phase of TBI (Hornyak *et al.*, 1997; Worzniak *et al.*, 1997; Plenger *et al.*, 1996). In animal studies too, advantageous effects of methylphenidate on neural function have been shown (Husson *et al.*, 2004; Forsyth & Jayamoni, 2003; Kajs-Wyllie, 2002).

The clinical safety of methylphenidate has been evaluated in several studies and has been safely administered to monitored patients with TBI (Alban *et al.*, 2004; Burke *et al.*, 2003). The risk of seizures in TBI patients receiving methylphenidate is not increased (Wroblewski *et al.*, 1992).

Clinical Trial

This prospective randomized double-blind clinical trial was conducted between June 2003 and February 2004 in two university trauma centers in Isfahan.

Subjects

Forty consecutive patients with severe TBI (post-resuscitation Glasgow Coma Scale (GCS) = 5–8, evaluated before intubation if possible) and 40 moderate TBI patients (GCS = 9–12), were randomly divided into treatment and control groups on the day of admission. Randomization was performed by using patients' hospital file numbers; that is, patients with odd numbers were assigned to one group and patients with even numbers were assigned to the other one. Informed consent was obtained from a first degree relative of each patient.

Children (age < 15 years), patients with very severe TBI (GCS = 3–4) or those with severe multiple trauma (i.e. concomitant chest and abdominal injuries), were excluded from the study. Patients who did not tolerate enteral feeding in the first 48 h of admission despite maximum medical treatment were also excluded. The excluded patients were replaced by new ones randomly.

Trial Methods

The treatment group received methylphenidate 0.3 mg/kg per dose (maximum 20 mg per dose) twice daily on the second day of admission when enteral (oral or tube) feeding started. Patients in the control group received placebo (starch pills, which were made in a similar fashion) in the same time course (twice daily).

Instruments/Measures

All patients underwent emergency computed tomography (CT) of the brain on admission and were transferred to the neurosurgical ICU, directly or after emergency craniotomy as dictated by the CT findings. All medical and surgical decisions including the timing of ICU and hospital discharge were adjudicated by the patients' attending physicians, who were blinded to the intervention. Main ICU discharge criteria used by the physicians were vital sign stability, GCS (especially the motor score which had to be six), and enteral feeding tolerance. Study intervention (methylphenidate or placebo treatment) continued until the time of discharge.

Primary and Secondary Outcomes

GCS on discharge time, length of ICU, and lengths of hospital stay were measured.

Analysis

Data regarding age, GCS on admission (post-resuscitation), GCS on discharge, and initial brain CT scan findings were analyzed between groups by using t-tests. Sex differences were analyzed by the chi-square test. Duration of ICU care and hospital admission were compared between the two groups by using paired t-tests (one way). Severe and moderate TBI patients were also analyzed separately.

Table 1. **Admission and Discharge Information in Patients with Severe and Moderate TBI in Treatment and Control Groups**

		AGE (SD) YEARS	SEX M/F	POST-RESUSCITATION GCS (SD)	GCS ON DISCHARGE (SD)
Severe head injury	Treatment	35 (17.9)	16/4	14.4 (1.1)	6.8 (1.01)
	Control	33.7 (13.1)	17/3	14.3 (0.8)	6.09 (1.02)
	p-value	0.4	0.3	0.37	0.38
Moderate head injury	Treatment	32.3 (15.9)	17/4	14.86 (0.36)	10.38 (1.12)
	Control	29.6 (15.4)	16/3	14.95 (0.23)	10.16 (1.12)
	p-value	0.3	0.4	0.18	0.27
Total	Treatment	33.6 (16.7)	33/8	14.63 (0.83)	8.63 (2.09)
	Control	31.7 (14.3)	33/6	14.62 (0.67)	8.49 (1.96)
	p-value	0.29	0.33	0.46	0.36

SD: standard deviation; M/F: male/female; GCS: Glasgow Coma Scale.

Table 2. **Initial CT Scan Findings and Craniotomy Operation in Patients with Severe and Moderate Head Injury, Treatment versus Control Groups**

		INITIAL CT SCAN (%)			CRANIOTOMY (%)
		DAI	CONT.	SOL	
Severe head injury	Treatment	9 (45%)	8 (40%)	3 (15%)	4 (20%)
	Control	8 (40%)	8 (40%)	4 (20%)	3 (15%)
	p-value	0.34			0.34
Moderate head injury	Treatment	11 (52%)	6 (29%)	4 (19%)	2 (9.5%)
	Control	11 (58%)	5 (26%)	3 (16%)	3 (15.7%)
	p-value	0.36			0.28
Total	Treatment	20 (49%)	14 (34%)	7 (17%)	6 (14.6%)
	Control	19 (49%)	13 (33%)	7 (18%)	6 (15.4%)
	p-value	0.32			0.46

DAI: diffuse axonal injury; Cont.: brain contusion; SOL: space occupying lesion.

Results

Admission data including mean age, sex distribution, and post-resuscitation GCS scores for each group (severe and moderate; treatment and control) are presented in Table 1. The number of craniotomies and initial CT scan findings are listed in Table 2. Demographic (i.e. age and sex) and trauma data (i.e. GCS on admission, the number of craniotomies, and the main CT scan findings) were comparable in treatment and control groups in both severe and moderate TBI groups, based on p-values in Tables 1 and 2.

Efficacy

Tables 1 and 2 list the admission information in both treatment and control groups showing no significant differences in major prognostic factors (age, sex, post-resuscitation GCS, and brain CT scan findings) between the two groups.

In patients with severe TBI, the mean ICU care required for the treatment group was 9.85 days versus 12.95 days for the control group, an ICU care duration decrease by 3 days (23%; $p = 0.06$; Figure 1). The mean hospital stay in the

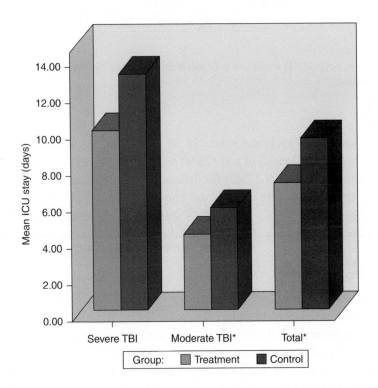

Fig. 1.
Mean ICU stay in patients with severe and moderate TBI receiving methylphenidate or placebo (*$p < 0.05$).

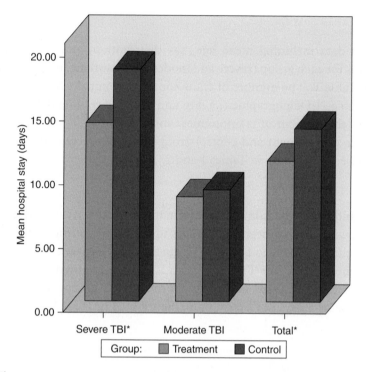

Fig. 2.
Mean hospital stay in patients with severe and moderate TBI receiving methylphenidate or placebo (*$p < 0.05$).

treatment group was 14.1 days versus 18.35 days in the control group, a 4.25 day reduction in hospital length of stay (23%; $p = 0.029$; Figure 2).

The average length of ICU stay for patients with moderate TBI were 4.09 days in the treatment, and 5.58 days in the control group's ICU stay was 1.5 days shorter, on average (26%; $p = 0.05$; Figure 1). Corresponding data for the length of hospital stay were 8.29 and 8.84 days (Figure 2), respectively.

Tolerability and Safety

There were four fatalities, all in patients with severe TBI (10%), two in the treatment and two in the control group. There were also five cases of post-traumatic seizure in the severely TBI patients: two in the treatment and three in the control group. No effect on sleep–wake cycle was observed (Al-Adawi *et al.*, 2006). This difference in ICU and hospital stay may be due to the main effect of methylphenidate on lower GCS states in which patients were admitted to ICU (Williams *et al.*, 1998).

Unique Aspects of Trial

Presuming that the timing of methylphenidate administration may play an important role (i.e. the earlier, the more effective) (Jin & Schachar, 2004), we examined its short-time effect on ICU and hospital length of stay in patients with severe and moderate TBI. To our knowledge, this study was the first to investigate the effect of methylphenidate in the very acute phase of TBI.

Translation to Clinical Practice

Methylphenidate has been known for several years as a neurostimulant drug, and there is recent evidence of neuroprotective effects (Husson *et al.*, 2004; Kajs-Wyllie, 2002; Challman & Lipsky, 2000). Several investigators have studied the effects of methylphenidate after TBI, mostly for its effects on attention, memory, and psychosocial performance, albeit with somewhat mixed results (Kim *et al.*, 2006; Siddall, 2005; Jin & Schachar, 2004; Rosati, 2002; Challman & Lipsky, 2000; Whyte *et al.*, 1997). All of these studies have investigated the effect during rehabilitation of the patients.

Our study investigates the effect of methylphenidate in acute stage of trauma and showed a 23% reduction in ICU and hospital length of stay in severe TBI and 26% in ICU stay in moderate TBI. This 23–26% reduction in ICU care need and hospital stay time may have clinical significance, especially in countries with limited ICU beds. One possibility is that this decrease may be due to the rapid response of GCS in the TBI patients receiving methylphenidate even though the underlying cause of these findings is still unknown and requires further study. The mean GCS of patients in the discharge time was not significantly different in the treatment and control groups, so patients were discharged with the same level of consciousness as measured by GCS. This effect of methylphenidate on arousal (but not on hospital length of stay) has been previously reported (Hornyak *et al.*, 1997; Worzniak *et al.*, 1997; Plenger *et al.*, 1996).

As mentioned earlier, methylphenidate shows neurostimulatory and some neuroprotective effects. Its reduction on the length of ICU treatment and hospitalization might be interpreted in several ways: first, by rapidly increasing arousal and GCS, which in turn results in faster discharge; second, by its neuroprotective effect which can lead to a more favorable neurocognitive outcomes. Which processes are most significant in bringing about the reduction in ICU and hospital stays, however, remain unknown. There were several major limitations in our study (including uncertain mechanism of drug action, limited sample and center size, and marginal statistical significance), and results should be constructive.

Summary

Methylphenidate was associated with reductions in ICU and hospital length of stay by 23% in severe TBI patients ($p = 0.06$ for ICU and $p = 0.029$ for hospital stay time). In moderate TBI patients who received methylphenidate, there was 26% fall ($p = 0.05$) in ICU length of stay only. Although not reaching statistical significance (perhaps because of the small sample size), these reductions are clinically significant (Figures 1 and 2). Further studies with a greater number of patients and a long-term follow up in order to evaluate the effects of methylphenidate in the acute phase of TBI are warranted.

Acknowledgment

This study has been supported by a grant from Isfahan University of Medical Sciences, Department of Research.

References

Al-Adawi, S., Burke, D.T., & Dorvlo, A.S. (2006). The effect of methylphenidate on the sleep–wake cycle of brain-injured patients undergoing rehabilitation. *Sleep Medicine,* 7(3), 287–291. Epub 2006 March 27.

Alban, J.P., Hopson, M.M., Ly, V., & Whyte, J. (2004). Effect of methylphenidate on vital signs and adverse effects in adults with traumatic brain injury. *American Journal of Physical Medicine and Rehabilitation,* 83(2), 131–137; quiz 138–141, 167.

Burke, D.T., Glenn, M.B., Vesali, F., Schneider, J.C., Burke, J., Ahangar, B., & Goldstein, R. (2003). Effects of methylphenidate on heart rate and blood pressure among inpatients with acquired brain injury. *American Journal of Physical Medicine and Rehabilitation,* 82(7), 493–497.

Challman, T.D., & Lipsky, J.J. (2000). Methylphenidate: its pharmacology and uses. *Mayo Clinic Proceedings,* 75(7), 711–721.

Forsyth, R., & Jayamoni, B. (2003). Noradrenergic agonists for acute traumatic brain injury. *Cochrane Database of Systematic Reviews,* Issue 1:CD003984 (review).

Hornyak, J.E., Nelson, V.S., & Hurvitz, E.A. (1997). The use of methylphenidate in paediatric traumatic brain injury. *Pediatric Rehabilitation,* 1(1), 15–17.

Husson, I., Mesples, B., Medja, F., Leroux, P., Kosofsky, B., & Gressens, P. (2004). Methylphenidate and MK-801, an *N*-methyl-D-aspartate receptor antagonist: shared biological properties. *Neuroscience,* 125(1), 163–170.

Jin, C., & Schachar, R. (2004). Methylphenidate treatment of attention-deficit/hyperactivity disorder secondary to traumatic brain injury: a critical appraisal of treatment studies. *CNS Spectrums,* 9(3), 217–226 (review).

Kajs-Wyllie, M. (2002). Ritalin revisited: does it really help in neurological injury? *Journal of Neuroscience Nursing,* 34(6), 303–313 (review).

Kim, Y.H., Ko, M.H., Na, S.Y., Park, S.H., & Kim, K.W. (2006). Effects of single-dose methylphenidate on cognitive performance in patients with traumatic brain injury: a double-blind placebo-controlled study. *Clinical Rehabilitation,* 20(1), 24–30.

Kline, A.E., Yan, H.Q., Bao, J., Marion, D.W., & Dixon, C.E. (2000). Chronic methylphenidate treatment enhances water maze performance following traumatic brain injury in rats. *Neuroscience Letters,* 280(3), 163–166.

Mahalick, D.M., Carmel, P.W., Greenberg, J.P., Molofsky, W., Brown, J.A., Heary, R.F., Marks, D., Zampella, E., Hodosh, R., & von der Schmidt III, E. (1998). Psychopharmacologic treatment of acquired attention disorders in children with brain injury. *Pediatric Neurosurgery*, 29(3), 121–126.

Moein, H., Khalili, H.A., Keramatian, K. (2006). Effect of methylphenidate on ICU and hospital length of stay in patients with severe and moderate traumatic brain injury. *Clinical Neurology and Neurosurgery*, 108(6), 539–542.

Plenger, P.M., Dixon, C.E., Castillo, R.M., Frankowski, R.F., Yablon, S.A., & Levin, H.S. (1996). Subacute methylphenidate treatment for moderate to moderately severe traumatic brain injury: a preliminary double-blind placebo-controlled study. *Archives of Physical Medicine and Rehabilitation*, 77(6), 536–540.

Rosati, D.L. (2002). Early polyneuropharmacologic intervention in brain injury agitation. *American Journal of Physical Medicine and Rehabilitation*, 81(2), 90–93.

Siddall, O.M. (2005). Use of methylphenidate in traumatic brain injury. *Annals of Pharmacotherapy*, 39(7–8), 1309–1313. Epub 2005 May 24 (review).

Speech, T.J., Rao, S.M., Osmon, D.C., & Sperry, L.T. (1993). A double-blind controlled study of methylphenidate treatment in closed head injury. *Brain Injury*, 7(4), 333–338.

Whyte, J., Hart, T., Schuster, K., Fleming, M., Polansky, M., & Coslett, H.B. (1997). Effects of methylphenidate on attentional function after traumatic brain injury. A randomized, placebo-controlled trial. *American Journal of Physical Medicine and Rehabilitation*, 76(6), 440–450.

Whyte, J., Hart, T., Vaccaro, M., Grieb-Neff, P., Risser, A., Polansky, M., & Coslett, H.B. (2004). Effects of methylphenidate on attention deficits after traumatic brain injury: a multidimensional, randomized, controlled trial. *American Journal of Physical Medicine and Rehabilitation*, 83(6), 401–420.

Williams, S.E., Ris, M.D., Ayyangar, R., Schefft, B.K., & Berch, D. (1998). Recovery in pediatric brain injury: is psychostimulant medication beneficial? *Journal of Head Trauma Rehabilitation*, 13(3), 73–81.

Worzniak, M., Fetters, M.D., & Comfort, M. (1997). Methylphenidate in the treatment of coma. *Jouranl of Family Practice*, 44(5), 495–498.

Wroblewski, B.A., Leary, J.M., Phelan, A.M., Whyte, J., & Manning, K. (1992). Methylphenidate and seizure frequency in brain injured patients with seizure disorders. *Journal of Clinical Psychiatry*, 53(3), 86–89.

Progress in Neurotherapeutics and Neuropsychopharmacology, 3:1, 199–209 © 2008 Cambridge University Press
DOI: 10.1017/S1748232107000109   Printed in the United Kingdom

Improvement in Speeded Cognitive Processing After Anti-epileptic Drug Withdrawal – A Controlled Study in Mono-therapy Patients

Erik Hessen

Helse Øst Health Services and Department of Neurology, Akershus University Hospital, Norway;
Email: erik.hessen@nevropsykologi.no

Morten I. Lossius

Helse Øst Health Services and Department of Neurology, Akershus University Hospital, Norway
National Center for Epilepsy, Rikshospitalet, University of Oslo, Norway; Email: morten.lossius@epilepsy.no

Ivar Reinvang

Department of Psychology, University of Oslo, Norway; Email: ivar.reinvang@psykologi.uio.no

Leif Gjerstad

Department of Neurology, Rikshospitalet, University of Oslo, Norway; Email: leif.gjerstad@medisin.uio.no

ABSTRACT

Background: Anti-epileptic drugs (AEDs) are associated with cognitive side effects. Doubt exists regarding the degree of cognitive effects primarily related to problems with design and methodology in many studies. The aim of the reported study was to assess the effect of AED withdrawal in patients on monotherapy using computerised measures of attention, reaction time and speed of information processing. *Methods*: One hundred and fifty patients seizure free >2 years on drug monotherapy went through a randomised, double blind, placebo controlled study. All patients were included for 12 months or until seizure relapse. Cognitive function was assessed with the California Computerized Assessment Package at baseline and 7 months after withdrawal. *Results*: The major finding was that discontinuation of major AEDs significantly improved performance on tests that require complex cognitive processing under time pressure. The difference in speed of cognitive processing between the withdrawal and non-withdrawal groups was between 24 and 43 ms.

Correspondence should be addressed to: Erik Hessen, Helse Øst Health Services and Department of Neurology, Akershus University Hospital, Norway; Email: erik.hessen@nevropsykologi.no

No significant difference emerged between the groups on simple tasks of attention and reaction time. Most of the patients in the study were treated with carbamazepine and valproate. The outcome of carbamazepine withdrawal was similar to the outcome for the total study population while discontinuation of valproate only revealed a non-significant tendency in the same direction. *Interpretation*: The results suggest that seizure-free epilepsy patients on monotherapy can obtain improvement in speeded cognitive processing if they withdraw anti-epileptic treatment.

Key words: AED, anti-epileptic drugs, CalCAP, carbamazepine, cognitive side effects, valproate.

Introduction

All major anti-epileptic drugs (AEDs) have been associated with adverse cognitive side effects (Aldenkamp, 2001). AEDs are usually given as persistent treatment and concern about their impact on cognitive function is an important aspect in the management of people with epilepsy (Vermeulen & Aldenkamp, 1995). The most important cognitive effects of AEDs include attention/vigilance, psychomotor speed and memory. About 100 studies have been published on this issue in the last 30 years. However, much uncertainty remains regarding the degree of cognitive effects of AEDs and regarding differences between the major AEDs. This uncertainty is primarily due to the fact that many studies do not adhere to basic standards of design, methodology and cognitive assessment (Brunbech & Sabers, 2002; Baker & Marson, 2001; Meador, 1998). The most important problems include different selection criteria of patients, inconsistent selection and administration of cognitive tests, lack of control groups or randomisation of treatment and lack of statistical power due to inclusion of few patients in many of the studies.

In selecting tests to evaluate the cognitive effects of AEDs it is vital to include tests representing functions believed to be sensitive to AEDs. In addition the tests must meet acceptable criteria of reliability, validity and sensitivity to change. In the present study we chose to focus on reported side effects of AEDs on attention/vigilance and psychomotor speed (Meador, 2001). Baker & Marson (2001) have recommended the use of computerised tests of attention and psychomotor speed in clinical trials of AEDs. On this basis we chose the California Computerized Assessment Package (CalCAP) (Miller, 1980), which has not previously been used in assessment of possible cognitive effects of AEDs. However, it incorporates a wide range of attention related speeded cognitive measures with different levels of complexity that are sensitive to important treatment effects in both epileptic and other patient categories. This has been revealed in studies of cognitive AED effects (Meador *et al.*, 1991; Gillham *et al.*, 1988) and in studies of HIV-seropositive patients receiving anti-retroviral therapy (Martin, 1999).

Purpose of the Trial

The aim of the reported study was to assess in a randomised, double blind, placebo controlled study of seizure-free epilepsy patients on monotherapy, the possible impact of withdrawal of major AEDs on attention, reaction time and speed of information processing.

Agents

Most of the patients in the study were treated with carbamazepine and valproate. Some were also treated with phenytoin, phenobarbital and lamotrigine (Table 3).

Clinical Trial

Subjects

The patients were selected from the epilepsy registry at the Akershus University Hospital and from six neurological outpatient clinics in the Oslo area; 241 appeared to fulfil the inclusion criteria (Table 1) and were invited. Of these 13 still had seizures, 20 were dismissed due to other exclusion criteria and 17 patients did not show up. Of the remaining 191 patients 23 did not want to participate in the study. Thus, only 168 patients were included. Before randomisation another 18 patients left the study. Of these, 12 changed their minds, 2 experienced seizures, 3 had generalised epileptiform activity on their EEG and 1 had an acute disease (subarachnoidal haemorrhage). These were withdrawn and 150 patients went through randomisation. Eleven of these patients had seizure relapse during the study period and went out of the study. Therefore, baseline- and retest results are only reported for the remaining 139 patients that completed the study.

Table 1. **Inclusion and Exclusion Criteria**

Inclusion criteria
Epilepsy (two unprovoked seizures or more)
2 years seizure freedom
Monotherapy
18–67 years
5 years seizure freedom if prior unsuccessful withdrawal

Exclusion criteria
Juvenile myoclonus epilepsy (JME)
Polypharmacy
Paroxysmal epileptiform activity in patients with primarily generalised epilepsy
Two prior withdrawal attempts
Pregnant or seeking pregnancy
Mental retardation
Progressive neurological disease
Other serious disease which may influence the health status of the patient in the study period
Co-medication (except post menopausal hormone substitution), ASA and thyroxin

Trial Methods

The study was prospective randomised controlled and double blinded. The patients were included in the study for 12 months or until seizure relapse. Criteria for breaking the code were seizure relapse or acute disease. The cognitive assessments were done prior to and after intervention (withdrawal/not withdrawal). Both assessments were conducted by an experienced specialist in clinical neuropsychology (Erik Hessen). The investigator was blinded during the whole study period.

Randomisation was done by a statistician. The withdrawal period lasted 12 weeks. Patients were then examined about possible seizure relapse and supplied with medication or placebo. Seven months after withdrawal start, the patients were reassessed with the same cognitive test; 12 months after the start of withdrawal the code was broken.

Instruments/Measures

Cognitive Testing

Cognitive function was tested with the CalCAP (Miller, 1980). The stimulus material includes both verbal and non-verbal stimuli. The tasks vary in complexity, and responses are precisely measured and include mean reaction times and total numbers of true positive responses (hits) and false positive responses (false alarms). The CalCAP test battery consists of four subtests of simple reaction time and six subtests measuring more complex aspects of attention, choice reaction time, psychomotor speed and rapid information processing.

The CalCAP has been shown to discriminate cognitively impaired cases from matched controls as well as or better than conventional cognitive tests (Worth *et al.*, 1993; Miller, 1992; Miller *et al.*, 1991; 1989). These data suggest sensitivity of the measures provided by CalCAP for detecting changes in different cognitive processes like attention, motor and psychomotor functioning, and support the use of reaction time procedures for evaluation and monitoring of conditions characterised by impairment of attention and cognitive slowing, including possible effects of AEDs. Order of administration of the 10 subtests and the different cognitive domains measured by the CalCAP is shown in Table 2.

Statistical Analysis

Two sets of statistical analyses were performed with the Statistical Package for Social Sciences for Windows (SPSS, version 11.0). First, descriptive statistics of the demographic, clinical and cognitive characteristics of the patient population were computed. Then a series of independent t-tests were performed comparing mean differences between the cognitive variables measured before and after withdrawal of AEDs. In order to adjust for multiple comparisons a strict significance criterion of $p < 0.01$ was chosen.

Table 2. **Order of Administration of Subtests and Cognitive Domains Measured by the CalCAP**

ORDER	SIMPLE REACTION TIME	COMPLEX TESTS OF ATTENTION/INFORMATION PROCESSING
1	Simple RT 1-DH	
2	Simple RT 2-Nond. H	
3		Choice RT for single digits
4		Sequential RT for similar digits in sequence
5		Language discrimination – rapid language processing
6	Simple RT 2-DH	
7		Degraded words distract – visual selective attention
8		Response reversal – rapid visual scanning
9		Form discrimination – comparison of non-nameable forms
10	Simple RT 3-DH	

Outcomes

Baseline characteristics of the two groups (withdrawal versus non-withdrawal) are shown in Table 3. The baseline test scores from the CalCAP are given as mean reaction time in milliseconds and as number of hits and false alarms on the different tasks.

Changes in scores on the CalCAP from baseline to 7 months after intervention are shown in Table 4 for the entire study group. Significant differences associated with drug withdrawal were evident on choice reaction time with digits (Choice RT-Digits) ($p < 0.001$), rapid language discrimination (Language discrimination) ($p = 0.003$) and form discrimination task (Form discrimination) ($p = 0.013$). On all the four tests of simple reaction time there were no significant changes in any of the groups. With regard to true and false positive responses there were no significant differences between the withdrawal and the non-withdrawal group. The results for the carbamazepine subgroup (Table 5) were similar: significant differences associated with drug withdrawal were found for choice reaction time with digits ($p < 0.001$), language discrimination ($p = 0.003$) and degraded words with distraction ($p = 0.012$). No significant differences in true or false positive responses appeared between the two groups. The results for the valproate subgroup (Table 6) revealed no significant changes related to drug withdrawal. A significant decrease in false positive responses ($p = 0.013$) appeared in the withdrawal group on the language discrimination task. Otherwise no significant differences were found regarding true or false positive responses.

Analysis

The major findings of the present study were that in epilepsy patients seizure free for more than 2 years on monotherapy, withdrawal of AEDs was associated with improved performance on tests that require complex cognitive processing under time pressure like divided attention, rapid language discrimination and rapid

Table 3. **Baseline Characteristics of Patients**

	NO WITHDRAWAL ($N = 79$)	WITHDRAWAL ($N = 71$)
Mean age (range)	37.4 (18–66)	39.2 (19–65)
Female (%)	40 (50.6)	40 (56.3)
Epilepsy onset 0–18 years (%)	32 (41)	26 (37)
Epilepsy onset 18–60 years (%)	47 (60)	45 (63)
Seizure free 2–5 years (%)	23 (29)	27 (39)
Seizure free >5 years (%)	56 (71)	44 (62)
Known aetiology (%)	23 (29)	20 (28)
MRI pathology (%)	21 (28)	16 (23)
Normal neurological status (%)	73 (92)	67 (94)
Carbamazepine (%)	52 (66)	41 (58)
Valproate (%)	18 (23)	15 (21)
Phenytoin (%)	6 (8)	7 (10)
Phenobarbital (%)	2 (3)	3 (4)
Lamotrigine (%)	1 (1)	5 (7)
Serum concentration within therapeutic range (%)	64 (82)	54 (76)
Epileptiform activity on EEG (%)	35 (44)	25 (35)
CalCAP – mean reaction time (milliseconds)		
Simple RT 1-DH ms (SD)	374.53 (117.70)	369.98 (96.67)
Simple RT-Nond. H ms (SD)	317.57 (58.4)	322.63 (65.17)
Choice RT-Digits ms (SD)	425.83 (49.77)	440.50 (64.75)
Sequential RT ms (SD)	553.13 (110.32)	542.78 (134.54)
Language discrimination ms (SD)	587.18 (81.47)	590.42 (84.74)
Simple RT 2-DH ms (SD)	349.18 (70.15)	347.14 (63.67)
Degraded words distract ms (SD)	537.46 (101.44)	561.38 (107.36)
Response reversal-words ms (SD)	672.28 (112.85)	692.98 (118.65)
Form discrimination ms (SD)	776.31 (158.59)	809.98 (167.48)
Simple RT 3-DH ms (SD)	340.40 (67.09)	334.45 (54.99)
CalCAP – true positive responses (N)		
Choice RT-Digits tp (SD)	14.69 (0.73)	14.41 (1.46)
Sequential RT tp (SD)	17.14 (4.01)	17.09 (4.06)
Language discrimination tp (SD)	21.44 (3.91)	21.52 (3.62)
Degraded words distract tp (SD)	13.64 (2.71)	13.42 (2.65)
Response reversal-words tp (SD)	12.01 (3.01)	11.44 (3.12)
Form discrimination tp (SD)	13.54 (4.71)	12.69 (4.95)
CalCAP – false positive responses (N)		
Choice RT-Digits fp (SD)	0.78 (0.92)	0.91 (1.17)
Sequential RT fp (SD)	1.44 (1.74)	1.17 (1.53)
Language discrimination fp (SD)	2.14 (1.93)	2.48 (4.02)
Degraded words distract fp (SD)	2.28 (2.91)	1.98 (2.34)
Response reversal-words fp (SD)	1.46 (2.43)	1.58 (2.17)
Form discrimination fp (SD)	5.11 (7.80)	3.77 (2.83)

form discrimination. Comparable results were achieved in the subgroup taking carbamazepine.

The main strength of the study is that it fulfils the design criteria of a randomised, double blind, placebo controlled withdrawal study of seizure-free epilepsy patients on monotherapy, tested after several months of steady state

Table 4. **Changes in CalCAP Scores from Baseline to 7 Months After Intervention**

	NO WITHDRAWAL (N = 75)	WITHDRAWAL (N = 64)	p VALUES
CalCAP – mean reaction time (milliseconds)			
Simple RT 1-DH ms (SD)	−13.38 (83.07)	−2.75 (100.27)	ns
Simple RT-Nond. H ms (SD)	5.35 (66.45)	0.38 (56.48)	ns
Choice RT-Digits ms (SD)	4.07 (33.29)	−24.02 (56.07)	<0.001
Sequential RT ms (SD)	−17.69 (93.88)	−9.28 (113.43)	ns
Language discrimination ms (SD)	6.99 (45.79)	−17.44 (46.58)	0.003
Simple RT 2-DH ms (SD)	2.19 (55.41)	1.94 (55.03)	ns
Degraded words distract ms (SD)	9.92 (65.78)	−14.11 (85.32)	0.067
Response reversal-words ms (SD)	−1.96 (66.22)	−26.19 (74.68)	0.047
Form discrimination ms (SD)	8.07 (93.37)	−34.98 (106.61)	0.013
Simple RT 3-DH ms (SD)	0.15 (54.67)	12.89 (40.33)	ns
CalCAP – true positive responses (N)			
Choice RT-Digits tp (SD)	0.11 (0.83)	0.36 (1.10)	ns
Sequential RT tp (SD)	0.67 (3.99)	0.70 (4.20)	ns
Language discrimination tp (SD)	0.04 (2.95)	0.94 (2.29)	0.050
Degraded words distract tp (SD)	0.31 (2.11)	0.63 (2.37)	ns
Response reversal-words tp (SD)	0.19 (2.35)	0.86 (2.11)	0.086
Form discrimination tp (SD)	−0.18 (2.93)	1.09 (3.37)	0.020
CalCAP – false positive responses (N)			
Choice RT-Digits fp (SD)	−0.33 (0.99)	−0.45 (1.17)	ns
Sequential RT fp (SD)	−0.57 (1.69)	−0.20 (1.58)	ns
Language discrimination fp (SD)	0.19 (2.71)	−0.02 (2.75)	ns
Degraded words distract fp (SD)	−0.71 (2.38)	−0.36 (2.55)	ns
Response reversal-words fp (SD)	−0.38 (2.17)	−0.25 (2.43)	ns
Form discrimination fp (SD)	−0.99 (5.97)	0.53 (3.08)	ns

Note: Lower scores on the mean reaction time-measures indicates improvement in milliseconds from baseline to retest. Increased true positive responses indicates improvement from baseline to retest. Decreased false positive responses indicates improvement from baseline to retest.

treatment. Secondly the study includes a large sample of subjects and therefore has good statistical power.

The present data are relevant for patients that fulfilled the described inclusion criteria: No seizures on AED-monotherapy for at least 2 years, no epileptiform activity on EEG in patients with generalised epilepsy and no patients with juvenile myoclonic epilepsy (JME). There is reason to believe that the selected group of patients is representative for the majority of seizure-free epilepsy patients (Kwan & Brodie, 2000; Lossius *et al.*, 1999). The findings however, cannot be extrapolated to all epilepsy patients, including patients with refractory epilepsy.

Unique Aspects of Trial

To our knowledge this is the first randomised, double blind, placebo controlled study to investigate the effect on attention, reaction time and speed of information processing after withdrawal of AEDs in seizure-free epilepsy patients. Also

Table 5. **Changes in CalCAP Scores for Subjects on Carbamazepine from Baseline to 7 Months After Intervention**

	NO WITHDRAWAL (N = 48)	WITHDRAWAL (N = 41)	p VALUES
CalCAP – mean reaction time (milliseconds)			
Simple RT 1-DH ms (SD)	−11.48 (97.58)	2.63 (114.34)	ns
Simple RT-Nond. H ms (SD)	21.02 (47.74)	2.93 (59.90)	ns
Choice RT-Digits ms (SD)	6.19 (36.95)	−26.29 (34.77)	<0.001
Sequential RT ms (SD)	−14.54 (91.32)	−37.95 (81.73)	ns
Language discrimination ms (SD)	11.15 (50.74)	−21.10 (48.25)	0.003
Simple RT 2-DH ms (SD)	2.42 (57.07)	−8.37 (54.88)	ns
Degraded words distract ms (SD)	10.63 (58.46)	−30.85 (91.99)	0.012
Response reversal-words ms (SD)	−8.79 (73.03)	−26.37 (80.30)	ns
Form discrimination ms (SD)	7.63 (104.53)	−33.63 (110.09)	0.074
Simple RT 3-DH ms (SD)	2.25 (62.48)	11.61 (36.89)	ns
CalCAP – true positive responses (N)			
Choice RT-Digits tp (SD)	0.08 (0.94)	0.32 (0.99)	ns
Sequential RT tp (SD)	0.58 (3.78)	1.51 (3.69)	ns
Language discrimination tp (SD)	−0.04 (3.34)	0.63 (2.02)	ns
Degraded words distract tp (SD)	−0.13 (1.04)	0.78 (2.69)	0.035
Response reversal-words tp (SD)	0.33 (2.65)	0.90 (2.11)	ns
Form discrimination tp (SD)	0.02 (3.29)	1.10 (3.51)	ns
CalCAP – false positive responses (N)			
Choice RT-Digits fp (SD)	−0.44 (1.70)	−0.49 (1.05)	ns
Sequential RT fp (SD)	−0.58 (1.74)	−0.32 (1.25)	ns
Language discrimination fp (SD)	0.27 (2.86)	0.17 (1.82)	ns
Degraded words distract fp (SD)	−0.88 (2.46)	−0.24 (2.58)	ns
Response reversal-words fp (SD)	−0.52 (2.54)	−0.05 (2.84)	ns
Form discrimination fp (SD)	−1.31 (7.06)	0.51 (3.03)	ns

Note: Lower scores on the mean reaction time-measures indicates improvement in milliseconds from baseline to retest. Increased true positive responses indicates improvement from baseline to retest. Decreased false positive responses indicates improvement from baseline to retest.

the use of the CalCAP test battery have previously not been employed in a similar study. As both research design and test-methods have been somewhat different from other reported studies, it is difficult to make direct comparison of the present results with results from other studies on cognitive influence of major AEDs.

It is interesting however, that in studies of healthy adult volunteers with similar research design and test-methods as in the reported study by Meador *et al.* (1993; 1991) of direct comparison of exposure to phenytoin and carbamazepine found that both drugs caused impairment on a choice reaction time task and that carbamazepine in addition impaired performance on tasks of conflict interference and memory (Story recall). In a later study of healthy volunteers Meador *et al.* (2001) found that carbamazepine impaired performance more than lamotrigine on tests of attention, cognitive speed, memory and graphomotor coding. Valproate has been shown to cause mild to moderate impairment of mental and psychomotor speed (Prevey *et al.*, 1996; Aldenkamp *et al.*, 1993; Craig & Tallis, 1994; Thompson & Trimble, 1981). Galassi *et al.* (1992) compared carbamazepine with

Table 6. **Changes in CalCAP Scores for Subjects on Valproate from Baseline to 7 Months After Intervention**

	NO WITHDRAWAL (N = 16)	WITHDRAWAL (N = 11)	p VALUES
CalCAP – mean reaction time (milliseconds)			
Simple RT 1-DH ms (SD)	−16.06 (46.41)	−33.00 (65.41)	ns
Simple RT-Nond. H ms (SD)	−30.00 (97.29)	−8.91 (56.98)	ns
Choice RT-Digits ms (SD)	−1.44 (20.42)	−23.36 (112.10)	ns
Sequential RT ms (SD)	−38.00 (75.43)	65.64 (191.13)	0.060
Language discrimination ms (SD)	−2.31 (34.85)	−20.00 (48.07)	ns
Simple RT 2-DH ms (SD)	−7.31 (47.09)	5.45 (53.52)	ns
Degraded words distract ms (SD)	−13.63 (51.96)	7.27 (46.64)	ns
Response reversal-words ms (SD)	11.44 (39.16)	−28.64 (59.05)	0.044
Form discrimination ms (SD)	10.75 (68.45)	−80.36 (121.30)	0.020
Simple RT 3-DH ms (SD)	−9.06 (25.42)	13.36 (48.99)	ns
CalCAP – true positive responses (N)			
Choice RT-Digits tp (SD)	0.13 (0.62)	0.18 (1.08)	ns
Sequential RT tp (SD)	1.56 (2.03)	−1.27 (5.39)	0.065
Language discrimination tp (SD)	0.31 (2.18)	1.82 (3.25)	ns
Degraded words distract tp (SD)	0.81 (1.56)	0.64 (1.36)	ns
Response reversal-words tp (SD)	−0.06 (1.53)	0.36 (1.91)	ns
Form discrimination tp (SD)	−0.81 (2.23)	2.00 (4.12)	0.030
CalCAP – false positive responses (N)			
Choice RT-Digits fp (SD)	−0.25 (0.78)	−0.45 (1.64)	ns
Sequential RT fp (SD)	−0.50 (1.75)	0.45 (1.86)	ns
Language discrimination fp (SD)	0.13 (1.82)	−2.18 (2.68)	0.013
Degraded words distract fp (SD)	−0.31 (2.65)	−0.45 (0.69)	ns
Response reversal-words fp (SD)	−0.19 (0.98)	−0.36 (1.03)	ns
Form discrimination fp (SD)	−0.50 (3.33)	0.27 (4.05)	ns

Note: Lower scores on the mean reaction time-measures indicates improvement in milliseconds from baseline to retest. Increased true positive responses indicates improvement from baseline to retest. Decreased false positive responses indicates improvement from baseline to retest.

valproate and found that subjects on valproate performed worse on tasks of visuomotor function and memory.

Translation to Clinical Practice

The major finding in the reported trial is that withdrawal of major AEDs improves performance on tests that require complex cognitive processing under time pressure. The difference in speed of cognitive processing between the withdrawal and non-withdrawal groups was between 24 and 43 ms. Elements of these cognitive processes are necessary in many daily life activities and even a slight slowing in processes that are repeated many times in daily life activities may have an important impact. The results indicate that performance of certain kinds of intellectual work, tasks requiring divided attention and fast information processing may be negatively affected by use of AEDs.

Withdrawal of AEDs in seizure-free patients is not without risks. In adults seizure relapse have been shown to have significant psychosocial costs (Sillanpaa & Schmidt, 2006). Thus, the decision to withdraw AEDs requires careful evaluation of risk factors for seizure recurrence versus expected cognitive benefits (Specchio & Beghi, 2004). Unless there is clear indication of drug related cognitive impairment in a patient, there may not be convincing reasons to withdraw medication in seizure-free patients, based on the expectation of cognitive improvement.

Summary

The results suggest that seizure-free epilepsy patients on monotherapy can obtain improvement in speeded cognitive processing if they withdraw anti-epileptic treatment. The difference in speed of cognitive processing between the withdrawal and non-withdrawal groups was between 24 and 43 ms. The outcome of carbamazepine withdrawal was similar to the outcome for the total study population while discontinuation of valproate only revealed a non-significant tendency in the same direction. Withdrawal of AEDs in seizure-free patients is not without risks, and unless there is clear indication of drug related cognitive impairment in a patient, there may not be convincing reasons to withdraw medication in seizure-free patients, based on the expectation of cognitive improvement.

References

Aldenkamp, A.P. (2001). Effects of antiepileptic drugs on cognition. *Epilepsia*, 42, 46–49.

Aldenkamp, A.P., Alpherts, W.C.J., Blennow, G., *et al. (1993). Withdrawal of antiepileptic medication: effects on cognitive function in children: the results of the multicentre "Holmfrid" study. *Neurology*, 43, 41–51.

Baker, G.A., & Marson, A.G. (2001). Cognitive and behavioural assessments in clinical trials: what type of measure? *Epilepsy Research*, 45, 163–167.

Brunbech, L., & Sabers, A. (2002). Effect of antiepileptic drugs on cognitive function in individuals with epilepsy. *Drugs*, 62, 593–604.

Craig, I., & Tallis, R. (1994). Impact of valproat and phenytoin on cognitive function in elderly patients. Results of a single blind randomised comparative study. *Epilepsia*, 35, 381–390.

Galassi, R., Morreale, A., Di Sarro, R., *et al. (1992). Cognitive effects of antiepileptic drug discontinuation. *Epilepsia*, 33, 41–44.

Kwan, P., & Brodie, M.J. (2000). Early identification of refractory epilepsy. *New England Journal of Medicine*, 342, 314–319.

Lossius, M.I., Stavem, K., & Gjerstad, L. (1999). Predictors for recurrence of epileptic seizures in a general epilepsy population. *Seizure*, 8, 476–479.

Martin, E.M., Pitrak, D.L., Novak, R.M., Pursell, K.J., & Mullane, K.M. (1999). Reaction times are faster in HIV-seropositive patients on antiretroviral therapy: a preliminary report. *Journal of Clinical and Experimental Neuropsychology*, 5, 730–735.

Meador, K.J. (2001). Cognitive effects of epilepsy and of antiepileptic medications. In: Wyllie, E. (ed.), *The Treatment of Epilepsy: Principles and Practice* (3rd ed.). Philadelphia: Lippincott Williams & Wilkins, pp. 1215–1225.

Meador, K.J. (1998). Cognitive and behavioural assessments in AED trials. *Antiepileptic Drug Development: Advances in Neurology*, 76, 231–238.

Meador, K., Loring, D.W., Ray, P.G., *et al.* (2001). Differential cognitive and behavioural effects of carbamazepine and lamotrigine. *Neurology*, 56, 1177–1182.

Meador, K.J., Loring, D.W., Abney, O.L., *et al.* (1993). Effects of carbamazepine and phenytoin on EEG and memory in healthy adults. *Epilepsia*, 34, 153–157.

Meador, K.J., Loring, D.W., Allen, M.E., *et al.* (1991). Comparative cognitive effects of carbamazepine and phenytoin in healthy adults. *Neurology*, 41, 1537–1540.

Miller, E.N. (1992). Use of computerized reaction time in the assessment of dementia (abstract). *Neurology*, 42, 220.

Miller, E.N. (1980). *California Computerized Assessment Battery (CalCAP) Manual*. Los Angeles: Norland Software.

Miller, E.N., Satz, P., & Visscher, B. (1991). Computerized and conventional neuropsychological assessment of HIV-1 infected homosexual men. *Neurology*, 41, 1608–1616.

Miller, E.N., Satz, P., & Visscher, B. (1989). Computerized neuropsychological assessment for HIV-related encephalopathy. Symposium on novel and traditional approaches for early detection of HIV-1 related dementia (Vancouver, Canada). *Journal of Clinical and Experimental Neuropsychology*, 11, 34–35.

Prevey, M.L., Delaney, R.C., Cramer, J.A., *et al.* (1996). Effect of valproate on cognitive function: comparison with carbamazepine: the Department of Veterans Affairs Epilepsy Cooperative Study 264 Group. *Archives of Neurology*, 53, 1008–1016.

Sillanpaa, A., & Schmidt, D. (2006). Prognosis of seizure recurrence after stopping antiepileptic drugs in seizure-free patients: a long-term population based study of childhood-onset epilepsy. *Epilepsy & Behavior*, 8, 713–719.

Specchio, L.M., & Beghi, E. (2004). Should antiepileptic drugs be withdrawn in seizure-free patients? *Drugs*, 18, 201–212.

Thompson, P.J., & Trimble, M.R. (1981). Sodium valproate and cognitive function in normal volunteers. *British Journal of Clinical Pharmacology*, 12, 819–824.

Vermeulen, J., & Aldenkamp, A.P. (1995). Cognitive side-effects of chronic antiepileptic drug treatment: a review of 25 years of research. *Epilepsy Research*, 22, 65–95.

Worth, J.L., Savage, C.R., Baer, L., Esty, E.K., & Navia, B.A. (1993). Computer-based neuropsychological screening for AIDS dementia complex. *AIDS*, 7, 677–681.

Progress in Neurotherapeutics and Neuropsychopharmacology, 3:1, 211–226 © 2008 Cambridge University Press
DOI: 10.1017/S1748232107000018   Printed in the United Kingdom

A Randomized-Controlled Trial of Bilateral rTMS for Treatment-Resistant Depression

Paul B. Fitzgerald

Alfred Psychiatry Research Centre, The Alfred and Monash University School of Psychiatry,
Psychology and Psychological Medicine, Commercial Road, Melbourne, Victoria, Australia;
Email: paul.fitzgerald@med.monash.edu.au

ABSTRACT

Background: Antidepressant effects have been demonstrated with both high-frequency left-sided repetitive transcranial magnetic stimulation (rTMS) (HFL-TMS) and low-frequency stimulation to the right prefrontal cortex (LFR-TMS). However, doubts remain about the extent of these reported treatment effects. *Design and Methods*: The study was a 6 week double-blind randomized sham-controlled trial of sequential bilateral rTMS (SBrTMS) in depression. The method consisted of 3 trains of LFR-TMS of 140 s duration at 1 Hz being applied daily followed immediately by 15 trains of 5 s duration of HFL-TMS at 10 Hz. Sham stimulation was applied using identical parameters, but with the coil angled at 45 degrees from the scalp resting on the side of one wing of the coil. *Results*: There was a significant difference in response between the two groups at the 2-week time-point ($F(1,25) = 25.5, p < 0.001$) and for the full duration of the study ($F(5,44) = 3.9, p = 0.005$). A significant proportion of the active study group met response (11/25) and remission criteria (9/25) by study end compared to the sham group (2 and 0/22). *Interpretation*: Bilateral rTMS treatment, involving the sequential application of both HFL-TMS and LFR-TMS, has substantial treatment efficacy in patients with treatment-resistant depression. The treatment response is clinically significant following 4–6 weeks of active treatment. Therefore this novel style of bilateral rTMS has the potential to become a substantive clinical intervention, although the study requires replication.

Key words: bilateral, depression, transcranial magnetic stimulation, treatment resistant.

Correspondence should be addressed to: Paul B. Fitzgerald, MBBS, MPM, PhD, FRANZCP, Alfred Psychiatry Research Centre, First Floor, Old Baker Building, The Alfred, Commercial Road, Melbourne, Victoria 3004, Australia; Ph: +61 3 9276 6552; Fax: +61 3 9276 6588; Email: paul.fitzgerald@med.monash.edu.au

Introduction and Overview

Major depressive disorder is a severe and highly prevalent illness which is often debilitating and results in considerable morbidity. Although a number of useful treatments exist for depression, a significant proportion of patients fail to benefit from these therapies (commonly considered ~30%, but potentially significantly more (Fava, 2003)). In the last decade, repetitive transcranial magnetic stimulation (rTMS) has emerged as an alternative option to combat the symptoms of treatment-resistant depression (TRD). A number of methods of rTMS administration have been assessed for their antidepressant properties. The majority of studies have applied high-frequency stimulation to the left dorsolateral prefrontal cortex (PFC) (HFL-TMS). A smaller number of studies have applied low-frequency stimulation (1 Hz) to the right PFC (LFR-TMS). These unilateral approaches have both been shown to have antidepressant activity (Fitzgerald, 2003) however doubts remain as to the degree of clinical response achieved and its clinical relevance (Mitchell & Loo, 2006). An alternative approach is the combination of these in a sequential manner. A number of small studies have investigated the use of sequential bilateral rTMS (SBrTMS), but the potential of this combination has not been rigorously investigated in studies with substantive sample sizes. We targeted this possibility by conducting a randomized, double-blind sham-controlled trial of the efficacy of SBrTMS; the administration of high-frequency left-sided stimulation followed by low-frequency right-sided rTMS (Fitzgerald *et al.*, 2006). We hypothesized that active bilateral rTMS would produce a greater therapeutic effect than sham stimulation and additionally, cause no significant cognitive side effects. Moreover, we provided extended treatment for up to 6 weeks and hypothesized that this would result in superior clinical effects to those seen in previous research conducted with more limited time duration.

Purpose of the Trial

To prospectively evaluate sequentially combined HFL-TMS and LFR-TMS in the therapy of treatment-resistant depression. Specifically, we sought to demonstrate the efficacy of active bilateral rTMS compared to sham stimulation and determine the effects of extended treatment. In addition, we aimed to investigate the impact of rTMS treatment on cognition.

Treatment Approach

rTMS is a non-invasive means of stimulating nerve cells in superficial areas of the brain. The site of the stimulation, its frequency and the intensity determine its effects. The ability of rTMS to affect mood was first noted in normal patients in the late 1980s. Studies using focal stimulation of the dorsolateral prefrontal cortex (DLPFC) appeared in 1995 and 1996. Since this time a considerable number of small clinical trials of rTMS have been conducted (for example, Fitzgerald *et al.*, 2003; Janicak *et al.*, 2002; Grunhaus *et al.*, 2000; George *et al.*, 2000; 1995). A majority of these trials have used high-frequency rTMS (between 5 and 20 Hz) applied to the left DLPFC. The antidepressant properties of this form of stimulation have been confirmed in a number of meta-analyses (Kozel & George, 2003; Martin *et al.*, 2003; Holtzheimer *et al.*, 2001). Recently the provision of low-frequency stimulation (typically 1 Hz) to the right DLPFC has been shown to have similar antidepressant activity (Isenberg *et al.*, 2004; Fitzgerald *et al.*, 2003; Klein *et al.*, 1999). Each variant of stimulation frequency is proposed to be clinically effective when applied to one particular hemisphere due to opposite effects on cortical activity induced by low and high-frequency stimulation (Fitzgerald *et al.*, 2003). In particular, it has been proposed that high-frequency stimulation increases activity in an underactive left prefrontal region and that low-frequency stimulation has the opposite effect (Hasey, 2001). The sum of these effects may be to correct a relative imbalance between the two hemispheres (Hasey, 2001) but this remains unconfirmed by empirical studies.

Despite the conduct of multiple trials of rTMS, doubts remain about the overall utility of the technique. For example, in a number of the meta-analyses performed of high-frequency stimulation, the clinical effects described were quite modest. For example, a mean overall improvement of only 23.8% on the Hamilton depression rating scale (HAMD) with active treatment compared to 7.3% with sham (Holtzheimer, 2001). Therefore, there remains a need to consider and test novel methods of administration of rTMS techniques. One possibility is the sequential combination of high-frequency left and low-frequency right-sided stimulation (SBrTMS). To date, this approach has been tested in only a limited way. The first trial of this technique compared HFL-TMS to SBrTMS and a condition with high (10 Hz) and low (1 Hz) frequency rTMS both applied to left DLPFC and showed no difference between the groups (Conca *et al.*, 2002). However, this study was small and only over 5 days of treatment, a duration now generally considered too short to show substantive rTMS treatment effects. A second study also showed no difference in response between SBrTMS and HFL-TMS, but interpretation of this study is confounded by the concurrent commencement of antidepressant medication with the rTMS treatment (Hausmann *et al.*, 2004). A third small study also compared SBrTMS and HFL-TMS but did not include a sham arm. This study showed no difference between the groups but this would have been unlikely given the small sample and overall very high response rates found, possibly related to the lack of a sham control (6/9 in SBrTMS and 5/9 in HFL-TMS) (Rybak *et al.*, 2005).

Clinical Trial

Subjects

Patients were recruited from the outpatient department of a public mental health service and by referral from a number of private psychiatrists between January 2003 and September 2004; all remained outpatients during the trial. Fifty patients with a diagnostic and statistical manual of mental disorder (DSM IV) diagnosis of major depression assigned by the treating and study psychiatrist participated in the study. Forty-two patients had a diagnosis of major depressive episode and 8 had a diagnosis of bipolar 1 disorder, depressive episode (4 in each group) (Table 1). Fifty-six patients were screened originally, 6 were excluded prior to randomization due to insufficient depression severity (3) or comorbidity (3).

To enter the study, all patients were required to score >20 on the Montgomery-Åsberg depression rating scale (MADRS; mean = 33.6, SD = 7.8). We excluded patients with significant medical illness, neurological disorder or other axis 1 psychiatric disorders. To meet inclusion criteria, all patients must have failed to respond to a minimum of two courses of antidepressant medication for at least 6 weeks (Stage II, Thase and Rush Definition (Thase & Rush, 1997)) (mean number of course = 5.9, SD = 3.0). Patients were not deliberately withdrawn from medication prior to the trial, however, medication type and dosage needed to remain stable for 4 weeks prior to commencement of the study and persist throughout the duration of the trial. Twenty-one patients were taking an SSRI, 9 an SNRI, 10 a tricyclic antidepressant, 4 a drug from another class and 6 no antidepressant medication. Eleven patients were taking mood stabilizers and 14 an antipsychotic. There was no difference between the proportion of patients taking any of

Table 1. **Demographic and Baseline Clinical Variables**

	ACTIVE		SHAM		SIGNIFICANT DIFFERENCE
	MEAN	SD	MEAN	SD	
Age	46.8	10.7	43.7	10.2	ns
Sex	10/15		9/16		ns
Age of onset	30.4	13.8	25.2	11.4	ns
Number of episodes	3.8	3.6	4.4	4.3	ns
Diagnosis (uni/bipolar)	21/4		21/4		ns
MADRS	34.0	5.6	34.2	5.2	ns
HAMD	22.5	7.4	19.8	4.4	ns
BDI	29.2	9.6	29.3	9.7	ns
BPRS	19.4	5.6	19.8	4.3	ns
GAF	48.8	8.2	49.0	4.9	ns
CORE	9.0	4.1	8.4	4.8	ns
Previous ECT	10		10		ns
Response to previous ECT	4		6		ns

the medication types between the 2 groups. Twenty patients reported at least one previous treatment course with ECT; half reported a previously favorable response. Three patients were left handed (2 in the active and 1 in the sham group, $p > 0.05$).

The study was approved by the Human Research Ethics Committee of the Alfred Hospital and written informed consent was obtained from all patients.

Trial Methods

The study consisted of a parallel double-blind randomized-controlled trial with an active rTMS and sham treatment arm (Figure 1). In addition, patients who received sham treatment were unblinded at the end of the study and offered open

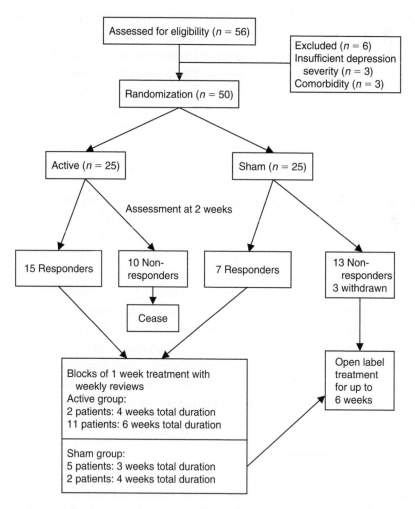

Fig. 1.
Study design showing number screened and randomized and entering extension phase.

label active treatment. All patients initially received 10 sessions of treatment on a daily basis, 5 days per week. After the 10th session, a blinded assessment was made. At this time patients were classified as "responding" if they had achieved a >20% reduction in MADRS score. If this was the case, they were offered a further week of rTMS. At week three patients were classified as continued responders if they achieved a further >10% reduction in MADRS score. If this was the case they were offered a 4th week of treatment. Weekly assessment of this sort continued and patients could receive a total of 6 weeks of treatment, dependent on consistent treatment response. At any review, patients who were not responding were withdrawn from the study and if they had received sham they were offered open label active rTMS under the same treatment conditions (review at 2 weeks and weekly thereafter).

Treatment was provided with a Medtronic Magpro30 magnetic stimulator (Medtronic Inc, Minneapolis, USA). It was applied through a stand held 70 mm figure of 8 coil. There was limited interaction between the patients and the rTMS administrator during the rTMS sessions. The coil was held tangential to the scalp with the handle pointing back and away from the midline at 45 degrees inducing a current flow that was posterior to anterior in the cortex perpendicular to the central sulcus. Stimulation occurred 5 cm anterior to the site found to be optimal for stimulation of the Abductor Pollicis Brevis muscle. The resting motor threshold (RMT) was measured bilaterally using standard EMG methods (Pridmore et al., 1998).

Treatment stimulation was sequentially administered to the right DLPFC and then the left DLPFC; patients received both stimulation conditions in each treatment session. Right-sided stimulation was applied at 1 Hz, in 3 trains of 140 s duration with a 30 s interval between trains. It was applied at 110% of the RMT. Left-sided stimulation was applied at 10 Hz, in fifteen 5 s trains with a 25 s inter-train interval. Left-sided stimulation was applied at 100% of the RMT. We chose a lower intensity on the left than on the right as in our previous experience right-sided stimulation is better tolerated at higher intensities. Therefore, we were attempting to maximize the tolerable dose to rTMS treatment with each condition.

Sham stimulation was applied with stimulation parameters identical to that for the active treatment (on both sides), but with the coil angled at 45 degrees off the head with the medial wing of the coil resting on the scalp. Some degree of scalp sensation was experienced by participants.

Instruments/Measures

Several clinical ratings were performed. At each assessment, patients were assessed with the MADRS, the 17 item version of the Hamilton Depression Rating Scale (HAMD) (Hamilton, 1967), the Beck Depression Inventory (BDI) (Beck et al., 1961), the Brief Psychiatric Rating Scale (BPRS) (Overall & Gorham, 1962), the

CORE rating of psychomotor disturbance (Parker *et al.*, 1990) and the Global Assessment of Function (GAF) (American Psychiatric Association, 1994). Ratings at follow up were conducted with these tools and additionally, the clinical global improvements (CGI) scale (Guy, 1976). Handedness was recorded with the Edinburgh Handedness Inventory (Oldfield, 1971). Ratings were conducted by clinical trained raters who were required to demonstrate adequate inter-rater reliability ($r^2 > 0.9$).

Cognition was assessed at each visit with the following tests: the Hopkins Verbal Learning Test (Shapiro *et al.*, 1999), Controlled Oral Word Association Test (Benton *et al.*, 1989), Digit Span (forwards and backwards) (Wechsler, 1939), the Brief Visuospatial Memory Test-Revised (Benedict *et al.*, 1996) and the Visuospatial Digit Span.

Primary and Secondary Outcomes

The primary outcome measure was the degree of change in individual scores on the MADRS (Montgomery & Asberg, 1979). Secondary outcomes were assessed for the remaining clinical scales, particularly the HAMD (Hamilton, 1967) and the BDI (Beck *et al.*, 1961).

Analysis

The *t*-tests and χ^2-squared tests were used to investigate differences between the groups on demographic and baseline clinical variables. The primary outcome analysis was conducted with intention to treat methods (last observation carried forward) on MADRS scores using a repeated measure analysis of variance (ANOVA). A secondary series of models were computed including potential covariates such as age, sex, diagnosis and medication status. *Post hoc* paired *t*-tests were used to analyze change scores between different study visits. In addition, the percentage of patients meeting response (>50% reduction in MADRS score) and remission (final MADRS score of <10 (Hawley *et al.*, 2002)) criteria were compared with Fisher's exact test. Analysis was also conducted using repeated measures ANOVA models for group differences in BDI and HAMD scores. Baseline to final study visit change scores were calculated for the BPRS, GAF and CGI and compared between the groups. The cognitive data were analyzed with paired *t*-tests comparing the baseline and end study scores. Separate analyses were conducted for the two groups as whole. Where a difference was seen in the basic analysis, a two-way ANOVA model was computed with time and group as the two factors. Pearson's correlation coefficients were calculated between change in MADRS and change in cognitive variables for the equivalent time periods if there was an effect of active treatment group on cognitive performance.

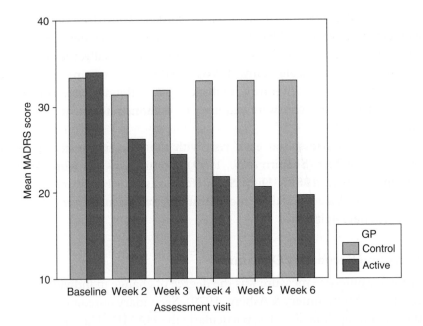

Fig. 2.
Mean MADRS total scores at each study assessment for the intention to treat, last observation carried forward data.

Results

EFFICACY
There were no significant baseline differences between the groups (Table 1). Three patients in the sham group did not complete the initial 2-week treatment period. One patient withdrew consent prior to undergoing the first treatment session and two patients withdrew during treatment, both had experienced no change or a mild degree of clinical deterioration prior to withdrawal.

Comparing outcomes in the active phase of the study, there was a significantly greater improvement in depression scores in the active compared to the sham (Figure 2) group. This difference was significant at the 2-week time period across the whole study period (group by time interaction ($F(5,44) = 3.9, p = 0.005$)). In the active group, 10 finished after 2 weeks, 2 after 3 weeks, 2 after 4 weeks and 11 completed all 6 weeks. In the sham group only 7 continued after 2 weeks and 2 of these continued into week 4 but none progressed further than week 4 in the study. In the active group, MADRS scores continued to fall across the entire study period: the reduction in MADRS scores was significant for the active group between baseline and week 2 ($p < 0.001$), week 3 and 4 ($p < 0.001$), week 4 and 5 ($p = 0.05$) and week 5 and 6 ($p = 0.01$). For the sham group, there was a reduction in MADRS scores significant at a trend level between baseline and week 2 ($p = 0.06$) but not between other study visits. The group differences in the primary analysis remained significant when controlling for age, sex, diagnosis and treatment with any antidepressant, mood stabilizer or antipsychotic medication as covariates.

Analysis of the other outcome variables revealed similar effects. For BDI scores there was a significant difference between the two groups (Group by Time interaction: ($F(5,44) = 3.2$, $p = 0.01$) favoring active treatment. For HAMD scores, there was a significantly greater improvement in the active group ($45.2 \pm 40.1\%$ versus $5.4 \pm 23.1\%$, $t(38.4) = 4.3$, $p < 0.001$). There was a significantly greater improvement in total BPRS scores in the active group ($41.5 \pm 38.5\%$ versus $8.2 \pm 30.7\%$, $t(45.7) = 3.4$, $p = 0.001$). There was also significant differences in end study scores on the CGI (illness severity) (3.4 ± 1.6 versus 4.4 ± 0.7, $t(33.0) = -2.9$, $p < 0.01$), CGI (improvement) (3.3 ± 1.2 versus 4.0 ± 1.4, $t(45) = -2.1$, $p < 0.05$) and the GAF (59 ± 16.5 versus 50.1 ± 10.3, $t(40.2) = 2.0$, $p < 0.05$).

In regards to analysis of response rates (Table 2), by study end, 11 patients in the active group and 2 patients in the sham group met criteria for clinical response ($p < 0.05$). Nine patients in the active group and no patients in the sham group met criteria for clinical remission ($p = 0.005$) and 5 of these patients had MADRS scores of 4 or below. Thirteen patients in the active and 2 patients in the sham group experienced a >50% reduction in HAMD scores ($\chi^2 = 11.5$, $p = 0.001$).

Eighteen of the patients in the sham group went on to receive active treatment (7 had 2 weeks, 1 had 3 weeks, 3 had 4 weeks, 2 had 5 weeks and 5 had 6 weeks). The mean improvement in MADRS scores was $37.0 \pm 43.7\%$ ($t(17) = 3.7$, $p < 0.005$) and 8 patients met response criteria.

Correlation analysis was conducted to study potential predictors of response. There was an inverse relationship between the severity of melancholic symptoms

Table 2. **Treatment Response**

	GROUP (n)	MADRS		BDI	
		MEAN	SD	MEAN	SD
Baseline	Active (25)	34.0	5.9	29.2	18.3
	Sham (25)	34.1	5.2	29.3	9.9
Week 2	Active (25)	26.2	10.2	18.3	10.3
	Sham (22)	30.9	8.2	21.6	13.7
Week 3	Active (15)	18.7	8.7	14.1	8.8
	Sham (7)	29.6	11.7	18.8	14.4
Week 4	Active (13)	11.7	7.1	10.5	8.3
	Sham (2)	34.5	12.0	21.0	19.8
Week 5	Active (11)	11.1	6.9	10.0	6.8
	Sham				
Week 6	Active (11)	8.9	7.9	9.2	6.7
	Sham				

and response (total CORE score: $r^2 = -0.33$, $p < 0.05$ ($n = 43$), non-interactiveness subscale: $r^2 = -0.34$, $p < 0.05$ ($n = 43$)). No other variables correlated with response.

TOLERABILITY

rTMS was generally tolerated quite well. Five patients in the active and two patients in the sham group reported a headache persisting for longer than 10 min after one or more treatment sessions. Three patients in the active group (none in the sham) reported feeling nausea after one or more treatment session. This was relatively brief in all cases.

SAFETY

There were no major adverse events. TMS treatment was not related to impaired cognitive performance. Performance decreased in the Hopkins Verbal Learning Test delayed recall for both active and sham groups with no group by time interaction ($F(1,45) = 0.09, p > 0.05$). Performance improved on several other tests.

Unique Aspects of Trial

There were a number of important features about the design of this trial. First, most published rTMS studies and all studies of SBrTMS have included very small sample populations; this study utilized a significantly larger cohort than similar published trials. Second, the trial was longer in treatment duration than any other published rTMS trial to date. In the year prior to publication, studies with durations as short as 1 week, but more typically 2–4 weeks, were published. We extended this to 6 weeks and significantly found improvement that continued across this time period. Third, we used a relatively unique combination of treatment parameters. All of the studies that have included an SBrTMS arm to date have applied considerably fewer 1 Hz right-sided pulses. This may in part be related to the use of only 120 pulses in the original study of LFR-TMS (Klein et al., 1999). However, our previous research clearly shows a greater number of pulses is well tolerated (Fitzgerald et al., 2003) and physiological effects of 1 Hz rTMS appear to be related to the number of pulses applied (Maeda et al., 2000).

The results of the trial clearly showed that SBrTMS is more effective than sham rTMS stimulation in patients with TRD. However, the most striking aspect of the results was not the degree of statistical significance but the magnitude of the effects seen. In particular, we found a response rate to rTMS of around 50% (depending on the scale used) which is markedly higher than that seen in almost all previous sham-controlled studies. It is not clear why this may be the case. As our methods, and especially our patient group, were similar to our previously reported trial of high-frequency left-sided and low-frequency right-sided rTMS alone (Fitzgerald et al., 2003) it is possible to make some interesting, although tentative comparisons with unilateral treatment. As shown in Table 3, bilateral treatment appears to be associated with greater effects than either of the unilateral approaches. Importantly, this difference is not just in end study scores, but apparent at 2 and 4 weeks. This implies the difference is not just due to the longer duration of treatment in the current study. There were some differences in the number and strength of pulses between the unilateral study and the conditions applied in this trial: we gave more right-sided pulses (420 versus 300) at higher intensity (110 versus 100% of RMT) and the left-sided stimulation was provided at the same intensity but in fewer trains (750 versus 1000 pulses). Therefore it is possible that our improved results compared to our previous study came about because of the greater degree of right-sided stimulation alone. However, given the well established antidepressant properties of high-frequency left-sided rTMS this seems doubtful. It seems more likely that the increased efficacy results specifically from the combination of the two treatment parameters.

Combining the two-treatment types could enhance response in several ways. First, this could be related to the "inclusion" in treatment of patients who are responsive to either left- or right-sided treatment. However, this should maximize the number of responders but not the degree of response (given the limited number of pulses given on either side). Alternatively, the two treatments may have a synergistic response in likely treatment responders. This is suggested by the significance of the overall degree of clinical response. This could occur through several mechanisms. For example, there may be a complementary effect of the different stimulation types on differing aspects of mood circuitry. Alternatively, as unilateral stimulation has bilateral effects (Nahas *et al.*, 2001; Peschina *et al.*, 2001), both stimulation types may be working through the modulation of a single hemisphere or part of mood regulation circuitry. Interestingly, more basic research suggests that combining stimulation with different rTMS frequencies may have additive effects (Iyer *et al.*, 2003) and it is possible that the initial 1 Hz stimulation activates circuitry in a way that allows an enhanced response to higher-frequency stimulation.

Table 3. **Treatment Response Rates**

	BASELINE	WEEK 2 (WHOLE GROUP)	WEEK 4 (CONTINUED RESPONDERS)	MADRS	
				REDUCTION BY 50% AT 4 WEEKS	REDUCTION BY 50% BY STUDY END
Left	36.1 ± 7.5	30.8 ± 7.5	20.9 ± 6.6	3/20	3/20
Right	37.7 ± 8.4	32.2 ± 9.0	19.0 ± 9.3	4/20	4/20
Bilateral	34.0 ± 5.9	26.2 ± 10.2	11.7 ± 7.1	10/25	11/25

Treatment response in active groups over two comparable trials. Left: high-frequency left-sided rTMS; Right: low-frequency right-sided rTMS; Bilateral: sequential combination of left and right-sided treatment.

Translation to Clinical Practice

OTHER RECENT ADVANCES

The other major advance in the evaluation of rTMS methods that is underway is the conduct of several large multi-site clinical trials. One of these, sponsored by a private company, Neuronetics Inc., recruited over 300 patients in sites in North America and Australia with completion of the main arms of the study in late 2005. A second investigator initiated NIH funded study is currently underway at a number of centers in the United States. Importantly, both of these studies have or are comparing a single treatment condition, high-frequency left-sided rTMS stimulation to sham controls. Given the results of the previous smaller single site trials, it is possible that these studies will demonstrate clinical effects of active treatment greater than sham and that this will be of sufficient magnitude to justify approval of the techniques by regulatory authorities, although these clinical effects may remain modest in nature. This is likely to have a considerable effect on the uptake of rTMS in clinical practice. Currently rTMS has been approved in at least one Western country, Canada, which approved its use in the therapy of TRD in 2003. Uptake in other jurisdictions is likely to require the type of data that is produced by large multi-site trials.

HOW THE TRIAL RESULTS FIT INTO THE EMERGING
TREATMENT AND RESEARCH FRAMEWORK

It is possible that the availability of large multi-site study evidence for the efficacy of HFL-TMS may actually place some limits on the further development of the field. Clearly the results of our trial suggest that the "original" method of rTMS administration (HFL-TMS) may not be the most effective, which should not necessarily be surprising. We certainly no longer apply electroconvulsive therapy in the way in which it was originally proposed. However, given the costs associated with large scale studies, once a market becomes available for rTMS treatment, it may become much harder to fund and conduct the very large studies that would be required to prove that a "new" rTMS modality is better than the established standard. Data from the current study suggests this should remain a priority, however.

Summary of How to Treat the Disorder Incorporating the Results of the New Trial Data

TRD remains a difficult and often persistent clinical problem. It is generally considered that there is a diminishing likelihood of response to antidepressant trials once patients have failed to respond to adequate trials of multiple drugs. Despite this there are a range of useful treatment strategies that may be employed for TRD. The initial step is a reappraisal of the diagnosis, contributing factors and the adequacy of previous treatment trials. A number of clinical factors such as psychosis, bipolarity, comorbid axis I and axis II disorders, alcohol or substance dependence and medical comorbidity may all influence outcome of antidepressant treatment (Fagiolini & Kupfer, 2003). Beyond these factors, there are a number of pharmacological, psychological and emerging biological options. In regards to pharmacotherapy, a variety of strategies have been suggested (see review in Nelson, 2003). However, only a few of these are supported by methodologically sound randomized trials with evidence for the use of lithium perhaps the most robust (Thase, 2004; Stimpson *et al.*, 2002). There is little research evidence supporting individual psychotherapeutic approaches (McIntyre, 2003; Stimpson *et al.*, 2002).

In regards to non pharmacological biological treatments, electroconvulsive therapy is clearly the "gold standard" intervention for TRD (McCall, 2001), although some doubts have been raised about its true efficacy in TRD (McIntyre, 2003). However, a considerable number of patients will wish to, or need to, avoid ECT for reasons including medical comorbidity, the experience of side effects in the past with ECT and general fear (Fox, 1993). A range of other biological interventions are also under active investigation. On the basis of a relatively small number of trials, vagal nerve stimulation was recently approved for use in TRD in the US (Carpenter *et al.*, 2006) and trials are currently underway of magnetic seizure therapy, direct current stimulation and deep brain stimulation (Fitzgerald, 2006). In this context it remains a little uncertain where rTMS, including SBrTMS, may fit into the therapeutic armamentarium. Given the safety of the technique, its acceptance to patients and its high degree of tolerability (Walter, 2001), if it can be proven to have adequate efficacy, it is likely to be a much more acceptable alternative to patients than ECT and the other more invasive treatment options. However, it seems most likely to complement the use of these techniques rather than replace them (Fitzgerald, 2004) and its widespread adoption depends on the conduct of further studies demonstrating adequate clinical responses. The results of the current study suggest that at least some of this effort should go into further evaluation of the role of SBrTMS rather than unilateral approaches alone.

Acknowledgments

PBF was supported by a Practitioner Fellowship grant from National Health and Medical Research Council (NHMRC) and a NARSAD Young Investigator award. I would like to acknowledge all the members of my research team who contributed to the trials described in this chapter and the patients who contributed their time and good will.

References

American Psychiatric Association (1994). Diagnostic and Statistical Manual of Mental Disorder (4th ed.). Washington, DC: American Psychiatric Association Press.

Beck, A., Ward, C., Mendelson, M., Mock, J., & Erbaugh, J. (1961). An inventory for measuring depression. *Archives of General Psychiatry*, 4, 561–571.

Benedict, R.H., Schretlen, D., Groninger, L., Dobraski, M., & Shpritz, B. (1996). Revision of the brief visuospatial memory test: Studies of normal performance, reliability, and validity. *Psychological Assessment*, 8, 145–153.

Benton, A., & Hamsher, K. (1989). *Multilingual Aphasia Examination*. Iowa City, IA: AJA Associates.

Carpenter, L.L., Friehs, G.M., Tyrka, A.R., Rasmussen, S., Price, L.H., & Greenberg, B.D. (2006). Vagus nerve stimulation and deep brain stimulation for treatment resistant depression. *Medical and Health Rhode Island*, 89, 137, 140–141.

Conca, A., Di Pauli, J., Beraus, W., Hausmann, A., Peschina, W., Schneider, H., Konig, P., & Hinterhuber, H. (2002). Combining high and low frequencies in rTMS antidepressive treatment: preliminary results. *Human Psychopharmacology*, 17, 353–356.

Fagiolini, A., & Kupfer, D.J. (2003). Is treatment-resistant depression a unique subtype of depression? *Biological Psychiatry*, 53, 640–648.

Fava, M. (2003). Diagnosis and definition of treatment-resistant depression. *Biological Psychiatry*, 53, 649–659.

Fitzgerald, P.B. (2003). Is it time to introduce repetitive transcranial magnetic stimulation into standard clinical practice for the treatment of depressive disorders? *Australian and New Zealand Journal of Psychiatry*, 37, 5–11.

Fitzgerald, P.B. (2004). Repetitive transcranial magnetic stimulation and electroconvulsive therapy: complementary or competitive therapeutic options in depression? *Australasian Psychiatry*, 12, 234–238.

Fitzgerald, P.B. (2006). A review of developments in brain stimulation and the treatment of psychiatric disorders. *Current Psychiatry Reviews*, 2, 199–205.

Fitzgerald, P.B., Brown, T., Marston, N.A.U., Daskalakis, Z.J., & Kulkarni, J. (2003). A double-blind placebo controlled trial of transcranial magnetic stimulation in the treatment of depression. *Archives of General Psychiatry*, 60, 1002–1008.

Fitzgerald, P.B., Benitez, J., de Castella, A., Daskalakis, Z.J., Brown, T.L., & Kulkarni, J. (2006). A randomized, controlled trial of sequential bilateral repetitive transcranial magnetic stimulation for treatment-resistant depression. *American Journal of Psychiatry*, 163, 88–94.

Fox, H.A. (1993). Patients' fear of and objection to electroconvulsive therapy. *Hospital & Community Psychiatry*, 44, 357–360.

George, M.S., Wassermann, E.M., Williams, W.A., Callahan, A., Ketter, T.A., Basser, P., Hallett, M., & Post, R.M. (1995). Daily repetitive transcranial magnetic stimulation (rTMS) improves mood in depression. *Neuroreport*, 6, 1853–1856.

George, M.S., Nahas, Z., Molloy, M., Speer, A.M., Oliver, N.C., Li, X.B., Arana, G.W., Risch, S.C., & Ballenger, J.C. (2000). A controlled trial of daily left prefrontal cortex TMS for treating depression. *Biological Psychiatry*, 48, 962–970.

Grunhaus, L., Dannon, P.N., Schreiber, S., Dolberg, O.H., Amiaz, R., Ziv, R., & Lefkifker, E. (2000). Repetitive transcranial magnetic stimulation is as effective as electroconvulsive therapy in the treatment of nondelusional major depressive disorder: an open study. *Biological Psychiatry*, 47, 314–324.

Guy, W. (1976). Clinical global impressions. In: *ECDEU Assessment Manual for Psychopharmacology Revised*. Rockville, MD: National Institute of Mental Health, pp. 218–222.

Hamilton, M. (1967). Development of a rating scale for primary depressive illness. *British Journal of Social and Clinical Psychology*, 6, 278–296.

Hasey, G. (2001). Transcranial magnetic stimulation in the treatment of mood disorder: a review and comparison with electroconvulsive therapy. *Canadian Journal of Psychiatry*, 46, 720–727.

Hausmann, A., Kemmler, G., Walpoth, M., Mechtcheriakov, S., Kramer-Reinstadler, K., Lechner, T., Walch, T., Deisenhammer, E.A., Kofler, M., Rupp, C.I., Hinterhuber, H., &

Conca, A. (2004). No benefit derived from repetitive transcranial magnetic stimulation in depression: a prospective, single centre, randomised, double blind, sham controlled "add on" trial. *Journal of Neurology, Neurosurgery & Psychiatry*, 75, 320–322.

Hawley, C.J., Gale, T.M., & Sivakumaran, T. (2002). Defining remission by cut off score on the MADRS: selecting the optimal value. *Journal of Affective Disorders*, 72, 177–184.

Holtzheimer III, P.E., Russo, J., & Avery, D.H. (2001). A meta-analysis of repetitive transcranial magnetic stimulation in the treatment of depression. *Psychopharmacology Bulletin*, 35, 149–169.

Isenberg, K., Downs, D., Pierce, K., Svarakic, D., Garcia, K., Jarvis, M., North, C., & Kormos, T.C. (2005). Low frequency rTMS stimulation of the right frontal cortex is as effective as high frequency rTMS stimulation of the left frontal cortex for antidepressant-free, treatment-resistant depressed patients. *Annals of Clinical Psychiatry*, 17, 153–159.

Iyer, M.B., Schleper, N., & Wassermann, E.M. (2003). Priming stimulation enhances the depressant effect of low-frequency repetitive transcranial magnetic stimulation. *Journal of Neuroscience*, 23, 10867–10872.

Janicak, P.G., Dowd, S.M., Martis, B., Alam, D., Beedle, D., Krasuski, J., Strong, M.J., Sharma, R., Rosen, C., & Viana, M. (2002). Repetitive transcranial magnetic stimulation versus electroconvulsive therapy for major depression: preliminary results of a randomized trial. *Biological Psychiatry*, 51, 659–667.

Klein, E., Kreinin, I., Chistyakov, A., Koren, D., Mecz, L., Marmur, S., Ben-Shachar, D., & Feinsod, M. (1999). Therapeutic efficiency of right prefrontal slow repetitive transcranial magnetic stimulation in major depression: a double blind controlled trial. *Archives of General Psychiatry*, 56, 315–320.

Kozel, A., & George, M.S. (2002). Meta-analysis of left prefrontal repetitive transcranial magnetic stimulation (rTMS) to treat depression. *Journal of Clinical Practice*, 8, 270–275.

Maeda, F., Keenan, J.P., Tormos, J.M., Topka, H., & Pascual-Leone, A. (2000). Interindividual variability of the modulatory effects of repetitive transcranial magnetic stimulation on cortical excitability. *Experimental Brain Research*, 133, 425–430.

Martin, J.L., Barbanoj, M.J., Schlaepfer, T.E., Thompson, E., Perez, V., & Kulisevsky, J. (2003). Repetitive transcranial magnetic stimulation for the treatment of depression. Systematic review and meta-analysis. *British Journal of Psychiatry*, 182, 480–491.

McCall, W.V. (2001). Electroconvulsive therapy in the era of modern psychopharmacology. *International Journal of Neuropsychopharmacology*, 4, 315–324.

McIntyre, R.S., Muller, A., Mancini, D.A., & Silver, E.S. (2003). What to do if an initial antidepressant fails? *Canadian Family Physician*, 49, 449–457.

Mitchell, P.B., & Loo, C.K. (2006). Transcranial magnetic stimulation for depression. *Australia and New Zealand Journal of Psychiatry*, 40, 406–413.

Montgomery, S.A., & Asberg, M. (1979). A new depression scale designed to be sensitive to change. *British Journal of Psychiatry*, 134, 382–389.

Nahas, Z., Lomarev, M., Roberts, D.R., Shastri, A., Lorberbaum, J.P., Teneback, C., McConnell, K., Vincent, D.J., Li, X., George, M.S., & Bohning, D.E. (2001). Unilateral left prefrontal transcranial magnetic stimulation (TMS) produces intensity-dependent bilateral effects as measured by interleaved BOLD fMRI. *Biological Psychiatry*, 50, 712–720.

Nelson, J.C. (2003). Managing treatment-resistant major depression. *Journal of Clinical Psychiatry*, 64(Suppl. 1), 5–12.

Oldfield, R.C. (1971). The assessment and analysis of handedness: the Edinburgh inventory. *Neuropsychologia*, 9, 97–113.

Overall, J.E., & Gorham, D. (1962). The brief psychiatric rating scale. *Psychological Reports*, 10, 799–812.

Parker, G., Hadzi-Pavlovic, D., Boyce, P., Wilhelm, K., Brodaty, H., Mitchell, P., Hickie, I., & Eyers, K. (1990). Classifying depression by mental state signs. *British Journal of Psychiatry*, 157, 55–65.

Peschina, W., Conca, A., Konig, P., Fritzsche, H., & Beraus, W. (2001). Low frequency rTMS as an add-on antidepressive strategy: heterogeneous impact on 99mTc-HMPAO and 18 F-FDG uptake as measured simultaneously with the double isotope SPECT technique. Pilot study. *Nuclear Medical Communication*, 22, 867–873.

Pridmore, S., Fernandes Filho, J.A., Nahas, Z., Liberatos, C., & George, M.S. (1998). Motor threshold in transcranial magnetic stimulation: a comparison of a neurophysiological method and a visualization of movement method. *Journal of ECT*, 14, 25–27.

Rybak, M., Bruno, R., Turnier-Shea, Y., & Pridmore, S. (2005). An attempt to increase the rate and magnitude of the antidepressant effect of transcranial magnetic stimulation. *German Journal of Psychiatry*, 8, 59–65.

Shapiro, A.M., Benedict, R.H., Schretlen, D., & Brandt, J. (1999). Construct and concurrent validity of the Hopkins Verbal Learning Test-revised. *Clinical Neuropsychology*, 13, 348–358.

Stimpson, N., Agrawal, N., & Lewis, G. (2002). Randomised controlled trials investigating pharmacological and psychological interventions for treatment-refractory depression. Systematic review. *British Journal of Psychiatry*, 181, 284–294.

Thase, M.E. (2004). Therapeutic alternatives for difficult-to-treat depression: a narrative review of the state of the evidence. *CNS Spectrums*, 9, 808–816, 818–821.

Thase, M.E., & Rush, A.J. (1997). When at first you don't succeed: sequential strategies for antidepressant nonresponders. *Journal of Clinical Psychiatry*, 58(Suppl. 13), 23–29.

Walter, G., Martin, J., Kirkby, K., & Pridmore, S. (2001). Transcranial magnetic stimulation: experience, knowledge and attitudes of recipients. *Australia and New Zealand Journal of Psychiatry*, 35, 58–61.

Wechsler, D. (1939). *The Measurement of Adult Intelligence*. Baltimore: Williams and Wilkins.

Progress in Neurotherapeutics and Neuropsychopharmacology, 3:1, 227–240 © 2008 Cambridge University Press
DOI: 10.1017/S1748232107000146   Printed in the United Kingdom

Serotonin Related Genes Affect Antidepressant Treatment in Obsessive–Compulsive Disorder

----

F. Van Nieuwerburgh
Laboratory of Pharmaceutical Biotechnology, Ghent University, Ghent, Belgium;
Email: Filip.VanNieuwerburgh@UGent.be

D. Deforce
Laboratory of Pharmaceutical Biotechnology, Ghent University, Ghent, Belgium;
Email: Dieter.Deforce@Ugent.be

D.A.J.P. Denys
AMC, University of Amsterdam, Amsterdam, The Netherlands; Email: D.Denys@amc.nl

ABSTRACT

Up to 60% of OCD patients do not respond to a regular serotonin reuptake inhibitor (SRI) treatment. The purpose of the present study was to determine whether polymorphisms of the serotonin transporter (5-HTT), $5\text{-HT}_{1D\beta}$, and 5-HT_{2A} receptor genes affect the efficacy of SRI treatment in OCD. Ninety-one outpatients with primary OCD according to DSM-IV criteria consented to the study were randomly assigned a 12-week, double-blind trial to receive dosages titrated upward to 300 mg/day of venlafaxine, or 60 mg/day of paroxetine. Primary efficacy was assessed by the change from baseline on the Yale-Brown obsessive–compulsive scale (Y-BOCS), and response was defined as a $\geq 25\%$ reduction on the Y-BOCS. All of the paroxetine treated patients, with the G/G genotype of the 5-HT_{2A} polymorphism were responders ($\chi^2 = 8.66$, df = 2, $p = 0.013$). In the venlafaxine treated patients, the majority of responders carried the S/L genotype of the 5-HTTLPR polymorphism ($\chi^2 = 9.71$, df = 2, $p = 0.008$). The small group of patients who both carried the S/L genotype of the 5-HTTLPR polymorphism and the G/G genotype of the 5-HT_{2A} polymorphism responded all to treatment.

The results of this study suggest that the response in paroxetine and in venlafaxine treated OCD patients is associated with the G/G genotype of the

Correspondence should be addressed to: Damiaan Denys, AMC, University of Amsterdam, PA.2-179, PO Box 75867, 1070 AW Amsterdam, The Netherlands; Email: D.Denys@amc.nl

5-HT$_{2A}$ polymorphism and with the S/L genotype of the 5-HTTLPR polymorphism, respectively.

Key words: 5-HT$_{1D\beta}$, 5-HT$_{2A}$, 5-HTT, 5-HTTLPR, association study, obsessive–compulsive disorder, pharmacogenetics, serotonin, serotonin reuptake inhibitor, SSRI.

Introduction and Overview

Although serotonin reuptake inhibitors (SRIs) are the mainstay of treatment for OCD, up to 40–60% of OCD patients do not respond to an initial medication trial (Hollander *et al.*, 2002; Goodman *et al.*, 1998). Moreover, patients who fail to respond to a treatment with a SRI have 25% less chance to achieve response with another SRI compared to a patient who previously responded to a SRI (Denys *et al.*, 2003a). It is often necessary to switch between different selective SRIs (SSRIs) to find a more suitable alternative. This trial and error approach, where patients often do not display a full therapeutic response until several weeks after initiation, is unfavorable. This makes SSRI treatment of OCD a classic example where pharmacogenetics could bring a solution.

Reviews by Veenstra-VanderWeele *et al.* (2000) and Mancama & Kerwin (2003) give an overview of the role of pharmacogenetics in individualizing treatment with SSRIs and possible genetic influences on therapeutic response to drugs affecting the serotonin system. In OCD, three studies have investigated the role of the 5-HTTLPR and treatment response. McDougle *et al.* (1998) found an association of the L-allele with poorer response to SRIs, whereas Billett *et al.* (1997) and Di Bella *et al.* (2000) failed to find a relation between response and 5-HTT genotypes. Other receptors that might be involved in the therapeutic efficacy of SRIs are the terminal 5-HT$_{1D\beta}$ auto-receptor and the postsynaptic 5-HT$_{2A}$ receptor. Except for Tot *et al.* who failed to find an association between the -1438G/A and T102C polymorphism of the 5-HT$_{2A}$ receptor in 52 OCD patients following a 12-week trial with fluvoxamine, fluoxetine, or sertraline, no further study has investigated the 5-HT$_{2A}$ or 5-HT$_{1D\beta}$ receptor genes with regard to treatment response of SRIs in OCD.

Purpose of the Trial

In this study we tested the hypothesis that polymorphisms of the 5-HTT (L-allele of the 5-HTTLPR), 5-HT$_{1D\beta}$, and 5-HT$_{2A}$ gene are associated with treatment response with SRIs in OCD. We report the results of 91 patients who participated in 12-week, double-blind trial with paroxetine and venlafaxine and were assessed for the 44 bp insertion/deletion 5-HTTLPR, the 5-HT$_{1D\beta}$ G861C, and the 5-HT$_{2A}$ 1438G/A polymorphism.

Agents

The usefulness of the tricyclic antidepressant (TCA) clomipramine and SSRIs in OCD has been well established. Like the other SSRIs, paroxetine is better tolerated than the TCAs, causing few anticholinergic adverse effects. Like clomipramine, venlafaxine, and its active metabolite O-desmethyl venlafaxine, are potent inhibitors of the neuronal uptake of both serotonin and norepinephrine, and weak inhibitors of the reuptake of dopamine. Contrary to clomipramine, venlafaxine lacks the anticholinergic, antihistaminergic, and alpha-adrenergic blocking effects. Therefore, venlafaxine is less likely to produce adverse side effects related to these pharmacological properties (Denys *et al.*, 2003b).

A randomized double-blind comparison study of paroxetine and venlafaxine in patients with obsessive–compulsive disorder showed no significant differences between venlafaxine and paroxetine with regard to response or responder rates. The incidence of adverse events for venlafaxine and paroxetine was comparable (Denys *et al.*, 2003b).

Clinical Trial

Subjects

Ninety-one outpatients gave written informed consent to participate in this study which had been approved by the University of Utrecht Medical Ethical Review committee (Utrecht, The Netherlands). All patients were diagnosed with OCD according to DSM-IV criteria and the M.I.N.I., a clinical and structured interview, was used to confirm the diagnosis (Sheehan *et al.*, 1998) Severity of obsessive–compulsive symptoms was rated with the Y-BOCS, depressive symptoms with the HAM-D, and anxiety with the HAM-A (Goodman *et al.*, 1989; Hamilton, 1959; 1960). Only patients with a score of at least 18 on the Y-BOCS, or at least 12, if only obsessions or only compulsions were present, were included. Patients with a major depressive disorder or patients with a total score of 15 or more on the 17-item Hamilton depression rating scale (HAM-D) on admission were excluded. Information on family history of OCD and other psychiatric disorders was obtained by direct interviews with the patients and the presence of vocal and/or motor tics was assessed during the clinical interview.

Trial Methods

Patients were randomly assigned to receive either paroxetine or venlafaxine XR for 12 weeks in a single-center, double-blind controlled, and parallel-group study design. Paroxetine treatment was initiated at a dose of 15 mg/day, and gradually increased to 60 mg/day using a fixed dosing schedule. Venlafaxine treatment was initiated at a dose of 75 mg/day and gradually increased to 300 mg/day. Psychotropic drugs or psychotherapy were not allowed. Obsessive–compulsive symptoms were measured with the Y-BOCS, and response to treatment was prospectively defined as a ≥25% decrease in Y-BOCS score. Three out of 91 patients dropped out during the study because of lack of motivation or side effects. A detailed description of the study has been published earlier (Denys *et al.*, 2003b; Sheehan *et al.*, 1998; Goodman *et al.*, 1989; Hamilton, 1959; 1960).

Genotyping

Blood samples were collected from each subject and frozen at −80°C. DNA was extracted from 10 μl of peripheral blood according to standard procedures. The total number of subjects genotyped for the genes in this study was 88. In seven cases, the genotyping of the 5-HT$_{1D\beta}$ polymorphism failed, and in one case the genotyping of the 5-HTT polymorphism. All subjects were genotyped at the University of Ghent (Belgium) based on a coded identification number. The 5-HTT, 5-HT$_{1D\beta}$, and 5-HT$_{2A}$ genotyping was performed following a standardized protocol.

5-HTT

For the detection of the 44 bp insertion/deletion 5-HTTLPR polymorphism, the oligonucleotide primers were 5′-6FAM-GGCGTTGCCGCTCTGAATGC-3′ and 5′-AGGGACTGAGCTGGACAAC.

CAC-3′ were used to amplify a 484/528 bp fragment comprising the 5-HTT-linked polymorphic region. The PCR reaction was performed according to following conditions: 94°C for 1 min, 60°C for 1 min, 72°C for 1 min 40 s per cycle, for a total of 35 cycles. The PCR products were analyzed by capillary electrophoresis on an Applied Biosystems 3100 Genetic Analyzer.

5-HT$_{1D\beta}$

For detection of the 5-HT$_{1D\beta}$ G861C polymorphism, the oligonucleotide primers 5′-GAAACAGACGCCCAACAGGAC-3′ and 5′-CCAGAAACCGC-GAAAGAAGAT-3′ were used to amplify a 548 bp region comprising the G861C polymorphism site. The PCR reaction was performed under the following conditions: 90°C for 1 min, 55°C for 2 min, 72°C for 3 min per cycle, for a total of 32 cycles. Digestion of 10 μl of PCR product was accomplished by incubation for 4 h with 10 units of Hinc II restriction enzyme at 37°C. Digestion with Hinc II yields either two fragments (452 bp and 96 bp) for the G-allele or three fragments (310 bp, 142 bp and 96 bp) for the C-allele. The fragments resulting from the digestion were resolved on a 1.5% agarose gel and visualized by ethidium bromide staining.

5-HT$_{2A}$

For the detection of the 5-HT$_{2A}$ 1438G/A polymorphism within the promoter region of the 5-HT$_{2A}$ receptor gene, the oligonucleotide primers 5'-6FAM-AAGCTGCAAGGTAGCAACAGC-3' and 5'-NED-AACCAACTTATTTC-CTACCAC-3' were used to amplify a 468 bp region comprising the 5-HT$_{2A}$ 1438G/A polymorphism site. The PCR reaction was performed under the following conditions: 95°C for 1 min, 47°C for 1 min, 72°C for 1 min 20 s per cycle, for a total of 40 cycles. Digestion of 10 μl of PCR product was accomplished by overnight incubation with 10 units of Msp I restriction enzyme at 37°C. After incubation with Msp I, the 1438A allele remains intact while the 1438G allele is cut into a 223 bp piece (6FAM-labelled) and a 243 bp piece (NED-labelled). The fragments resulting from the digestion were analyzed by capillary electrophoresis on an Applied Biosystems 3100 Genetic Analyzer.

Analysis

The following statistical procedure was pursued. Firstly, the genotypic pattern of distribution and the allele frequencies of the 5-HTT, 5-HT$_{1D\beta}$, and 5-HT$_{2A}$ polymorphisms were analyzed in the whole sample ($n = 88$). Secondly, an analogous analysis was performed in the paroxetine treated patients ($n = 40$), and in the venlafaxine treated patients ($n = 44$) separately. Medication use and dose was uncertain in four patients and they were excluded from the treatment groups. The association between the distribution of the genotypes and allele frequencies with the responders and non-responders were assessed by cross-tabulation and χ^2 analyses. One way ANOVAs were calculated to determine whether significant differences were present between genotypes in mean decrease of Y-BOCS scores. Considering a partial Bonferroni's correction, the *p*-value for statistical significance would be 0.020 with an alpha of 0.05, 6 tests, 2 degrees of freedom, and a correlation correction factor of 0.5. The data are presented as mean ± SD, and performed at 5% level of significance. All statistical analyses were conducted with the SPSS statistical package version 11.5.

Results

Demographic variables and outcome measures are presented in Table 1. The patient sample was slightly skewed towards the female population (63%). Fifty-six out of 88 patients (63%) were rated as responders, 31 out of 40 patients in the paroxetine group, and 24 out of 44 patients in the venlafaxine group. Four patients were not assigned to a particular treatment group (see Methods section). There were no statistically significant differences between responders and non-responders as regards gender, age, age of onset, family history, and baseline Y-BOCS, HAM-A, or HAM-D measures.

Table 1. **Demographic and Clinical Characteristics of the Patients Sample**

	NON-RESPONDERS ($n = 32$)	RESPONDERS ($n = 56$)
Gender (male/female)	14/18	20/36
Age on admission	31.7 ± 12.0	34.1 ± 11.3
Positive family history	11	19
Mean age of onset	14.7 ± 9.3	17.2 ± 7.4
≤15 years age of onset	12	33
>20 years age of onset	20	23
Y-BOCS baseline	26.8 ± 5.8	25.2 ± 5.2
Y-BOCS endpoint	24.8 ± 5.7	13.2 ± 5.4
Y-BOCS mean % decrease	6.8 ± 11.0	48.6 ± 18.0
HAM-D	5.6 ± 10.7	7.8 ± 10.8
HAM-A	7.4 ± 6.7	9.8 ± 7.5
Paroxetine ($n = 40$)	9	31
Venlafaxine ($n = 44$)	20	24

In the whole sample (Table 2), a difference in genotype distribution of the 5-HTTLPR polymorphism was found between responders and non-responders. Sixty-four percent of the responders carried the S/L genotype of the 5-HTTLPR polymorphism compared to 18% carrying the S/S genotype and 18% carrying the L/L genotype. The difference just failed to be statistically significant after Bonferroni's correction ($\chi^2 = 7.17$, df $= 2$, $p = 0.028$). When the mean Y-BOCS decrease was stratified by 5-HTTLPR genotype, a superior response was observed in the S/L genotype (37% decrease) versus the S/S genotype (28%) and the L/L genotype (29%), but the ANOVA failed to reach statistical significance ($F_{2,84} = 1.2$, $p = 0.30$). Allele frequencies of the 5-HTTLPR polymorphism between responders and non-responders were not statistically significant different ($\chi^2 = 0.05$, df $= 1$, $p = 0.71$), and there were no significant differences between responders and non-responders in allele or genotype frequencies for the 5-HT$_{1D\beta}$ and 5-HT$_{2A}$ poly-morphisms in the whole sample.

In the paroxetine treated patients (Table 3 and Figure 1), the majority of respon-ders carried the G/G genotype of the 5-HT$_{2A}$ polymorphism ($\chi^2 = 8.66$, df $= 2$, $p = 0.013$). The association of a superior response with the G/G genotype was confirmed in the ANOVA when the mean Y-BOCS decrease was broken down according to the genotypes. Patients carrying the G/G genotype of the 5-HT$_{2A}$ polymorphism had a mean decrease of 51% on the Y-BOCS compared to 34% with the A/A genotype and 29% with the A/G genotype ($F_{2,39} = 4.95$, $p = 0.012$). In general, responders carried predominantly the G-allele compared to non-responders ($\chi^2 = 8.43$, df $= 1$, $p = 0.004$) (OR 4.89 95% CI 1.59–15.02).

In the venlafaxine treated patients (Table 4 and Figure 2), the majority of responders carried the S/L genotype of the 5-HTTTLPR polymorphism ($\chi^2 = 9.72$, df $= 2$, $p = 0.008$). The ANOVA showed a difference in favor of the S/L genotype with a mean Y-BOCS decrease of 38% compared to 24% in patients

Table 2. **Allele Frequencies and Genotype Distribution of the 5-HT$_{1D\beta}$-, 5-HT$_{2A}$ Receptor, and 5-HTT Polymorphisms in the Whole Sample (n = 88)**

	n	ALLELE FREQUENCES		p-VALUE	GENOTYPES			p-VALUE
5-HT$_{1D\beta}$		**C**	**G**		**CC**	**CG**	**GG**	
Non-responders	30	0.23	0.74	0.273	1 (3.3%)	12 (40.0%)	17 (56.7%)	0.510
Responders	51	0.31	0.69		4 (7.8%)	24 (47.1%)	23 (45.1%)	
5-HT$_{2A}$		**A**	**G**		**AA**	**AG**	**GG**	
Non-responders	32	0.48	0.52	0.418	5 (15.6%)	21 (65.6%)	6 (18.8%)	0.144
Responders	56	0.42	0.58		11 (19.6%)	25 (44.6%)	20 (35.7%)	
5-HTT		**L**	**S**		**LL**	**L/S**	**SS**	
Non-responders	32	0.55	0.45	0.551	12 (37.5%)	11 (34.4%)	9 (28.1%)	0.028
Responders	55	0.50	0.50		10 (18.2%)	35 (63.6%)	10 (18.2%)	

Table 3. **Allele Frequencies and Genotype Distribution of the 5-HT$_{1D\beta}$-, 5-HT$_{2A}$ Receptor, and 5-HTT Polymorphisms in the Paroxetine Treated Group (n = 40)**

	n	ALLELE FREQUENCIES		p-VALUE	GENOTYPES			p-VALUE
5-HT$_{1D\beta}$		**C**	**G**		**CC**	**CG**	**GG**	
Non-responders	8	0.19	0.81	0.513	0 (0.0%)	3 (37.5%)	5 (62.50%)	0.625
Responders	28	0.27	0.73		3 (10.7%)	9 (32.1%)	16 (57.1%)	
5-HT$_{2A}$		**A**	**G**		**AA**	**AG**	**GG**	
Non-responders	9	0.67	0.33	0.004	3 (33.3%)	5 (66.7%)	0 (0.0%)	0.013
Responders	31	0.29	0.71		4 (12.9%)	10 (32.3%)	17 (54.8%)	
5-HTT		**L**	**S**		**LL**	**L/S**	**SS**	
Non-responders	9	0.56	0.44	0.772	3 (33.3%)	4 (44.4%)	2 (22.2%)	0.787
Responders	30	0.52	0.48		7 (23.3%)	17 (56.7%)	6 (20.0%)	

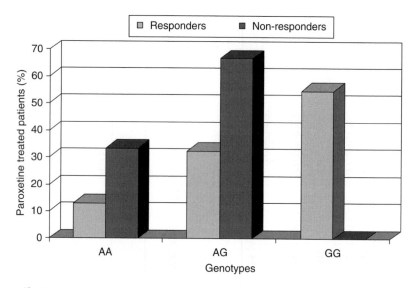

Fig. 1.

In the paroxetine treated patients ($n = 37$), the majority of responders (green) carried the GG genotype of the 5-HT$_{2A}$ polymorphism ($\chi^2 = 8.66$, df = 2, $p = 0.013$).

with the S/S genotype and 15% in patients with the LL genotype, who had the worst outcome, but failed to be statistically significant after correction ($F_{2,43} = 3.27$, $p = 0.04$).

Since the number of responders appeared to be correlated to the G/G genotype of the 5-HT$_{2A}$ polymorphism in the paroxetine treated patients, and to the S/L genotype of the 5-HTTLPR polymorphism in the venlafaxine treated patients, we analyzed thereupon responder rates in patients who had either one of the genotypes in the full sample. More than 81% of the responders (45 out of 55) carried either the G/G genotype of the 5-HT$_{2A}$ polymorphism or the S/L genotype of the 5-HTTLPR polymorphism ($\chi^2 = 8.1$, df = 1, $p = 0.004$). All of patients ($n = 9$) who carried both the G/G genotype of the 5-HT$_{2A}$ polymorphism and to the S/L genotype of the 5-HTTLPR polymorphism were responders. There was a statistically significant difference between the mean Y-BOCS decrease of 49% in these patients compared to the remainder of patients ($\chi^2 = 16.0$, df = 8, $p = 0.01$).

Conclusion and Translation to Clinical Practice

The main finding of this study is that in paroxetine treated OCD patients, the majority of responders carried the G/G genotype of the 5-HT$_{2A}$ polymorphism, whereas in the venlafaxine treated patients, the majority of responders carried the S/L genotype of the 5-HTTLPR polymorphism. The small group of patients ($n = 9$) who both carried the S/L genotype of the 5-HTTLPR polymorphism and the G/G genotype of the 5-HT$_{2A}$ polymorphism responded all to treatment.

Table 4. **Allele Frequencies and Genotype Distribution of the 5-HT$_{1D\beta}$, 5-HT$_{2A}$ Receptor, and 5-HTT Polymorphisms in the Venlafaxine Treated Group ($n = 44$)**

	n	ALLELE FREQUENCIES		p-VALUE	GENOTYPES			p-VALUE
5-HT$_{1D\beta}$		**C**	**G**		**CC**	**CG**	**GG**	
Non-responders	19	0.24	0.76	0.214	1 (5.3%)	7 (36.8%)	11 (57.9%)	0.221
Responders	22	0.36	0.64		1 (4.5%)	14 (63.6%)	7 (31.8%)	
5-HT$_{2A}$		**A**	**G**		**AA**	**AG**	**GG**	
Non-responders	20	0.40	0.60	0.087	2 (10.0%)	12 (60.0%)	6 (30.0%)	0.165
Responders	24	0.58	0.42		7 (29.2%)	14 (58.3%)	3 (12.5%)	
5-HTT		**L**	**S**		**LL**	**L/S**	**SS**	
Non-responders	21	0.55	0.45	0.393	8 (40.0%)	6 (30.0%)	6 (30.0%)	0.008
Responders	23	0.46	0.54		2 (8.3%)	18 (75.0%)	4 (16.7%)	

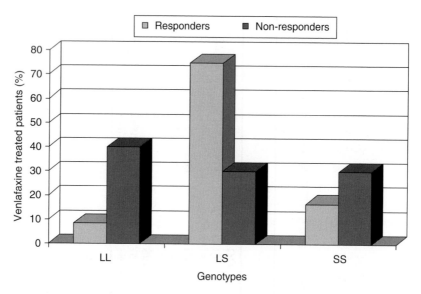

Fig. 2.

In the venlafaxine treated patients ($n = 44$), the majority of responders (green) carried the S/L genotype of the 5-HTTLPR polymorphism ($\chi^2 = 9.71$, df $= 2$, $p = 0.008$).

Three previous studies have investigated the role of the 5-HTTLPR and treatment response in OCD. Our results are in line with the findings of McDougle *et al.* who found a trend for an association of the L-allele with poorer response to SRIs (clomipramine, fluvoxamine, fluoxetine, sertraline, and paroxetine) in a sample of 33 patients (McDougle *et al.*, 1998). Billett *et al.* (1997) and Di Bella *et al.* (2000) failed to find an association between SRI response and 5-HTTLPR genotypes (Di Bella *et al.*, 2000; Billett *et al.*, 1997).

Our results are in contradiction with the majority of reports in mood disorders in which the presence of the L variant of the 5-HTTLPR has been associated with a more favorable and faster response to SRIs (Smits *et al.*, 2004). It is possible that this discrepancy is due to pathophysiologic and neurobiological dissimilarities between OCD and mood disorders. It has been suggested that SRIs exert their beneficial effects with their typical delay of 6–8 weeks in OCD by down regulating 5-HT$_{1D\beta}$ receptors in the orbito-frontal whereas in MDD, a faster response is observed probably due 5-HT auto-receptor desensitization in other brain areas such as the hippocampus and hypothalamus (Elmansari *et al.*, 1995). This supposition is appealing, but still needs to be confirmed.

It is unclear exactly why the S/L genotype of the 5-HTTLPR could cause a better response with SRIs in OCD. The L/L genotype has been related to higher 5-HTT densities and hence an increased efficacy of SRIs. However, it still needs to be clarified whether or not the 5-HTTLPR determines the number of 5-HTT in the human brain *in vivo* (Smith *et al.*, 2004; Williams *et al.*, 2003). Some studies have reported that L/L homozygous individuals had higher 5-HTT availability compared to S/L or S/S homozygous individuals in the raphe area, but others failed to find an association in the diencephalon, brainstem, and the thalamus (Van Dyck *et al.*, 2004; Shioe *et al.*, 2003; Willeit *et al.*, 2001; Heinz *et al.*, 2000). Equally, postmortem studies did not detect any significant influence of 5-HTTLPR on 5-HTT density in the hippocampus or frontal cortex (Mann *et al.*, 2000; Naylor *et al.*, 1998). For these reasons, it would be premature to relate superior response of the S/L genotype carriers in OCD to altered 5-HTT densities.

Only one study by Tot *et al.* has investigated the 5-HT_{2A} receptor gene with regard to treatment response in OCD. They failed to find an association between the -1438G/A and T102C polymorphism of the 5-HT_{2A} receptor in 52 OCD patients following a 12-week trial with fluvoxamine, fluoxetine, or sertraline (Tot *et al.*, 2003). It is unclear whether the -1438A/G promoter polymorphism results in functional effects (Veenstra-VanderWeele *et al.*, 2000). Meyer *et al.* have reported increased densities of the 5-HT_{2A} receptor after paroxetine treatment. On the other hand, Massou *et al.* have found the opposite (Meyer *et al.*, 2001; Massou *et al.*, 1997). A recent study in 54 Japanese patients with MDD failed to find a major role for the -1438G/A promoter polymorphism in therapeutic response to fluvoxamine (Sato *et al.*, 2002) Spurlock *et al.* (1998) found no effect of the -1438A/G promoter polymorphism on basal or cAMP- and protein kinase C induced gene transcription in HeLa cells, and found no difference in lymphocyte 5-HT_{2A} receptor mRNA expression between 1438A/A and G/G homozygotes (Spurlock *et al.*, 1998). Turecki *et al.* in a small postmortem study, reported higher prefrontal 5-HT_{2A} receptor binding in subjects with the -1438A allele, but Bray *et al.* (2004) failed to find a significant effect on 5-HT_{2A} receptor mRNA expression in postmortem brain tissue (Nakamura *et al.*, 1999; Turecki *et al.*, 1999).

It is singular why response in paroxetine treated patients is related to the 5-HT_{2A} receptor genotype and response in venlafaxine treated patients to the 5-HTTLPR. The 5-HTT and 5-HT_{2A} receptor are intimately linked. The constitutive lack of the 5-HTT alters the density of the 5-HT_{2A} receptor in a brain region specific manner, with an increase in the hypothalamus and decrease in the striatum (Rioux *et al.*, 1999; Li *et al.*, 1997). Thus, the apparent specific association of paroxetine and venlafaxine might be a spurious finding as result of a type two error due to the small sample sizes. Further investigation in larger samples might clarify this issue.

Summary

In summary, this study suggests a better outcome in OCD after treatment with venlafaxine for patients carrying the S/L genotype of the 5-HTTLPR polymorphism. Response to paroxetine was associated with the G/G genotype of the

5-HT$_{2A}$ polymorphism. The small group of patients who both carried the S/L genotype of the 5-HTTLPR polymorphism and the G/G genotype of the 5-HT$_{2A}$ polymorphism responded all to treatment. Our results indicate that 5-HT$_{2A}$ and 5-HTTLPR polymorphisms may be markers for treatment outcome in OCD.

References

Billett, E.A., Richter, M.A., King, N., Heils, A., Lesch, K.P., & Kennedy, J.L. (1997). Obsessive compulsive disorder, response to serotonin reuptake inhibitors and the serotonin transporter gene. *Molecular Psychiatry*, 2(Suppl. 5), 403–406.

Bray, N.J., Buckland, P.R., Hall, H., Owen, M.J., & O'Donovan, M.C. (2004). The serotonin-2A receptor gene locus does not contain common polymorphism affecting mRNA levels in adult brain. *Molecular Psychiatry*, 9, 109–114.

Denys, D., Burger, H., van Megen, H., de Geus, F., & Westenberg, H. (2003a). A score for predicting response to pharmacotherapy in obsessive–compulsive disorder. *International Clinical Psychopharmacology*, 18(Suppl. 6), 315–322.

Denys, D., van der Wee, N., van Megen, H.J.G.M., & Westenberg, H.G.M. (2003b). A double blind comparison of venlafaxine and paroxetine in obsessive–compulsive disorder. *Journal of Clinical Psychopharmacology*, 23(Suppl. 6), 568–575.

Denys, D., van Megen, H.J.G.M., van der Wee, N., & Westenberg, H.G.M. (2004). A double-blind switch study of paroxetine and venlafaxine in obsessive–compulsive disorder. *Journal of Clinical Psychiatry*, 65(Suppl. 1), 37–43.

Di Bella, D., Erzegovesi, S., Cavallini, M.C., d'Annucci, A., & Bellodi, L. (2000). Obsessive–compulsive disorder, treatment response and the 5htt gene. *American Journal of Medical Genetics*, 96(Suppl. 4), 536–536.

Elmansari, M., Bouchard, C., & Blier, P. (1995). Alteration of serotonin release in the guinea-pig orbitofrontal cortex by selective serotonin reuptake inhibitors – relevance to treatment of obsessive–compulsive disorder. *Neuropsychopharmacology*, 13(Suppl. 2), 117–127.

Goodman, W.K., Price, L.H., Rasmussen, S.A., Mazure, C., Fleischmann, R.L., Hill, C.L., Heninger, G.R., & Charney, D.S. (1989). The yale-brown obsessive compulsive scale. 1. Development, use, and reliability. *Archives of General Psychiatry*, 46(Suppl. 11), 1006–1011.

Goodman, W.K., Ward, H.E., & Murphy, T.K. (1998). Biologic approaches to treatment-refractory obsessive–compulsive disorder. *Psychiatric Annals*, 28(Suppl. 11), 641–649.

Hamilton, M. (1959). The assessment of anxiety states by rating. *British Journal of Medical Psychology*, 32, 50–55.

Hamilton, M. (1960). A rating scale for depression. *Journal of Neurology, Neurosurgery and Psychiatry*, 23, 56–62.

Heinz, A., Jones, D.W., Mazzanti, C., Goldman, D., Ragan, P., Hommer, D., Linnoila, M., & Weinberger, D.R. (2000). A relationship between serotonin transporter genotype and *in vivo* protein expression and alcohol neurotoxicity. *Biological Psychiatry*, 47(Suppl. 7), 643–649.

Hollander, E., Bienstock, C.A., Koran, L.M., Pallanti, S., Marazziti, D., Rasmussen, S.A., Ravizza, L., Benkelfat, C., Saxena, S., Greenberg, B.D., Sasson, Y., & Zohar, J. (2002). Refractory obsessive–compulsive disorder: state-of-the-art treatment. *Journal of Clinical Psychiatry*, 63, 20–29.

Li, Q., Muma, N.A., Battaglia, G., & Van der Kar, L.D. (1997). Fluoxetine gradually increases [i-125]doi-labelled 5-ht2a/2c receptors in the hypothalamus without changing the levels of g(q)- and g(11)-proteins. *Brain Research*, 775(Suppl. 1–2), 225–228.

Mancama, D., & Kerwin, R.W. (2003). Role of pharmacogenomics in individualising treatment with ssris. *CNS Drugs*, 17(Suppl. 3), 143–151.

Mann, J.J., Huang, J.Y., Underwood, M.D., Kassir, S.A., Oppenheim, S., Kelly, T.M., Dwork, A.J., & Arango, V. (2000). A serotonin transporter gene promoter polymorphism (5-httlpr) and prefrontal cortical finding in major depression and suicide. *Archives of General Psychiatry*, 57(Suppl. 8), 729–738.

Massou, J.M., Trichard, C., AttarLevy, D., Feline, A., Corruble, E., Beaufils, B., & Martinot, J.L. (1997). Frontal 5-ht2a receptors studied in depressive patients during chronic treatment by selective serotonin reuptake inhibitors. *Psychopharmacology*, 133(Suppl. 1), 99–101.

McDougle, C.J., Epperson, C.N., Price, L.H., & Gelernter, J. (1998). Evidence for linkage disequilibrium between serotonin transporter protein gene (slc6a4) and obsessive compulsive disorder. *Molecular Psychiatry*, 3(Suppl. 3), 270–273.

Meyer, J.H., Kapur, S., Eisfeld, B., Brown, G.M., Houle, S., DaSilva, J., Wilson, A.A., Rafi-Tari, S., Mayberg, H.S., & Kennedy, S.H. (2001). The effect of paroxetine on 5-ht2a receptors in depression: an [f-18]setoperone pet imaging study. *American Journal of Psychiatry*, 158(Suppl. 1), 78–85.

Nakamura, T., Matsushita, S., Nishiguchi, N., Kimura, M., Yoshino, A., & Higuchi, S. (1999). Association of a polymorphism of the 5ht2a receptor gene promoter region with alcohol dependence. *Molecular Psychiatry*, 4(Suppl. 1), 85–88.

Naylor, L., Dean, B., Pereira, A., Mackinnon, A., Kouzmenko, A., & Copolov, D. (1998). No association between the serotonin transporter-linked promoter region polymorphism and either schizophrenia or density of the serotonin transporter in human hippocampus. *Molecular Medicine*, 4(Suppl. 10), 671–674.

Rioux, A., Fabre, V., Lesch, K.P., Moessner, R., Murphy, D.L., Lanfumey, L., Hamon, M., & Martres, M.P. (1999). Adaptive changes of serotonin 5-ht2a receptors in mice lacking the serotonin transporter. *Neuroscience Letters*, 262(Suppl. 2), 113–116.

Sato, K., Yoshida, K., Takahashi, H., Ito, K., Kamata, M., Higuchi, H., Shimizu, T., Itoh, K., Inoue, K., Tezuka, T., Suzuki, T., Ohkubo, T., Sugawara, K., & Otani, K. (2002). Association between-1438g/a promoter polymorphism in the 5-ht2a receptor gene and fluvoxamine response in Japanese patients with major depressive disorder. *Neuropsychobiology*, 46(Suppl. 3), 136–140.

Sheehan, D.V., Lecrubier, Y., Sheehan, K.H., Amorim, P., Janavs, J., Weiller, E., Hergueta, T., Baker, R., & Dunbar, G.C. (1998). The mini-international neuropsychiatric interview (mini): The development and validation of a structured diagnostic psychiatric interview for dsm-iv and icd-10. *Journal of Clinical Psychiatry*, 59, 22–33.

Shioe, K., Ichimya, T., Suhara, T., Takano, A., Sudo, Y., Yasuno, F., Hirano, M., Shinohara, M., Kagami, A., Okubo, Y., Nankai, M., & Kanba, S. (2003). No association between genotype of the promoter region of serotonin transporter gene and serotonin transporter binding in human brain measured by pet. *Synapse*, 48(Suppl. 4), 184–188.

Spurlock, G., Heils, A., Holmans, P., Williams, J., D'Souza, U.M., Cardno, A., Murphy, K.C., Jones, L., Buckland, P.R., McGuffin, P., Lesch, K.P., & Owen, M.J. (1998). A family based association study of t102c polymorphism in 5ht2a and schizophrenia plus identification of new polymorphisms in the promoter. *Molecular Psychiatry*, 3(Suppl. 1), 42–49.

Smith, G.S., Lotrich, F.E., Malhotra, A.K., Lee, A.T., Ma, Y.L., Kramer, E., Gregersen, P.K., Eidelberg, D., & Pollock, B.G. (2004). Effects of serotonin transporter promoter polymorphisms on serotonin function. *Neuropsychopharmacology*, 29(Suppl. 12), 2226–2234.

Smits, K.M., Smits, L.J.M., Schouten, J.S.A.G., Stelma, F.F., Nelemans, P., & Prins, M.H. (2004). Influence of sertpr and stin2 in the serotonin transporter gene on the effect of selective serotonin reuptake inhibitors in depression: a systematic review. *Molecular Psychiatry*, 9(Suppl. 5), 433–441.

Tot, S., Erdal, M.E., Yazici, K., Yazici, A.E., & Metin, O. (2003). T102c and -1438 g/a polymorphisms of the 5-ht2a receptor gene in turkish patients with obsessive–compulsive disorder. *European Psychiatry*, 18(Suppl. 5), 249–254.

Turecki, G., Briere, R., Dewar, K., Antonetti, T., Lesage, A.D., Seguin, M., Chawky, N., Vanier, C., Alda, M., Joober, R., Benkelfat, C., & Rouleau, G.A. (1999). Prediction of level of serotonin 2a receptor binding by serotonin receptor 2a genetic variation in postmortem brain samples from subjects who did or did not commit suicide. *American Journal of Psychiatry*, 156(Suppl. 9), 1456–1458.

Van Dyck, C.H., Malison, R.T., Staley, J.K., Jacobsen, L.K., Seibyl, J.P., Laruelle, M., Baldwin, R.M., Innis, R.B., & Gelernter, J. (2004). Central serotonin transporter availability measured with [i-123]beta-cit spect in relation to serotonin transporter genotype. *American Journal of Psychiatry*, 161(Suppl. 3), 525–531.

Veenstra-VanderWeele, J., Anderson, G.M., & Cook, E.H. (2000). Pharmacogenetics and the serotonin system: initial studies and future directions. *European Journal of Pharmacology*, 410(Suppl. 2–3), 165–181.

Willeit, M., Stastny, J., Pirker, W., Praschak-Rieder, N., Neumeister, A., Asenbaum, S., Tauscher, J., Fuchs, K., Sieghart, W., Hornik, K., Aschauer, H.N., Brucke, T., & Kasper, S. (2001). No evidence for *in vivo* regulation of midbrain serotonin transporter availability by serotonin transporter promoter gene polymorphism. *Biological Psychiatry*, 50(Suppl. 1), 8–12.

Williams, R.B., Marchuk, D.A., Gadde, K.M., Barefoot, J.C., Grichnik, K., Helms, M.J., Kuhn, C.M., Lewis, J.G., Schanberg, S.M., Stafford-Smith, M., Suarez, E.C., Clary, G.L., Svenson, I.K., & Siegler, I.C. (2003). Serotonin-related gene polymorphisms and central nervous system serotonin function. *Neuropsychopharmacology*, 28(Suppl. 3), 533–541.

Progress in Neurotherapeutics and Neuropsychopharmacology, 3:1, 241–257 © 2008 Cambridge University Press
DOI: 10.1017/S1748232107000067   Printed in the United Kingdom

Night Eating Syndrome and Results from the First Placebo-Controlled Trial of Treatment, with the SSRI Medication, Sertraline: Implications for Clinical Practice

John P. O'Reardon

Weight & Eating Disorders Program, Department of Psychiatry, University of Pennsylvania, Philadelphia, PA, USA; Email: oreardon@mail.med.upenn.edu

Karen E. Groff

Weight & Eating Disorders Program, Department of Psychiatry, University of Pennsylvania, Philadelphia, PA, USA

Albert J. Stunkard

Weight & Eating Disorders Program, Department of Psychiatry, University of Pennsylvania, Philadelphia, PA, USA; Email: stunkard@mail.med.upenn.edu

Kelly C. Allison

Weight & Eating Disorders Program, Department of Psychiatry, University of Pennsylvania, Philadelphia, PA, USA; Email: kca@mail.med.upenn.edu

ABSTRACT

Objective: The goal of the study was to assess the efficacy of sertraline in the treatment of the night eating syndrome (NES). *Method*: Thirty-four outpatients diagnosed with NES were randomly assigned to receive either sertraline ($n = 17$) or placebo ($n = 17$) in an 8-week, double-blind, flexible-dose (50–200 mg/day) study. We used the mixed effects linear regression model to analyze change in the primary outcome measure, the Clinical Global Impression of Improvement Scale (CGI-I). Secondary outcomes included changes in the Night Eating Symptom Scale (NESS), the number of nocturnal awakenings and ingestions, total daily calorie intake after the evening meal, Clinical Global Impression of Severity Scale (CGI-S), Quality of Life Enjoyment and Satisfaction Scale (Q-LES), and weight. *Results*: Sertraline was associated with statistically significantly greater improvements than placebo in the CGI-I scale. As determined by a CGI-I score of $\leqslant 2$ (much or very much improved), 12 subjects in the sertraline group (71%) were classified as responders versus only 3 in the placebo group (18%). There were also

Correspondence should be addressed to: John P. O'Reardon, MD, Room 4005, 3535 Market Street, Philadelphia, PA 19104, USA; Email: oreardon@mail.med.upenn.edu

significant improvements in the NESS, CGI-S scales, Q-LES, frequency of nocturnal ingestions and awakenings, and calorie intake after supper. Overweight and obese subjects in the sertraline group ($n = 14$) lost a significant amount of weight by week 8 (mean $= -2.9$, SD $= 3.8$ kg) compared to those in the placebo arm ($n = 13$) (mean $= -0.3$, SD $= 2.7$ kg). *Conclusions:* In this 8-week trial, sertraline was effective in the treatment of NES and was well tolerated.

Key words: night eating syndrome, placebo-controlled trial, sertraline.

Introduction and Overview

The night eating syndrome (NES) is an eating disorder characterized by morning anorexia, evening hyperphagia, and insomnia with awakenings followed by nocturnal ingestions (Stunkard *et al.*, 1955; Birketvedt *et al.*, 1999). In addition, mood is usually low (Gluck *et al.*, 2001), with a pattern of worsening in the latter half of the day (Birketvedt *et al.*, 1999). The core feature of NES appears to be delay in the circadian timing of food intake (O'Reardon *et al.*, 2004). Food intake is lower in the first half of the day and increased in the evening and nighttime. Sleep is often disrupted in the service of food ingestion. In the largest controlled study to date of overweight and obese outpatients with NES ($n = 46$), energy intake in the first 8 h of the day (06:00–14:00 h) averaged only 575 kcals in NES subjects versus 1082 kcals in the control group ($n = 43$), while energy intake averaged 591 kcals in the last 8 h (22:00–06:00 h) in NES subjects compared to only 118 kcals in controls. The total energy intake over 24 h was not different between individuals with NES and those in a healthy obese control group (O'Reardon *et al.*, 2004).

The NES is of clinical importance as it is associated both with obesity and psychological distress. Its prevalence has been estimated at 1.5% in the general population (Rand *et al.*, 1997), between 8.9% (Stunkard *et al.*, 1996) and 14% in obesity clinics (Gluck *et al.*, 2001), and rates of up to 27% in severely obese persons (Rand *et al.*, 1997). NES appears to be more common in obese persons than in non-obese persons and to increase in prevalence with increasing adiposity. In a Danish study, obese women night eaters gained 5 kg over a 6-year period compared to a weight gain of 1 kg among obese non-night eaters (Andersen *et al.*, 2004). About half of individuals with NES report that they were of normal weight before the NES developed, suggesting that NES may be an important pathway to obesity (Marshall *et al.*, 2004).

There have been few reports of the treatment of NES. Case reports have suggested benefit from a variety of strategies including *d*-fenfluramine (Spaggiari *et al.*, 1994), phototherapy (Friedman *et al.*, 2002), progressive muscle relaxation (Pawlow *et al.*, 2003), and topiramate (Winkelman, 2003). The first clinical trial of pharmacotherapy was a 12-week open-label one ($n = 17$) with sertraline, a serotonin selective reuptake inhibitor (SSRI). It showed a significant reduction of symptoms in obese subjects with NES, with about half ($n = 8$) of the sample responding to sertraline. Those responders who achieved remission of NES ($n = 5$), also lost a significant amount of weight (-4.8 ± 2.6 kg) (Beck *et al.*, 1988).

This study sought to follow up our previous open-label trial with a double-blind, randomized, placebo-controlled trial. This time we also included a small number of normal weight subjects with NES to determine if sertraline might relieve their distress associated with the syndrome.

Method

Subjects were recruited from a study which characterized the psychological and behavioral aspects of NES (O'Reardon *et al.*, 2004). These patients were recruited through a combination of print advertisements, television programming, and a website. The characterization study included: (1) a structured clinical interview designed to assess the presence or absence of NES, performed by a trained clinician; (2) ten day sleep and food diary assessment; (3) the Structured Clinical Interview for the DSM-IV (SCID) to assess the presence of past or current psychiatric disorders; and (4) the Eating Disorder Examination to assess the presence of concomitant eating disorders.

Participants

Eligible subjects were ≥ 18 years, met standard criteria for NES based on assessment at the structured clinical interview, and had a body mass index (BMI) ≥ 18 kg/m^2. Applicants were excluded if they: (1) were severely depressed, as determined on assessment by DSM-IV criteria (with several symptoms present in excess of those required to make the diagnosis *and* symptoms markedly interfering with occupational functioning or with usual social activities or relationships); (2) had a lifetime diagnosis of bipolar disorder or any psychotic disorder; (3) reported substance abuse or dependence within the last 6 months; (4) were currently taking psychotropic medications (including hypnotics); (5) were working a night-shift or swing-shift schedule; (6) were in a weight reduction program; (7) were currently diagnosed with anorexia nervosa or bulimia nervosa, but not binge eating disorder (BED); or (8) lacked awareness of their night eating episodes. The latter criterion was used to exclude subjects with nocturnal sleep-related eating disorder (SRED), a parasomnia in which nocturnal eating is accompanied by a lack of awareness at the time and subsequent amnesia for the behavior.

Procedures and Measures

Baseline NES symptomatology was assessed as part of the characterization of NES study (O'Reardon *et al.*, 2004). Each subject collected data in a food and sleep diary during a 10-day 24-h prospective monitoring period, with the first 2 days discarded as practice days and the last day discarded because of incomplete data. The diary included a record of all meals, snacks and beverages consumed. Awakenings (during which the subject got out of bed), nocturnal ingestions as well as the timing of bedtime and getting up in the morning were all recorded. A research dietitian analyzed diaries for calorie intake and macronutrient content. Subjects were paid for the baseline diary data collection but not for participation in the treatment trial itself. Of the 65 subjects with NES who completed the diary assessment, 28 who were eligible to participate in the trial decided not to. Reasons for not participating included inability to schedule ($n = 16$), not wanting to be in a placebo-controlled study ($n = 7$), and not wanting a medication ($n = 5$). This left a total of 37 subjects who entered the treatment trial. Three subjects attended the baseline visit but did not return for any subsequent visits, leaving a total of 34 subjects whose data were included in the analyses.

Subjects were randomly assigned to 8 weeks of double-blind treatment with sertraline or placebo. Psychotropic agents other than the study medication were prohibited during the study. The 8-week duration of the trial was based on the results of our earlier 12-week trial. Subjects took tablets, identical in appearance, containing either 50 mg of sertraline or placebo. Subjects commenced with one tablet daily taken with the evening meal. Subjects were seen every other week for 30 min visits at which medication dosage could be adjusted up to a maximum of four tablets daily. Tolerance of and adherence to prescribed medication were recorded at each visit.

Subjects were weighed at each visit and completed three self-report scales: (1) the Night Eating Symptom Scale (NESS) (O'Reardon *et al.*, 2004); (2) Beck Depression Inventory (BDI) (Beck *et al.*, 1988); (3) the Quality of Life Enjoyment and Satisfaction Scale (Q-LES) (Endicott *et al.*, 1993). The study physician recorded the number of nighttime awakenings (defined as when the subject got up out of bed for reasons other than solely to use the bathroom) and ingestions. The study physician also administered the Clinical Global Impression of Improvement (CGI-I) and Severity (CGI-S) scales and the 17-item Hamilton Depression Rating Scales (HDRS) at each visit. The HDRS and BDI were used to track changes in depressive symptoms. Outcome was categorized at week 8 on the basis of the score on the CGI-I scale, which is scored in a range from 1 to 7. Ratings on the CGI-I were considered a primary outcome measure, with a priori standards applied as follows; subjects with scores of $\leqslant 2$ were categorized as responders (2 = much improved, 1 = very much improved, as compared to baseline) and those responders with scores of 1 were categorized as remitters.

The frequencies of ingestions and awakenings were derived by assessing carefully the results of the NESS for the previous week with the subject. The NESS is a self-report scale that measures the range and severity of symptoms of night eating over the past week (O'Reardon *et al.*, 2004). It measures the degree of morning anorexia, evening hyperphagia, sleep disturbance, nocturnal eating episodes and associated cravings or compulsions to eat, and level and pattern of mood disturbance in a series of 13 items. Each item is scored from 0 to 4 providing a possible range of scores from 0 to 52.

Evening hyperphagia was assessed by reviewing with the subject the proportion of their daily calorie intake that occurred between the end of the evening meal and bedtime plus any nocturnal ingestions that occurred, and it was expressed as a percentage of total 24 h caloric intake. As some subjects with NES delay their supper considerably as part of the circadian delay in the food intake rhythm, a cut-off of 8 pm was used. Any food intake commencing after this time was considered to be calorie intake after the evening meal.

Data Analysis

Means and standard deviations (SD) of the outcome variables at each time point were used for descriptive statistics as well as for the depiction of trends over the 8 weeks. The analyses were conducted on an intent-to-treat basis for all subjects who completed at least one follow-up visit following the baseline visit. The repeated measures outcome variables over the 8-week period were analyzed by a mixed effects linear regression model in the form of: outcome variable = intercept + group + week + group $\times$ week. The intercept was assumed to be random in order to take within-subject correlations of the dependent variables into account for statistical inference. Group and time variables were taken as fixed and discrete; two sided $p < 0.05$ was considered significant. This mixed effects modeling approach with available cases using a maximum likelihood method is valid in the presence of observations which are missing at random (Verbeke & Molenberghs, 1997).

The effects of particular interest were the main group effect and the interaction between group and week, with this interaction representing differences in trends of the outcome variables over time between the NES and control groups. Omnibus interaction significance tests are reported in the text. *Post hoc* testing of the main group effects at each time point on the outcome variables was followed by testing of the corresponding parameter contrasts in the mixed effects model with Wald *t*-tests. For this purpose, we used a Bonferroni-corrected significance level $0.05/4 = 0.0125$ (correcting for the number of treatment visits after baseline), except when testing for correlations. Significant differences for these *post hoc* analyses are presented in the figures. Main group effects at any week with *p* values lower than this corrected significance level were declared to be significant even if overall either the main group effect or interaction effect was not significant.

Three subjects who met criteria for BED in addition to NES were included as part of the sample. In line with recent evidence, BED and NES appear to be two distinct disorders rather than variable expressions of the same underlying psychopathology (Allison *et al.*, 2005b; Allison & Stunkard, 2005). In this respect, BED was treated as a psychiatric co-morbidity in NES subjects which was not viewed as exclusionary for study participation. All three BED plus NES subjects were randomly assigned to the placebo group. We tested for the significance of BED by including BED status in the above mixed effects models. BED status did not have a significant effect on any of the outcomes except for caloric intake after the evening meal. Thus, caloric intake after the evening meal was the only variable for which BED status was controlled. Pearson's correlations were used to assess the association of changes at week 2 with those at week 8 in the SSRI group. We used SAS v8.2 for statistical analyses.

Results

Characteristics of the sertraline and placebo groups at baseline are presented in Table 1. No significant differences for these variables between the groups were found at baseline.

Outcome Data

CGI-I and CGI-S Scales

The CGI-I score classified 12 of the 17 subjects receiving sertraline as responders (CGI-I $\leq$ 2) and 7 of these 12 achieved remission or complete resolution of NES symptoms (interaction $F = 6.7$, df $= 4,113$, $p < 0.001$). Of those receiving placebo, only three subjects were classified as responders, a response rate significantly lower than obtained with sertraline (Chi square $= 9.66$, df $= 1$, $p = 0.0019$), with one

Table 1. **Baseline Characteristics for the Sertraline and Placebo Groups. No Significant Differences Between Groups Were Present at Baseline**

	SERTRALINE ($N = 17$)		PLACEBO ($N = 17$)	
	MEAN	SD	MEAN	SD
Age (years)	45.1	11.0	44.2	10.6
BMI (kg/m^2)	32.4	6.5	32.9	9.0
NESS	31.7	5.6	30.5	6.2
Duration of NES (years)	17.6	15.5	15.3	12.7
BDI	14.4	9.7	12.1	9.5
HDRS	9.9	4.5	9.6	5.2
Q-LES	47.1	11.2	47.4	9.3
	N	%	N	%
Female	11	64.7	12	70.6
Normal weight	3	17.6	4	23.5
Race				
Caucasian	12	70.6	15	88.2
African American	5	29.4	2	11.8

of the 3 placebo responders achieving remission status. Of the 3 normal weight subjects in the sertraline group, 2 were responders, while none of the 4 normal weight subjects in the placebo group were responders.

Figure 1a shows that the largest reduction in symptoms occurred between baseline and week 2, indicating an early and robust effect of sertraline. Overall a subject on sertraline had a 30% chance of responding by week 2. On the CGI-I scale, 5 of the 12 who ultimately responded to sertraline had responded as early as week 2, and 4 of these 5 achieved remission status by week 2. The lack of early improvement with sertraline did not preclude ultimate response, as 50% of all responses occurred between weeks 4 and 8.

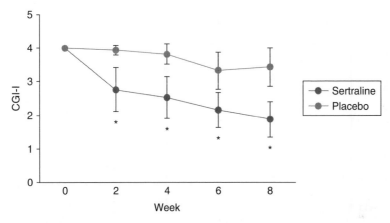

Fig. 1a.
Clinical Global Impression of Improvement (CGI-I) trends over 8 weeks in the sertraline and placebo groups. p value is significant (<0.0125) for weeks 2, 4, 6, and 8.

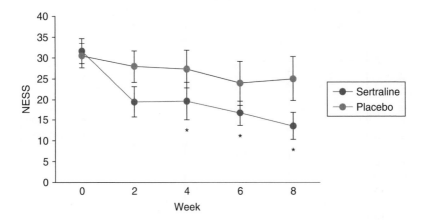

Fig. 1b.
Night Eating Symptom Scale (NESS) trends over 8 weeks in the sertraline and placebo groups. p value is significant (<0.0125) for weeks 2, 4, 6, and 8.

The CGI-S scale is a further index of overall change in NES symptoms. The sertraline group had a reduction of two points in symptom severity from a baseline score of 4.2 (moderate severity) to an endpoint score of 2.2 (borderline ill) whereas there was a much more modest reduction in the placebo group, from 4.2 to 3.4 (interaction $F = 4.1$, df $= 4,107$, $p = 0.004$).

NESS

Changes in NES symptomatology were significantly greater in the sertraline group, as assessed by the NESS over the course of the 8-week study (Figure 1b).

By week 8 the NESS score in the sertraline group dropped by 18.1 points (57%) from a baseline score of 31.7 as compared to a reduction of only 5 points

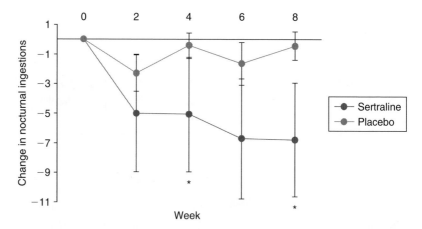

Fig. 2a.
Change in frequency of awakenings per week from the baseline in the sertraline and placebo groups over 8 weeks. *p* value = 0.0137 (NS) at week 8.

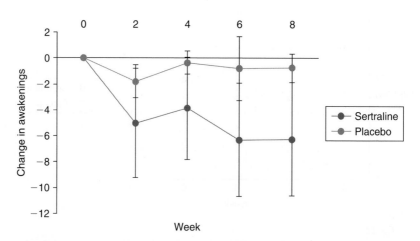

Fig. 2b.
Change in frequency of nocturnal ingestions per week from the baseline in the sertraline and placebo groups over 8 weeks. *p* value is significant (<0.0125) for weeks 2 and 8.

(16%) from a baseline score of 30.5 in the placebo group (interaction $F = 8.0$, df $= 4,112, p < 0.0001$). A significant correlation was found between the change in NESS score from baseline to week 2 and the change from baseline to week 8 for subjects receiving sertraline ($r = 0.68, p = 0.01$), indicating that early improvement with sertraline was predictive of ultimate response. Additionally, in terms of the speed of response, the dose at the first observed response (CGI-I $\leqslant 2$) in the sertraline group was correlated with the week of response, suggesting that early responders improved at lower doses than later responders ($r = 0.836, p < 0.001$). However, the probability of response by the study endpoint at week 8 was not correlated with dose, indicating that dose, *per se*, was not an important predictor of ultimate response to sertraline ($r = 0.516, p = 0.086$).

Ingestions and Awakenings

Figure 2a shows a significant reduction in the frequency of nocturnal ingestions in the sertraline group as compared to the placebo group. The number of nocturnal ingestions in the sertraline group fell by 81% (from a mean at baseline of 8.3, SD $= 8.5$/week to 1.6, SD $= 2.6$/week) versus only 14% (from a mean of 6.4, SD $= 4.9$–5.5, SD $= 4.9$/week) for the placebo group (interaction $F = 3.7$, df $= 4,80, p = 0.01$). Figure 2b indicates that the number of awakenings fell by 74% (from a mean of 8.8, SD $= 8.6$ to mean $= 2.3$, SD $= 4.7$/week) in the sertraline group versus only 14% (from a mean of 6.4, SD $= 4.6$–5.5, SD $= 5.0$) in the placebo group. This drop failed to reach significance in the overall interaction effect ($F = 0.9$, df $= 4,80, p = 0.4$), but it yielded a difference in main effect between groups ($F = 4.7$, df $= 1,32, p = 0.03$). In *post hoc* testing, after adjustment for multiple comparisons, the difference in awakenings at week 8 was not significant ($t = -2.52$, df $= 80, p = 0.0137$, NS).

Calorie Intake After the Evening Meal

Figure 3a shows that caloric intake after the evening meal in the sertraline group fell by about two-thirds, from 47.3% of total daily calories at baseline to 14.8% at week 8. In the placebo group caloric intake after the evening meal fell by less than one-third from 44.7% at baseline to 31.6% at week 8 (interaction $F = 3.5$, df $= 4,106, p = 0.009$). Comparisons of individual time points were not significant (week 8 $t = 2.0$, df $= 106, p = 0.047$, NS).

Weight Change

Among overweight subjects the sertraline group ($n = 14$) lost 2.9 (SD $= 3.8$) kg versus 0.3 (SD $= 2.8$) kg in the placebo group ($n = 13$) (interaction $F = 2.3$, df $= 4,59, p = 0.086$). The difference in main effect for weight between groups at week 8 ($t = -2.56$, df $= 59$, uncorrected $p = 0.0131$) was not significant, with the Bonferroni correction ($p = 0.052$). However, this Bonferroni correction does not take into consideration the within-subject correlation of the repeatedly measured weight losses, which was estimated to be 0.62 from the mixed effects model. Therefore, when the James correction (James, 1991; Leon & Heo, 2005) for multiple correlated observations is applied, the sertraline effect on weight loss at week 8 was significant ($p = 0.041$) (Figure 3b).

Mood Measures

Mood measures showed only a modest level of depressive symptoms in both groups at baseline (HDRS score of 9.9, SD $= 4.5$ in the sertraline group and a

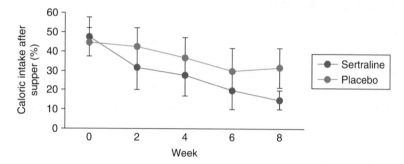

Fig. 3a.
Trends in caloric intake after the evening expressed as a percentage of the total daily caloric intake in the sertraline and placebo groups. *p* value = 0.047 (NS) at week 8.

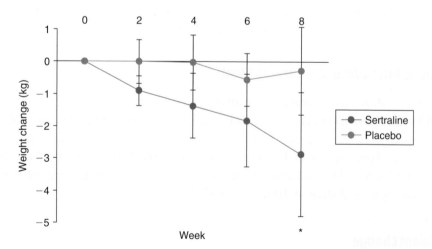

Fig. 3b.
Weight change (kg) from baseline in overweight subjects in the sertraline and placebo groups over 8 weeks. *p* value is significant (0.041) at week 8.

score of 9.6, SD = 5.2 in the placebo group, BDI score of 14.4, SD = 9.3 in the sertraline group and a score of 12.1, SD = 9.5 in the placebo group), and they did not differ over time (HDRS change; $F = 1.5$, df = 4,110, $p = 0.2$, BDI change; $F = 1.9$, df = 4,100, $p = 0.1$).

The reduction in depressive symptoms in the sertraline group did not significantly correlate with change in the NESS as reflected by Pearson correlation coefficients of $r = 0.26$ with change in the BDI and 0.08 with change in the HDRS. When the two depression items were removed from the full NESS, the score on the modified NESS still correlated strongly with the full NESS score (Pearson's $r = 0.98$, $p < 0.001$), implying that change in depressive symptoms is not the principal driver of change in NES symptoms.

Quality of Life Outcome

In the sertraline group there was an increase in the Q-LES score from 47.1 (SD = 12.0) points at baseline to 54.3 (SD = 9.6) points at week 8. Those on placebo remained essentially unchanged (mean = 47.6, SD = 9.9 at baseline and mean = 47.4, SD = 7.3 at week 8; interaction $F = 2.5$, df = 4,108, $p = 0.045$). No differences were noted at specific time points.

Dosing and Adverse Events

The mean dose of sertraline at study endpoint was 126.5 ± 50.4 mg. In contrast, the average dose of placebo attained would have translated to 173.5 ± 40.0 mg indicating that dose was appropriately increased when a suboptimal response was observed ($t = 3.0$, df = 32, $p = 0.005$). Sertraline was well tolerated and no subject withdrew because of adverse events. Common side-effects were mild and included dry mouth, fatigue, diminished libido, and sweating. Nausea as an adverse event was infrequent and transient (affecting two subjects on placebo and one on sertraline). There were two dropouts in the study, each related to lack of efficacy, one from the sertraline group at week 6, and one from the placebo group at week 4.

Discussion of Trial

The results of this, the first randomized placebo-controlled trial in the treatment of the NES, show that sertraline, an SSRI medication, reduced the symptoms of NES and most subjects (71%) met responder criteria at the end of 8 weeks. The extent of improvement in core NES symptoms was striking. The number of nocturnal ingestions in the sertraline group was reduced by about 80% by study endpoint. The caloric intake after supper dropped from 47.3% of the total daily calories at baseline to 14.8% at week 8, thus approaching the normative levels of intake found in our previous study in non-NES obese controls (O'Reardon *et al.*, 2004).

Consistent with the reduction in evening and nocturnal hyperphagia are the weight losses (about a pound a week), which are similar to those in our earlier, open-label trial with sertraline (O'Reardon *et al.*, 2004). This finding is the more striking in that no advice or behavioral guidance regarding weight loss was given. It suggests that sertraline may have a restraining effect on the tendency to gain weight in persons with NES.

Two patterns of improvement with sertraline were evident. Five subjects experienced an early and robust improvement on sertraline, meaning that close to half of the ultimate responders ($n = 12$) were evident after only 2 weeks on active medication. Improvement in the seven other responders occurred more gradually, between weeks 4 and 8. The fact that there was only a weak, non-significant, correlation ($r = 0.08$ for the HDRS) between the improvement in depressive symptoms in NES subjects on sertraline and the improvement in NES symptoms more generally implies strongly that the improvement on sertraline was independent of its antidepressant effect.

Subjects on sertraline had the NES for a prolonged period of time (average duration of 17.6 years) before entering the study but, nevertheless, four of the five fast responders achieved a full remission of the syndrome after only 2 weeks on sertraline at a dose of 50 mg daily. This indicates that, despite chronicity of symptoms, a rapid and robust improvement is possible for some NES patients. A similar finding has been reported in another eating disorder, bulimia nervosa. When treated with the SSRI fluoxetine, a significant reduction was noted in both the binge eating and vomiting episodes after a single week of active treatment (Goldstein *et al.*, 1995). It is possible that the nocturnal ingestions in NES, while not actual binges, share the psychological component of disinhibition with the binges of bulimia, and that serotonergic medications such as fluoxetine and sertraline have the potential to quickly ameliorate the loss of control present in both disorders.

As indicated earlier, the core feature of NES appears to be a delay in the circadian timing of energy intake with intake suppressed in the morning and increased in the evening and night. In an earlier study of carefully monitored outpatients with NES and weight matched controls we found dissociation between the sleep and eating rhythms in the NES group, with a delay in the food intake rhythm but not in the sleep rhythm (O'Reardon *et al.*, 2004).

The maintenance of normal circadian rhythms is the task of the suprachiasmatic nucleus (SCN) of the hypothalamus and serotonergic neurons are known to have inputs into the SCN (Miller *et al.*, 1996). It is possible that sertraline may act by modulating SCN function to restore a more normal food intake pattern in subjects with NES. The SCN may be a site of action for promoting a rapid improvement in NES symptoms in some individuals.

Limitations of this study include its short duration and small sample size. Future studies of sertraline and other pharmacotherapy agents in treating NES should determine if positive results are sustained over the longer term. If so, sertraline may be able to control both the core NES symptoms and the obesity that is a frequent and distressing complication of the syndrome.

Unique Aspects of the Trial

The most unique aspect of this trial is the fact that it is the first randomized placebo-controlled trial in the treatment of NES. Prior to this study, treatment of NES has been essentially anecdotal. A case series of four patients with nocturnal eating improved with topiramate (Winkelman, 2003) and a case report described successful treatment with morning light therapy (Friedman *et al.*, 2002). However, there had been no randomized placebo-controlled trials addressing this often debilitating disorder. The study was designed to have flexible dosing enabling the clinician to titrate the dose to as much as 200 mg of sertraline daily, thus emulating normal clinical practice (adjusting for side-effects, titrating for efficacy). This study had an excellent retention rate with only one active and one placebo dropout, both due to lack of efficacy.

This study included normal-weight subjects, who also appeared to benefit from sertraline but their numbers were too small for this conclusion to be definitive. This is a provocative clinical observation, as more than half of NES patients with obesity report normal weight status before the onset of the syndrome (Marshall *et al.*, 2004). Proactive treatment with an agent such as sertraline may have the potential to prevent onset of obesity in normal weight NES sufferers.

This study included measurements of depression to help determine if NES symptoms were reduced as a function of mood. Results showed that reduction in NES symptoms did not correlate with a reduction in mood symptoms indicating that sertraline is effective independent of its antidepressant action.

Translation to Clinical Practice

Obesity is one of the most important public health issues that clinicians and patients face today. The search for causes of obesity beyond lifestyle issues such as portion control and lack of exercise continues (Nestle & Jacobson, 2000). NES represents a treatable illness that has been associated with obesity. The results of this study are promising in this regard and may suggest the advent of a straightforward treatment, an SSRI, for this illness, with an acceptable number of side-effects. A recent open-label study with sertraline in NES ($n = 50$) demonstrated that the treatment delivered feasibly and effectively in primary care practice settings (Stunkard *et al.*, 2006).

There may be a class effect regarding pharmacotherapy of NES. With six serotonin reuptake inhibitors available to the clinician (citalopram, *S*-citalopram, fluoxetine, fluvoxamine, paroxetine, in addition to sertraline), there may be significant flexibility in treatment options if a patient fails to respond to or is unable to tolerate sertraline. A case series has been published suggesting efficacy with other SSRI agents (paroxetine, fluvoxamine) in NES (Miyaoka *et al.*, 2003). It is clearly reasonable for the clinician to try other medications in this class if a patient with NES fails to respond to sertraline. In major depression for instance, switching within the class between SSRIs has been found to be equivalent in efficacy to switching out of the class to a different antidepressant agent (Rush *et al.*, 2006). Further randomized placebo-controlled trials will be necessary, however, before a class effect for SSRIs in the treatment of NES is established.

It is important for clinicians to be diligent and precise when investigating causes of obesity, as treatment varies among disorders. A degree of confusion persists with regard to distinguishing between BED, SRED, and NES. Although, they share similarities, diagnostic clarity is important especially as different treatment strategies emerge. Although both NES and SRED are associated with sleep disturbances, NES is generally thought of as an eating disorder with related insomnia while SRED is more appropriately described as a primary sleep disorder, distinguished by partial or complete amnesia for eating episodes and specific polysomnographic findings (Auger, 2006). BED patients tend to manifest daytime problematic eating and do not seem to have the associated sleep disturbance that NES and SRED patients have (O'Reardon *et al.*, 2005). The pattern of abnormal eating in NES consists of repeated episodes of compulsive ingestion of relatively small amounts of food or snacks at inappropriate times, rather than the larger scale binges of BED.

NES has been recognized as a clinical entity for many years following the original report by Stunkard *et al.* (1955). Many patients, however, remain undiagnosed and therefore untreated likely due to lack of clinician recognition. A recent report surveyed the prevalence of NES in two psychiatric clinic settings ($n = 399$), one at an academic medical center in the North East of the US and the second in the Mid West (Lundgren *et al.*, 2006). It found an overall prevalence of 12.3% of NES, a rate much higher than would be expected for other eating disorders such as Anorexia Nervosa (0.3%) and Bulimia Nervosa (1%) in this setting.

A significant association was found between the diagnosis of NES and prescription of atypical antipsychotic agents, such as quetiapine and olanzapine. This raises the possibility that psychiatrists might be mistakenly prescribing sedative agents such as these in an attempt to treat insomnia when the more correct diagnosis is NES. Since agents like olanzapine and quetiapine are clearly associated with the adverse event of significant weight gain, this might well have the effect of worsening the obesity already present due to NES. It is important for psychiatrist to screen for NES when assessing insomnia. Simple screening questions include: "Are you troubled by overeating in the evening or nighttime?" and "Do you get up at nighttime to eat?" For more formal assessment of NES symptomatology the Night Eating Questionnaire is also helpful (Marshall *et al.*, 2004).

Integration of Study Results Within a Treatment Framework

In summary, a rational treatment approach to NES would be to screen first for the disorder using the screening questions above, especially in patients who are obese or have sleep disturbances. If the screen is positive, proceed to the more formal Night Eating Questionnaire, in the context of further clinical inquiry. Based on the study results, an evidence-based first-line treatment is to prescribe sertraline and titrate to effect. If a patient does not tolerate or respond to sertraline, use of another SSRI is logical, although there are no data yet that establishes a class effect. Second-line treatment, based on limited available evidence, would be topiramate, the anticonvulsant agent, which has demonstrated efficacy in BED and holds promise in NES. Preliminary evidence is now emerging to support the use of cognitive behavioral therapy as an alternative or adjunct to pharmacotherapy (Allison *et al.*, 2005a). Additional studies with both medication and non-pharmacologic approaches will be needed to elucidate a more complete evidence-based treatment algorithm.

Acknowledgment

Study supported from grant R01 DK56735 (the National Institutes of Health) and by a grant from Pfizer Pharmaceuticals.

References

Allison, K.C., & Stunkard, A.J. (2005). Obesity and eating disorders. *Psychiatric Clinics of North America*, 28, 55–67.

Allison, K.C., Martino, N.S., O'Reardon, J.P., & Stunkard, A.J. (2005a). CBT treatment of night eating syndrome: a pilot study. *Obesity Research*, 13, A83.

Allison, K.C., Grilo, C.M., Masheb, R.M., & Stunkard, A.J. (2005b). Binge eating disorder and night eating syndrome: a comparative study of disordered eating. *Journal of Consulting and Clinical Psychology*, 73(6), 1107–1115.

Andersen, G.S., Stunkard, A.J., Sorensen, T.I., Petersen, L., & Heitmann, B.L. (2004). Night eating and weight change in middle-aged men and women. *International Journal of Obesity and Related Metabolic Disorder*, 28, 1338–1343.

Auger, R. (2006). Sleep-related eating disorder. *Psychiatry*, 11, 64–69.

Beck, A.T., Steer, R.A., & Garbin, M.G. (1988). Psychometric properties of the Beck Depression Inventory: twenty-five years of evaluation. *Clinical Psychology Review*, 8, 77–100.

Birketvedt, G.S., Florholmen, J., Sundsfjord, J., Osterud, B., Dinges, D., Bilker, W., & Stunkard, A.J. (1999). Behavioral and neuroendocrine characteristics of the night eating syndrome. *Journal of the American Medical Association*, 282, 657–663.

Endicott, J., Nee, J., Harrison, W., & Blumenthal, R. (1993). Quality of Life Enjoyment and Satisfaction Questionnaire (Q-LES-Q): a new measure. *Psychopharmacology Bulletin*, 29, 321–326.

Friedman, S., Even, C., Dardennes, R., & Guelfi, J.D. (2002). Light therapy, obesity, and night-eating syndrome. *The American Journal of Psychiatry*, 159, 875–876.

Gluck, M.E., Geliebter, A., & Satov, T. (2001). Night eating syndrome is associated with depression, low self-esteem, reduced daytime hunger, and less weight loss in obese outpatients. *Obesity Research*, 9, 264–267.

Goldstein, D.J., Wilson, M.G., Thompson, J.H., Potvin, J.H., & Rampey Jr., A.H. (1995). Long-term treatment of bulimia nervosa. Fluoxetine bulimia nervosa research group. *The British Journal of Psychiatry*, 166, 660–666.

James, S. (1991). The approximate multinormal probabilities applied to correlated multiple endpoints in clinical trials. *Statistics in Medicine*, 10, 1123–1135.

Leon, A.C., & Heo, M. (2005). A comparison of multiplicity adjustment strategies for correlated binary endpoints. *Journal of Biopharmaceutical Statistics*, 15, 839–855.

Lundgren, J.D., *et al.* (2006). Prevalence of the night eating syndrome in a psychiatric population. *American Journal of Psychiatry*, 163(1), 156–158.

Marshall, H.M., Allison, K.C., O'Reardon, J.O., Birketvedt, G., & Stunkard, A.J. (2004). The night eating syndrome among nonobese persons. *International Journal of Eating Disorders*, 35, 217–222.

Miller, J.D., Morin, L.P., Schwartz, W.J., & Moore, R.Y. (1996). New insights into the mammalian circadian clock. *Sleep*, 19, 641–667.

Miyaoka, T., *et al.* (2003). Successful treatment of nocturnal eating/drinking syndrome with selective serotonin reuptake inhibitors. *International Clinical Psychopharmacology*, 18 (3), 175–177.

Nestle, M., & Jacobson, M. (2000). Halting the obesity epidemic: a public health policy approach. *Public Health Reports*, 115, 12–24.

O'Reardon, J.P., Allison, K.C., & Stunkard, A.J. (2004). A clinical trial of sertraline in the treatment of the night eating syndrome. *International Journal of Eating Disorders*, 35, 16–26.

O'Reardon, J.P., Ringel, B.L., Dinges, D.F., Allison, K.C., Rogers, N.L., Martino, N.S., & Stunkard, A.J. (2004). Circadian eating and sleeping patterns in the night eating syndrome. *Obesity Research*, 12, 1789–1796.

O'Reardon, J.P., Peshek, A., & Allison, K. (2005). Night eating syndrome: diagnosis, epidemiology, and management. *CNS Drugs*, 19(12), 997–1008.

Pawlow, L.A., O'Neil, P.M., & Malcolm, R.J. (2003). Night eating syndrome: effects of brief relaxation training on stress, mood hunger and eating patterns. *International Journal of Obesity Related Metabolic Disorders*, 27, 970–978.

Rand, C.S., MacGreggor, A.M.C., & Stunkard, A.J. (1997). The night eating syndrome in the general population and among postoperative obesity surgery patients. *International Journal of Eating Disorders*, 22, 65–69.

Rush, A.J., *et al.* (2006). Bupropion-SR, sertraline, or venlafaxine-XR after failure of SSRIs for depression. *New England Journal of Medicine*, 354 (12), 1231–1242.

Spaggiari, M.C., Granella, F., Parrino, L., Marchesi, C., Melli, I., & Terzano, M.G. (1994). Nocturnal eating syndrome in adults. *Sleep*, 17, 339–344.

Stunkard, A.J., Grace, W.J., & Wolff, H.G. (1955). The night eating syndrome: a pattern of food intake in certain obese patients. *American Journal of Medicine*, 19, 78–86.

Stunkard, A.J., Berkowitz, R., Wadden, T., Tanrikut, C., Reiss, E., & Young, L. (1996). Binge eating disorder and the night eating syndrome. *International Journal of Obesity of Related Metabolic Disorders*, 20, 1–6.

Stunkard, A.J., Allison, K.C., Lundgren, J.D., Martino, N., Heo, M., Etemad, B., & O'Reardon, J.P. (2006). A paradigm for facilitating pharmacotherapy at a distance: treatment of the night eating syndrome. *Journal of Clinical Psychiatry*, 67, 1568–1572.

Verbeke, G., & Molenberghs, G. (1997). *Linear Mixed Models in Practice. A SAS-oriented Approach*. New York: Springer, pp. 222–233.

Winkelman, J.W. (2003). Treatment of nocturnal eating syndrome and sleep-related eating disorder with topiramate. *Sleep Medicine*, 4, 243–246.

Progress in Neurotherapeutics and Neuropsychopharmacology, 3:1, 259–274 © 2008 Cambridge University Press
DOI: 10.1017/S1748232107000134   Printed in the United Kingdom

Modafinil: A Candidate for Pharmacotherapy of Negative Symptoms in Schizophrenia

John H. Peloian

Department of Psychiatry, VA Greater Los Angeles Healthcare System; Email: jpeloian@ucla.edu

Joseph M. Pierre

Department of Psychiatry, VA Greater Los Angeles Healthcare System
Department of Psychiatry and Biobehavioral Sciences, Geffen School of Medicine at the University of California,
Los Angeles, USA; Email: joseph.pierre2@va.gov

ABSTRACT

Background: Although historically neglected in clinical research, negative symptoms of schizophrenia are now considered distinct targets of pharmacotherapy. While second-generation antipsychotic treatments were heralded as having a greater therapeutic impact on negative symptoms than their conventional antipsychotic counterparts, the size of this effect is modest. Adjunctive medications such as antidepressants offer limited efficacy, while stimulants have a poor risk–benefit profile. More recently, promising results have been demonstrated with pro-glutamatergic agents such as glycine or D-cycloserine, although a larger trial found no advantage with either agent compared with placebo. Modafinil, a novel wakefulness-promoting agent, is an intriguing candidate for adjunctive pharmacotherapy to treat negative symptoms in schizophrenia. We explored this therapeutic potential through a placebo-controlled trial of patients with prominent negative symptoms. *Methods*: We randomly assigned patients with schizophrenia or schizoaffective disorder to treatment with either modafinil or placebo for 8 weeks. Double-blind assessments of clinical symptoms and neurocognition were administered at baseline and every 2 weeks thereafter. *Results*: Twenty subjects were enrolled ($N = 10$ modafinil, $N = 10$ placebo). There were no significant differences between modafinil and placebo for changes in negative symptom ratings, the primary study endpoint. However, modafinil treatment was associated with a greater rate and degree of global improvement at study endpoint compared with placebo. No significant worsening of psychopathology was observed and modafinil was well-tolerated. *Interpretation*: Although no effect on negative symptoms was found, adjunctive therapy with modafinil may result in global improvements in patients with

Correspondence should be addressed to: Joseph M. Pierre, M.D., Co-chief, Schizophrenia Treatment Unit, VA West Los Angeles Healthcare Center, Los Angeles, USA; Associate Clinical Professor, Department of Psychiatry and Biobehavioral Sciences, David Geffen School of Medicine at UCLA, Los Angeles, USA; Email: joseph.pierre2@va.gov

schizophrenia who have prominent negative symptoms. These findings support additional research into a potential role for modafinil in the treatment of negative symptoms in schizophrenia.

Key words: cognition, deficit syndrome, modafinil, negative symptoms, schizophrenia.

Introduction and Overview

Negative symptoms of schizophrenia reflect reductions in aspects of higher cognitive, emotional, and psychological functioning. These symptoms may consist of avolition (loss of motivation, diminished drive, and apathy), alogia (impoverished thinking and speech), and affective flattening (resulting in a loss of facial expression, eye contact, and expressive gestures or vocal inflections). Negative symptoms were recognized as core features of schizophrenia by both Emil Kraepelin and Eugen Bleuler nearly a century ago. Since at least the early 1970s, this aspect of schizophrenia has been proposed as a separate domain with unique pathophysiological and therapeutic implications. Despite the clinical relevance of these symptoms, no drug has ever received a specific Food and Drug Administration (FDA) indication for the treatment of negative symptoms in schizophrenia (Kirkpatrick et al., 2006).

Negative symptoms have been observed to be functionally debilitating, associated with poor overall outcome, and only modestly responsive to antipsychotic treatment (Kirkpatrick et al., 2006; Milev et al., 2005; Tamminga et al., 1998; Arndt et al., 1995; Fenton & McGlashan, 1991; Carpenter et al., 1985). Although second-generation antipsychotic medications may have benefits over first-generation agents in terms of negative symptom response, there is controversy as to whether such effects are attributable to the improvement of primary negative symptoms or the remediation of secondary negative symptoms (Leucht et al., 1999; Carpenter, 1995). The separation of primary versus secondary negative symptoms is intended to distinguish between core aspects of schizophrenia (primary) and those symptoms which are caused by another process (secondary), such as positive symptoms or comorbid medical illness, extrapyramidal side effects (EPS), depression, or environmental factors. For example, the reduction of hallucinations or paranoia may cause a patient to appear better related and less distracted such that rated negative symptoms improve. Likewise, if a patient is switched from a conventional antipsychotic to a second-generation drug with a reduced EPS burden, improvements in bradykinesia or hypomimia could be rated as negative symptom improvement.

Patients with primary negative symptoms can be distinguished from other patients with considerable reliability (Kirkpatrick et al., 2006). Enduring primary negative symptoms are key features of the "deficit syndrome," a concept that has been proposed as a distinct subtype of schizophrenia (Kirkpatrick *et al.*, 2001). Studies indicate that patients with the deficit syndrome differ from non-deficit patients on measures of premorbid adjustment, illness outcome, depression, and brain structure and function (Amador *et al.*, 1999). In terms of antipsychotic response, it appears that second-generation antipsychotics are no better than conventional agents at treating primary negative symptoms amongst patient samples meeting criteria for the deficit syndrome (Kopelowicz *et al.*, 2000; Rosenheck *et al.*, 1999; Buchanan *et al.*, 1998; Breier *et al.*, 1994).

The efficacy of antipsychotic medications for negative symptoms is therefore disappointing in two respects. First, antipsychotic medications as a class do not appear to impact negative symptoms to any great degree (Erhart *et al.*, 2006; Kirkpatrick *et al.*, 2006; Laughren & Levin, 2006). Second, a substantial proportion of negative symptom improvements that are observed in acute antipsychotic trials are likely due to secondary negative symptom changes resulting from remediation of positive symptoms. Likewise, much of the apparent benefit on negative symptoms of the second-generation antipsychotics over their conventional counterparts can be attributed to their reduced EPS risk such that primary negative symptoms remain largely refractory to antipsychotic therapy. These conclusions support the need for the development of adjunctive medication strategies specifically targeting negative symptoms. Furthermore, a clinical trial design that employs prominent negative symptom sufferers with positive symptoms already stabilized through antipsychotic therapy is required to allow detection of primary negative symptom change (Kirkpatrick *et al.*, 2006).

Purpose of Our Trial

Historically, drug development has targeted "positive" psychotic symptoms (hallucinations, delusions, and disorganization) hoping that antipsychotic efficacy will extend to other aspects of schizophrenia, including negative symptoms. This presupposes that positive and negative symptoms share neurological mechanisms, leading to a shared treatment response. Due to the lack of success in treating primary negative symptoms with conventional and second-generation antipsychotics, it seems likely that distinct pathophysiologies underlie positive and negative symptoms. In fact, enduring explanatory models suggest that while positive symptoms arise from dopaminergic hyperactivity in mesolimbic pathways, negative symptoms are associated with dopaminergic hypofunction in the prefrontal cortex (Stone *et al.*, 2007; Davis *et al.*, 1991). Other findings have also implicated derangements in muscarinic, serotonergic, glutamatergic neurotransmission as underlying negative symptom pathology (Stone *et al.*, 2007; Goff & Evins, 1998). Such discoveries have stimulated investigation of novel pharmacotherapies targeting negative symptoms, although no robust effects have yet been detected.

Although selective serotonin-reuptake inhibitors (SSRIs) are routinely used in clinical practice for negative symptoms, studies exploring SSRI augmentation have yielded only modest and inconsistent results (Rummel *et al.*, 2005; Möller, 2004; Silver, 2003). A recent meta-analysis failed to support a role for SSRI's in the treatment of negative symptoms in schizophrenia (Sepehry *et al.*, 2007). While several promising trials have suggested potential efficacy with the pro-glutamatergic agents D-cycloserine and glycine (Evins *et al.*, 2002; Heresco-Levy *et al.*, 2002; Goff *et al.*, 1999; Heresco-Levy *et al.*, 1999; Javitt *et al.*, 1994), no advantage with either agent compared with placebo was found in a more recent, larger, multicenter trail (Buchanan *et al.*, 2007). A significant need for a viable therapy for negative symptoms in schizophrenia therefore remains.

Modafinil

Modafinil is a wakefulness-promoting agent that is currently approved for the treatment of excessive daytime sleepiness associated with narcolepsy, obstructive sleep apnea, and shift-work sleep disorder. Its mechanism of action is unclear with negligible affinity for dopaminergic, adrenergic, or serotonergic receptors. Several theories exist to account for the therapeutic actions of modafinil. First, laboratory studies have demonstrated modafinil's ability to activate the hypocretin-orexin system and the tuberomammillary nucleus (TMN) of the hypothalamus. Both cell groups are implicated in the regulation of wakefulness (Scammell *et al.*, 2000; Ferraro *et al.*, 1997). Second, Minzenberg and Carter (2007) hypothesized that modafinil's ability to elevate extracellular histaminergic neurons contained in the TMN of the anterior hypothalamus may be another cause of increased arousal. Data from animal studies have also raised the possibility that modafinil may regulate wakefulness by altering extracellular brain catecholamines such as serotonin and dopamine (Murillo-Rodriguez *et al.*, 2007; de Saint Hilaire *et al.*, 2001) or by impacting glutamatergic and GABAergic systems in brain areas that govern alertness, motivation, and arousal such as the cortex and hypothalamus (Ferraro *et al.*, 1999). That modafinil might facilitate glutamatergic transmission is of particular interest given increasing evidence supporting a theory of gluta-matergic hypofunction in schizophrenia (Stone *et al.*, 2007; Coyle, 2006). For these reasons, modafinil, with its possible hypothalamic, dopaminergic, and pro-glutamatergic activities, makes an intriguing candidate for pharmacotherapy of negative symptoms.

Clinically, modafinil has been shown to improve daytime sleepiness, fatigue, mood, short-term memory, reaction time, and quality of life in patients with nar-colepsy (Beusterien *et al.*, 1999; US Modafinil in Narcolepsy Multicenter Study Group, 1998; Pigeau *et al.*, 1995). Other reports have observed modafinil to improve fatigue and sedation in a variety of off-label conditions including neurologic disorders, antipsychotic-induced sedation, and major depression (Makela *et al.*, 2003; Rammohan *et al.*, 2002; Damian *et al.*, 2001; Teitelman, 2001; Menza *et al.*, 2000). More rigorously designed trials suggest that the clinical effects of modafinil in major depression are limited. A 6-week placebo-controlled study involving 118 depressed subjects revealed short-term improvements in fatigue and daytime sleepiness, but no differences compared to placebo in those symptoms or depression ratings by study endpoint (DeBattista *et al.*, 2003). Likewise, a multicenter trial evaluating partial SSRI responders treated with adjunctive modafinil demonstrated significant overall clinical improvement at endpoint compared to placebo, but no significant difference in primary outcome measures including fatigue, sleepiness, and depression (Fava *et al.*, 2005). On the other hand, encouraging results have recently emerged for suggesting a role for adjunctive modafinil in the treatment of bipolar depression. In a 6-week placebo-controlled trial of modafinil augmentation, both response and remission rates for depression were significantly greater compared to placebo by week 2 and extending through study endpoint (Frye *et al.*, 2007).

Within schizophrenia, modafinil has been suggested to have benefit for fatigue and possibly neurocognitive deficits (Sevy *et al.*, 2005; Spence *et al.*, 2005; Turner *et al.*, 2004). Yu and Maguire (2002) reported a single case in which the addition of modafinil improved the chronic negative symptoms (alogia, affect, anergia, and asociality) of a patient with schizophrenia within a week of administration. These improvements allowed the patient to effectively participate in a weight loss program and social groups. In a 4-week, uncontrolled, open-label, pilot study that evaluated adjunctive modafinil in patients with schizophrenia or schizoaffective disorder, significant improvement was seen in global functioning, as well as fatigue, negative symptoms, and cognitive function, while maintaining positive symptom stability (Rosenthal & Bryant, 2004).

Given these promising but exploratory lines of evidence suggesting a role for modafinil in negative symptoms, we performed a clinical trial to test the efficacy of modafinil for the treatment of negative symptoms in schizophrenia. This randomized, placebo-controlled study included patients with schizophrenia or schizoaffective disorder with prominent negative symptoms and positive symptoms stabilized with antipsychotic therapy. The patients were treated with either modafinil or placebo for 8 weeks.

Clinical Trial

Subjects

Trial subjects were outpatients of the VA West Los Angeles Medical Center. The inclusion criteria were: (1) age 18–65, (2) a diagnosis of schizophrenia or schizoaffective disorder based on the structured clinical interview for DSM-IV

(SCID; First *et al.*, 1996), (3) prominent negative symptoms as defined by a scale for the assessment of negative symptoms (SANS; Andreasen, 1982) total score $\geqslant 20$, (4) stability of antipsychotic medication (no change in dose in the preceding 4 weeks), (5) well-controlled positive symptoms defined by a brief psychiatric rating scale (BPRS; Overall & Gorham, 1962) psychosis factor (sum of 4 items: suspiciousness, unusual thought content, hallucinatory behavior, conceptual disorganization) $\leqslant 14$, (6) no substance dependence in the 6 month prior to the study, (7) no serious medical illness, (8) no concomitant use of monoamine oxidase inhibitors, and (9) no women of child bearing potential. The study was approved by an institutional review board approval and was conducted from March 2002 through March 2006.

Modafinil Dose

Subjects were randomly assigned to either modafinil or placebo, initiated at 1 tablet daily of either modafinil 100 mg or placebo. After the 1st week, the dose was increased to a maximum dose of either 2 tablets daily of modafinil 100 mg or placebo. Thereafter, doses could be reduced back to 1 tablet daily of modafinil 100 mg or placebo in the event of tolerability issues. Anecdotal case reports that emerged prior to and after the start of our trial have raised the potential for modafinil to cause psychotic exacerbation (Mariani & Hart, 2005; Narendran *et al.*, 2002) or manic induction (Wolf *et al.*, 2006; Ranjan & Chandra, 2005; Vorspan *et al.*, 2005). On the other hand, no liability has emerged from larger samples or controlled studies (Frye *et al.*, 2007; Nasr *et al.*, 2006; Fava *et al.*, 2005; Rosenthal & Bryant, 2004; Turner *et al.*, 2004). Nevertheless, in order to minimize risk, we chose to limit the maximum dose of modafinil to 200 mg/day, since manic or psychotic worsening has typically been reported at doses greater than 300 mg/day.

Trial Methods and Instruments

Double-blind assessments were performed at baseline and every 2 weeks thereafter. The primary outcome measure was a change in negative symptoms, as rated by the total SANS score. In addition, secondary outcomes included SANS subscales, the BPRS, clinical global impression-severity of illness (CGI-S) and CGI-improvement (CGI-I), and QOLI (quality of life inventory) scores. The schedule for the deficit syndrome (SDS) (Kirkpatrick *et al.*, 1989) was administered at baseline so that *post-hoc* analyses could examine whether modafinil exerted a differential effect on patients with or without the deficit syndrome. The SDS was administered by an independently trained rater with all other ratings made by raters blinded to deficit syndrome status.

Several neurocognitive measures were selected based on their association with negative symptoms (Buchanan *et al.*, 1994): the California Verbal Learning Test (CVLT) (Delis *et al.*, 1987), measuring repetition learning and memory, Degraded

Stimulus-Continuous Performance Test (DS-CPT) (Nuechterlein *et al.*, 1986), used to measure sustained attention and Trail-Making Test-B (TMT-B) (s) (Army Individual Test Battery, 1944), which evaluates visuomotor tracking and motor speed.

Ratings for EPS were performed every 2 weeks. Given the possibility that modafinil might reduce weight and affect sleep, weight, and self-reported sleep (both day and night) were monitored weekly, along with vital signs and other subjective side effects.

Analyses

Baseline characteristics of the two treatment groups were compared using either *t*-test or χ^2 tests, as appropriate (Table 1). Between-group comparisons were performed using last observation-carried forward (LOCF) repeated-measures analysis of variance, testing for the interaction of time and treatment group. For the CGI-I score (not measured at baseline), between-group comparison was analyzed using the *t*-test. Subjects were also dichotomized into those with and without clinical improvement, based on a CGI-I score ≤3, with between-group comparisons performed using χ^2 analysis. *Post-hoc* analyses using analysis of covariance were performed on SANS outcomes, with SDS results and concomitant antidepressant status as covariates.

Results

Attrition: Of the 20 subjects who started study medication, 17 (85%) completed double-blind treatment. All study drop-outs occurred at the discretion of the investigator, rather than a patient's request to stop the medication.

Efficacy: Change in total SANS score, the primary study outcome, improved modestly in both treatment groups, but showed no significant difference between modafinil and placebo (Table 2). There were likewise no significant group differences on any secondary outcomes, including change in BPRS, CGI-S, QOLI, or neurocognitive measures (Table 3). No significant covariant effect of deficit syndrome status or antidepressant status was found on SANS scores.

The main significant group difference of this trial was found with the endpoint CGI-I score. This single-item scale is designed to make a global assessment of overall illness improvement. The mean endpoint CGI-I score for modafinil-treated subjects was 3.2 ± 0.6, while mean CGI-I for placebo-treated patients was 4.1 ± 0.6

Table 1. **Baseline Characteristics**

VARIABLE	PLACEBO	MODAFINIL
Age (mean ± S.D.)	49.8 ± 7.0	49.7 ± 6.8
Sex (m/f)	9/1	10/0
Antidepressant Rx (*N*)	6 (60%)	6 (60%)
Deficit syndrome	5 (50%)	5 (50%)

Table 2. **Primary Outcomes by Treatment Group**

	PRIMARY OUTCOMES				EFFECT SIZE
	PLACEBO		MODAFINIL		
	BASELINE MEAN ± S.D.	ENDPOINT MEAN ± S.D.	BASELINE MEAN ± S.D.	ENDPOINT MEAN ± S.D.	
Negative symptoms					
SANS total	38.5 ± 8.4	36.1 ± 7.7	38.2 ± 7.6	36.0 ± 7.7	0.02
SANS alogia	2.2 ± 1.3	2.0 ± 1.1	2.4 ± 1.1	2.4 ± 1.2	0.14
SANS affective flattening	3.0 ± 0.82	2.6 ± 0.52	2.8 ± 0.79	2.6 ± 0.97	0.27
SANS avolition-apathy	3.1 ± 0.75	2.6 ± 0.70	3.6 ± 0.70	2.9 ± 0.74	0.33
SANS anhedonia-asociality	3.4 ± 0.70	3.3 ± 0.95	3.3 ± 0.67	3.0 ± 0.82	0.25

Adapted from *The Journal of Clinical Psychiatry.*

Table 3. **Secondary Outcomes by Treatment Group**

	SECONDARY OUTCOMES				EFFECT SIZE
	PLACEBO		MODAFINIL		
	BASELINE MEAN ± S.D.	ENDPOINT MEAN ± S.D.	BASELINE MEAN ± S.D.	ENDPOINT MEAN ± S.D.	
Psychopathology					
BPRS	40.6 ± 4.5	37.8 ± 4.2	37.6 ± 8.2	34.4 ± 7.0	0.07
CGI-severity	4.0 ± 0.7	4.1 ± 0.6	3.9 ± 0.7	3.6 ± 0.8	0.64
CGI-change (*t*-test)[a]	–	4.1 ± 0.6	–	3.2 ± 0.6	1.5
QOLI-SV	4.4 ± 1.2	4.2 ± 1.3	3.9 ± 1.4	4.0 ± 0.9	0.22
Cognition					
CVLT (words)	36.6 ± 14.6	39.7 ± 21.1	39.2 ± 9.9	43.2 ± 9.5	0.11
DS-CPT (A')	0.94 ± 0.05	0.93 ± 0.05	0.92 ± 0.08	0.92 ± 0.08	0.14
TMT-B (s)	150 ± 82.5	122 ± 55.9	140 ± 46.6	134 ± 73.6	0.74

[a]*t*-test: $t = 3.35$, df $= 18$, $p = 0.004$.

($t = 3.35$, $p = 0.004$). In addition, when a cut-off score of ≤ 3 on the CGI-I scale was used to dichotomize clinical improvement (≥ 4 or more indicates no improvement or worsening), there was a significantly greater proportion of responders in the modafinil group compared with placebo (Figure 1). The response rate was 7/10 for modafinil-treated subjects compared to 1/10 treated with placebo ($\chi^2 = 7.5$, $p = 0.006$). This was a robust finding that stood in contrast to the lack of significant differences among the primary and other secondary outcomes.

Safety and Tolerability: Modafinil was well-tolerated. Reported adverse events are shown in Table 4. A few modafinil-treated patients complained of edema ($N = 1$), tinnitus ($N = 1$), and a bitter taste ($N = 1$). Psychotic worsening occurred in 3 patients (1 on modafinil and 2 on placebo) and resulted in premature study discontinuation. Modafinil-treated subjects reported greater reductions in mean

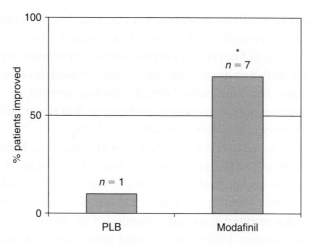

Fig. 1.
Clinical improvement (CGI-I-change ⩽3) at study endpoint by treatment group. $^{*}\chi^{2} = 7.5$, df $= 1, p = 0.006$. CGI-I = clinical global impression-improvement scale.

Table 4. **Miscellaneous Outcomes**

	PLACEBO		MODAFINIL		
Endpoint dose (mg)	180 ± 42		180 ± 42		
Drop-outs (*N*)	2 (20%)		1 (10%)		
Psychosis worsening (*N*)	2 (20%)		1 (10%)		
	BASELINE	ENDPOINT	BASELINE	ENDPOINT	EFFECT SIZE
Somatic side effects					
– Weight (lbs)	204.4 ± 29.8	205.2 ± 31.9	218.4 ± 45.3	215.5 ± 40.2	0.49
– Sleep night (h)	7.1 ± 1.3	7.1 ± 1.2	8.2 ± 2.1	7.9 ± 2.2	0.24
– Sleep day (h)	1.0 ± 0.8	0.64 ± 0.7	1.15 ± 1.0	0.3 ± 0.4	0.52

hours of daytime and nighttime sleep and experienced a greater degree of mean weight loss compared with placebo-treated patients, but these differences failed to reach statistical significance.

Novel Study Findings

Our trial was designed to be an exploratory, but randomized, prospective, and double-blinded study of modafinil for the treatment of negative symptoms in schizophrenia. Although other open-label reports and case studies of modafinil in schizophrenia with encouraging results have emerged (Rosenthal & Bryant,

2004; Yu & Maguire, 2002), no other placebo-controlled trials examining negative symptoms have been published to date. In contrast to these other uncontrolled reports, our trial did not reveal a greater impact on negative symptoms for
modafinil. These negative findings echo other studies of modafinil for fatigue in a
variety of conditions, in which well-designed, blinded, and placebo-controlled
trials failed to replicate more encouraging preliminary but uncontrolled reports
(Ondo *et al.*, 2005; Sevy *et al.*, 2005; Stankoff *et al.*, 2005).

Several explanations may account for these negative findings. First, modafinil
may simply not be effective for negative symptoms in schizophrenia. In our study,
this lack of effect was demonstrated in both patients with and without deficit
syndrome. On the other hand, it is possible that our decision to limit dosing to
modafinil 200 mg/day resulted in an undershooting of the therapeutic window for
modafinil in schizophrenia. Higher doses could prove more effective in future
studies.

Although we found no significant treatment advantage for modafinil with
regard to negative symptom outcomes, we did detect a significant difference in
overall illness improvement as measured by the endpoint CGI-I. In addition, a
sizeable advantage for modafinil was seen with 70% of modafinil-treated subjects
rated as CGI-I responders in contrast to only 10% of placebo-treated subjects.
Reinforced by several patient's subjective reports of enhanced well-being on
modafinil, we believe this is a "real" finding (and not simply type I error), albeit
one that in the face of no other associated symptomatic improvements is somewhat puzzling. Modafinil-treated subjects enjoyed greater overall improvement,
but our data gives no indication as to what specific symptomatic change resulted
in this global improvement.

One potential explanation for this discrepancy is that modafinil treatment
improved some symptoms that were not captured in our rating scales. In order to
explore an effect on depressive symptoms, we performed a *post-hoc* analysis of
extracted BPRS depressive items, but still found no significant effects. Also, only
three subjects had active depression diagnosed according to the DSM-IV. In
addition, the CGI-I was not influenced by deficit syndrome status, suggesting
that improvement was not limited to those with secondary negative symptoms
(e.g. due to comorbid depression). Therefore, global improvements did not seem
to be mediated by an effect on depressive symptoms.

An alternate possibility is that modafinil-treated patients did in fact experience
negative symptom improvements, but that they were not detected by the SANS,
where rateable improvement often depends on an actual change in behavior or
level of activity. Despite the established validity of the SANS, this and other existing negative symptom scales may be limited in their ability to detect subtle or very
specific negative symptom changes (Horan *et al.*, 2006). For example, improvements in alertness and arousal could be associated with a sense of subjective and

objective improvement that was captured in the CGI, but not the SANS. This possibility of subtle modafinil associated improvements in mood and arousal is supported by findings in major depression (Fava *et al.*, 2005) and in normal subjects (Taneja *et al.*, 2007). In addition, our study sample was mostly comprised of chronically ill men living in board and care settings with limited financial resources. Perhaps circumstances such as lack of money, social skills, or opportunities to be more active, prevented subjects from acting upon core negative symptom improvements. Finally, we noted that patients may sometimes be unaware that negative symptom improvements have occurred. At least one of our subjects reported no negative symptom change, but upon inadvertent discussion with his caretakers, it was discovered that he was in fact demonstrably more energetic and socially engaged.

Clinical Implications and Future Research

Although our study did not produce any effect on negative symptoms of schizophrenia with modafinil, our robust finding of global improvement suggests that there may yet be a role for modafinil in schizophrenia. Likewise, though we detected no change within a limited cognitive battery, there remains an interest in modafinil's potential as a cognitive enhancer (Mizenberg & Carter, 2007; Morein-Zamir *et al.*, 2007). Further investigation should include larger sample sizes to avoid the potential for type II errors, as well as exploration of modafinil beyond 200 mg/day. With regard to negative symptom ratings, taking greater care to obtain collateral or objective reports of improvement could be helpful. More importantly, we suspect that negative symptom *behaviors* may not improve to any large degree without the incorporation of psychosocial interventions with pharmacotherapy. While modafinil may prove useful in some patients with schizophrenia (e.g. those with iatrogenic over sedation or hypersomnia, etc.), it is likely that producing meaningful change in activity or sociality among patients who have been plagued by negative symptoms for years will require more than pharmacotherapy. There is increasing evidence that psychosocial treatments such as social skills training, cognitive remediation, employment, and family or cognitive therapies may be useful in treating negative symptoms (Shean, 2007; Greenwood *et al.*, 2005; Bark *et al.*, 2003; Bustillo *et al.*, 2001; Roder *et al.*, 2001). To the degree that symptoms of schizophrenia are largely independent (positive symptoms, negative symptoms, cognitive impairments), it is not surprising that multiple treatment modalities might be required to target all aspects of the disease and optimize outcome (Bark *et al.*, 2003). We suggest that future studies pair modafinil versus placebo with a psychosocial intervention in a 2×2 design that would provide subjects who experience pharmacologic improvement in negative symptoms with an avenue to facilitate the enactment of measurable changes in behavior.

References

Amador, X.F., Kirkpatrick, B., Buchanan, R.W., Carpenter, W.T., Marcinko, L., *et al.* (1999). Stability of the diagnosis of deficit syndrome in schizophrenia. *American Journal of Psychiatry*, 156, 637–639.

Andreasen, N.C. (1982). Negative symptoms in schizophrenia. *Archives of General Psychiatry*, 39, 784–788.

Arndt, S., Andreasen, N.C., Flaum, M., Miller, D., & Nopoulos, P. (1995). A longitudinal study of symptom dimensions in schizophrenia: prediction and pattern of change. *Archives of General Psychiatry*, 52, 352–360.

Army Individual Test Battery (1994). *Manual of Directions and Scoring*. Washington, DC: War Department, Adjutant General's Office.

Bark, N., Revheim, N., Huq, F., Khalderov, V., Ganz, Z.W., & Medalia, A. (2003). The impact of cognitive remediation on psychiatric symptoms of schizophrenia. *Schizophrenia Research*, 63, 229–235.

Beusterien, D.M., Rogers, A.E., Walsleben, J.A., Emsellem, H.A., Reblando, J.A., Wang, L., *et al.* (1999). Health-related quality of life effects of modafinil for treatment of narcolepsy. *Sleep*, 22, 757–765.

Breier, A., Buchanan, R.W., Kirkpatrick, B., Davis, O.R., Irish, D., Summerfelt, A., *et al.* (1994). Effects of clozapine on positive and negative symptoms in outpatients with schizophrenia. *American Journal of Psychiatry*, 151, 20–26.

Buchanan, R.W., Strauss, M.E., Kirkpatrick, B., Holstein, C., Breier, A., & Carpenter, W.T. Jr. (1994). Neuropsychological impairments in deficit vs nondeficit forms of schizophrenia. *Archives of General Psychiatry*, 51, 804–811.

Buchanan, R.W., Breier, A., Kirkpatrick, B., Ball, P., & Carpenter, W.T. Jr. (1998). Positive and negative symptom response to clozapine in schizophrenia patients with or without the deficit syndrome. *American Journal of Psychiatry*, 155, 751–760.

Buchanan, R.W., Javitt, D.C., Marder, S.R., Schooler, N.R., Gold, J.M., McMahon, R.P., *et al.* (2007). The cognitive and negative symptoms in schizophrenia trial (CONSIST): The efficacy of glutamatergic agents for negative symptoms and cognitive impairments. *American Journal of Psychiatry*, 10, 1593–1602.

Bustillo, J.R., Lauriello, J.R., Horan, W.P., & Keith, S.J. (2001). The psychosocial treatment of schizophrenia: an update. *American Journal of Psychiatry*, 158, 163–175.

Carpenter, W.T. (1995). Serotonin–dopamine antagonists and treatment of negative symptoms. *Journal of Clinical Psychopharmacology*, 15, 30S–35S.

Carpenter, W.T., Heinrichs, D.W., & Alphs, L.D. (1985). Treatment of negative symptoms. *Schizophrenia Bulletin*, 11, 440–452.

Coyle, J.T. (2006). Glutamate and schizophrenia: beyond the dopamine hypothesis. *Cell Molecular Neurobiology*, 26, 365–384.

Damian, M.S., Gerlach, A., Schmidt, F., Lehmann, E., & Reichmann, H. (2001). Modafinil for excessive daytime sleepiness in myotonic dystrophy. *Neurology*, 56, 794–796.

Davis, K.L., Kahn, R.S., Ko, G., & Davidson, M. (1991). Dopamine in schizophrenia: a review and reconceptualization. *American Journal of Psychiatry*, 148, 1474–1486.

DeBattista, C., Doghramji, K., Menza, M.A., Rosenthal, M.H., & Fieve, R.R. (2003). Adjunct modafinil for the short-term treatment of fatigue and sleepiness in patients with major depressive disorder: a preliminary double-blind, placebo-controlled study. *Journal of Clinical Psychiatry*, 64, 1057–1064.

Delis, D.C., Dramer, J.H., Kaplan, E., *et al.* (1987). *The California Verbal Learning Test (manual)*. San Antonio, TX: The Psychological Corporation.

de Saint Hilaire, Z., Orosco, M., & Rouch, C. (2001). Variation in extracellular monoamines in the prefrontal cortex and medial hypothalamus after modafinil administration: a microdialysis study in rats. *Neuroreport*, 12, 3533–3537.

Erhart, S.M., Marder, S.R., & Carpenter, W.T. (2006). Treatment of schizophrenia negative symptoms: future prospects. *Schizophrenia Bulletin*, 32, 234–237.

Evins, A.E., Amico, E., Posever, T.A., Posever, T.A., Toker, R., & Goff, D.C. (2002). D-cycloserine added to risperidone in patients with primary negative symptoms of schizophrenia. *Schizophrenia Research*, 56, 19–23.

Fava, M., Thase, M.E., & DeBattista, C. (2005). A multicenter, placebo-controlled study of modafinil augmentation in partial responders to selective serotonin reuptake inhibitors with persistent fatigue and sleepiness. *Journal of Clinical Psychiatry*, 66, 85–93.

Fenton, W.S., & McGlashan, T.H. (1991). Natural history of schizophrenia subtypes: positive and negative symptoms and long-term course. *Archives of General psychiatry*, 48, 978–986.

Ferraro, L., Antonelli, T., O'Connor, W.T., Tanganelli, S., Rambert, F., & Fuxe, K. (1997). The antinarcoleptic drug modafinil increases glutamate release in thalamic areas and hippocampus. *Neuroreport*, 8, 2883–2887.

Ferraro, L., Antonelli, T., Tanganelli, S., O'Connor, W.T., Perez de la Mora, M., Mendez-Franco, J., et al. (1999). The Vigilance promoting drug modafinil increases extracellular glutamate levels in the medial preoptic area and the posterior hypothalamus of the conscious rat: prevention by local $GABA_A$ receptor blockade. *Neuropsychopharmacology*, 4, 346–356.

First, M.B., Spitzer, R.L., Gibbon, M., & Williams, J.B.W. (1996). *Structured Clinical Interview for DSM-IV Axis I Disorders, Patient Edition (Version 2.0)*. New York, NY: Biometrics Research, New York State Psychiatric Institute.

Frye, M.A., Grunze, H., Suppes, T., McElroy, S.L., Keck, P.E. Jr., Walden, J., et al. (2007). A placebo-controlled evaluation of adjunctive modafinil in the treatment of bipolar depression. *American Journal of Psychiatry*, 164, 1242–1249.

Goff, D.C., & Evins, A.E. (1998). Negative symptoms in schizophrenia: neurobiological model and treatment response. *Harvard Review of Psychiatry*, 6, 59–77.

Goff, D.C., Tsai, G., Levitt, J., Amico, E., Manoach, D., Schoenfeld, D.A., et al. (1999). A placebo-controlled trial of D-cycloserine added to conventional neuroleptics in patients with schizophrenia. *Archives of General Psychiatry*, 56, 21–27.

Greenwood, K.E., Landau, S., & Wykes, T. (2005). Negative symptoms and specific cognitive impairments as combined targets for improved functional outcome within cognitive remediation therapy. *Schizophrenia Bulletin*, 31, 910–921.

Heresco-Levy, U., Javitt, D.C., Ermilov, M., Mordel, C., Silipo, G., & Lichtenstein, M. (1999). Efficacy of high-dose glycine in the treatment of enduring negative symptoms of schizophrenia. *Archives of General Psychiatry*, 56, 21–27.

Heresco-Levy, U., Ermilov, M., Shimoni, J., Shapira, B., Silipo, G., & Javitt, D.C. (2002). Placebo-controlled trial of D-cycloserine added to conventional neuroleptics, olanzapine, or risperidone in schizophrenia. *American Journal of Psychiatry*, 159, 480–482.

Horan, W.P., Kring, A.M., & Blanchard, J.J. (2006). Anhedonia in schizophrenia: a review of assessment strategies. *Schizophrenia Bulletin*, 32, 259–273.

Javitt, D.C., Zylberman, I., Zukin, S.R., Heresco-Levy, U., & Lindenmayer, J.P. (1994). Amelioration of negative symptoms in schizophrenia by glycine. *American Journal of Psychiatry*, 151, 1234–1236.

Kirkpatrick, B., Buchanan, R.W., Mckenney, P.D., Alphs, L.D., & Carpenter, W.T. (1989). The schedule for the deficit syndrome: an instrument for research in schizophrenia. *Psychiatry Research*, 30, 119–124.

Kirkpatrick, B., Buchanan, R.W., Ross, D.E., & Carpenter, W.T. Jr. (2001). A separate disease within the syndrome of schizophrenia. *Archives of General Psychiatry*, 58, 165–171.

Kirkpatrick, B., Fenton, W.S., Carpenter, W.T., & Marder, S.R. (2006). The NIMH-MATRICS consensus statement on negative symptoms. *Schizophrenia Bulletin*, 32, 214–219.

Kopelowicz, A., Zarate, R., Tripodis, K., Gonzalez, V., & Mintz, J. (2000). Differential efficacy of olanzapine for deficit and nondeficit negative symptoms in schizophrenia. *American Journal of Psychiatry*, 157, 987–993.

Laughren, T., & Levin, R. (2006). Food and drug administration perspective on negative symptoms in schizophrenia as a target for a drug treatment claim. *Schizophrenia Bulletin*, 32, 220–222.

Lehman, A.F. (1988). A quality of life interview for the chronically mentally ill (QOLI). *Evaluation and Program Planning*, 11, 51–62.

Leucht, S., Pitschel-Walz, G., Abraham, D., & Kissling, W. (1999). Efficacy and extrapyramidal side-effects of the new antipsychotics olanzapine, quetiapine, risperidone, and sertindole compared to conventional antipsychotics and placebo: a meta-analysis of randomized controlled trials. *Schizophrenia Research*, 35, 51–68.

Makela, E.H., Miller, K., & Cutlip, W.D. (2003). Three case reports of modafinil use in treating sedation induced by antipsychotic medications. *Journal of Clinical Psychiatry*, 61, 378–381.

Mariani, J.J., & Hart, C.L. (2005). Psychosis associated with modafinil and shift work. *American Journal of Psychiatry*, 10, 1983.

Menza, M.A., Kaufman, K.R., & Castellanos, A. (2000). Modafinil augmentation of antidepressant treatment in depression. *Journal of Clinical Psychiatry*, 61, 378–381.

Milev, P., Ho, B.C., Arndt, S., & Andreasen, N.C. (2005). Predictive values of neurocognition and negative symptoms on functional outcome in schizophrenia: a longitudinal first-episode study with 7-year follow-up. *American Journal of Psychiatry*, 162(2005), 495–506.

Mizenberg, M.J., & Carter, C.S. (2007). Modafinil: A review of neurochemical actions and effects on cognition. *Neuropsychopharmacology* (in press).

Möller, H.J. (2004). Non-neuroleptic approaches to treating negative symptoms in schizophrenia. *European Archives of Psychiatry and Clinical Neuroscience*, 254, 108–116.

Morein-Zamir, S., Turner, D., & Shakian, B.J. (2007). A review of the effects of modafinil on cognition in schizophrenia. *Schizophrenia Bulletin* (in press).

Murillo-Rodriguez, E., Haro, R., Palomero-Rivero, M., Millan-Aldaco, D., & Drucker-Colin, R. (2007). Modafinil enhances extracellular levels of dopamine in the nucleus accumbens and increases wakefulness in rats. *Behavioural Brain Research*, 176, 353–357.

Narendran, R., Young, C.M., Valenti, A.M., Nickolova, M.K., & Pristach, C.A. (2002). Is psychosis exacerbated by modafinil? *Archives of General Psychiatry*, 59, 292–293.

Nasr, S., Wendt, B., & Steiner, K. (2006). Absence of mood switch with and tolerance to modafinil: a replication study from a large private practice. *Journal of Affective Disorders*, 95, 111–114.

Nuechterlein, K.H., Edell, W.S., Norris, M., & Dawson, M.E. (1986). Attentional vulnerability indicators, thought disorder, and negative symptoms. *Schizophrenia Bulletin*, 12, 408–426.

Ondo, W.G., Fayle, R., Atassi, F., & Jankovic, J. (2005). Modafinil for daytime somnolence in Parkinson's disease: double blind, placebo controlled parallel trial. *Journal of Neurology Neurosurgery and Psychiatry*, 76, 1636–1639.

Overall, J.E., & Gorham, D.R. (1962). The brief psychiatric rating scale. *Psychological Report*, 10, 799–812.

Pierre, J.M., Peloian, J.H., Wirshing, D.A., Wirshing, W.C., & Marder, S.R. (2007). A randomized, double-blind, placebo-controlled trial of modafinil for negative symptoms in schizophrenia. *The Journal of Clinical Psychiatry*, 68, 705–710. Copyright 2007, Physicians Postgraduate Press. Adapted or reprinted by permission.

Pigeau, R., Naitoh, P., Buguet, A., McCann, C., Baranski, J., Taylor, M., et al. (1995). Modafinil, D-amphetamine and placebo during 64 hours of sustained mental work, 1: effects of mood, fatigue, cognitive performance and body temperature. *Journal of Sleep Research*, 4, 212–228.

Rammohan, K.W., Rosenberg, J.H., Lynn, D.J., Blumenfeld, A.M., Pollack, C.P., & Nagaraja, H.N. (2002). Efficacy and safety of modafinil (provigil) for the treatment of fatigue in multiple sclerosis: a two centre phase 2 study. *Journal of Neurology Neurosurgery and Psychiatry*, 72, 179–183.

Ranjan, S., & Chandra, P.S. (2005). Modafinil-induced irritability and aggression? A report of 2 bipolar patients. *Journal of Clinical Psychopharmacology*, 25, 628–629.

Roder, V., Zorn, P., Muller, D., & Brenner, H.D. (2001). Improving recreational, residential, and vocational outcomes for patients with schizophrenia. *Psychiatric Services*, 52, 1439–1441.

Rosenheck, R., Dunn, L., Peszke, M., Cramer, J., Xu, W., Thomas, J., et al. (1999). Impact of clozapine on negative symptoms and on the deficit syndrome in refractory schizophrenia. *American Journal of Psychiatry*, 156, 88–93.

Rosenthal, M.H., & Bryant, S.L. (2004). Benefits of adjunct modafinil in an open-label, pilot study in patients with schizophrenia. *Clinical Neuropharmacology*, 27, 38–43.

Rummel, C., Kissling, W., & Leucht, S. (2005). Antidepressants as add-on treatment to antipsychotics for people with schizophrenia and pronounced negative symptoms: a systematic review of randomized trials. *Schizophrenia Research*, 80, 85–97.

Scammell, T.E., Estabrooke, I.V., McCarthy, M.T., Chemelli, R.M., Yanagisawa, M., Miller, M.S., et al. (2000). Hypothalamic arousal regions are activated during modafinil-induced wakefulness. *Journal of Neuroscience*, 20, 8620–8628.

Sepehry, A.A., Potvin, S., Elie, R., & Stip, E. (2007). Selective serotonin reuptake inhibitor (SSRI) add-on therapy for the negative symptoms of schizophrenia: a meta-analysis. *Journal of Clinical Psychiatry*, 68, 604–610.

Sevy, S., Rosenthal, M.H., Alvir, J., Meyer, S., Visweswaraiah, H., Gunduz-Bruce, H., et al. (2005). Double-blind, placebo-controlled study of modafinil for fatigue and cognition in schizophrenia patients treated with psychotropic mediations. *Journal of Clinical Psychiatry*, 66, 839–843.

Shean, G.D. (2007). Recent developments in psychosocial treatments for schizophrenic patients. *Expert Reviews on Neurotherapy*, 7, 817–827.

Silver, H. (2003). Selective serotonin reuptake inhibitor augmentation in the treatment of negative symptoms of schizophrenia. *International Clinical Psychopharmacology*, 18, 305–313.

Spence, S.A., Green, R.D., Wilkinson, I.D., & Hunter, M.D. (2005). Modafinil modulates anterior cingulated function in chronic schizophrenia. *British Journal of Psychiatry*, 187, 55–61.

Stankoff, B., Waubant, E., Confavreux, C., Edan, G., Debouverie, M., Rumbach, L., et al. (2005). Modafinil for fatigue in MS: a randomized placebo-controlled double-blind study. *Neurology*, 64, 1139–1143.

Stone, J.M., Morrison, P.D., & Pilowsky, L.S. (2007). Glutamate and dopamine dysregulation in schizophrenia – a synthesis and selective review. *Journal of Psychopharmacology*, 21, 440–452.

Tamminga, C.A., Buchanan, R.W., & Gold, J.W. (1998). The role of negative symptoms and cognitive dysfunction in schizophrenia outcome. *International Clinical Psychopharmacology*, 13, S21–S26.

Taneja, I., Haman, K., Shelton, R.C., & Robertson, D. (2007). A randomized, double-blind, crossover trial of modafinil on mood. *Journal of Clinical Psychopharmacology*, 27, 76–79.

Teitelman, E. (2001). Off-label uses of modafinil. *American Journal of Psychiatry*, 158, 1341.

Turner, D.C., Clark, L., Pomarol-Clotet, E., McKenna, P., Robbins, T.W., & Sahakian, B.J. (2004). Modafinil improves cognition and attention set shifting in patient with chronic schizophrenia. *Neuropsychopharmacology*, 29, 1363–1373.

US Modafinil in Narcolepsy Multicenter Study Group (1998). Randomized trial of modafinil for the treatment of pathological somnolence in narcolepsy. *Annals of Neurology*, 43, 88–97.

Vorspan, F., Warot, D., Consoli, A., Cohen, D., & Mazet, P. (2005). Mania in a boy treated with modafinil for narcolepsy. *American Journal of Psychiatry*, 162, 813–814.

Wolf, J., Fiedler, U., Anghelescu, I., & Schwertferger, N. (2006). Manic switch in a patient with treatment-resistant bipolar depression treated with modafinil. *Journal of Clinical Psychiatry*, 67, 1817.

Yu, B.P., & Maguire, G.A. (2002). Can a wakefulness-promoting agent augment schizophrenia treatment? *Current Psychiatry*, 1, 52–57.

Progress in Neurotherapeutics and Neuropsychopharmacology, 3:1, 275–289 © 2008 Cambridge University Press
DOI: 10.1017/S1748232107000055   Printed in the United Kingdom

New Approaches to Treatment of Schizophrenia by Enhancing *N*-methyl-D-aspartate Neurotransmission

Guochuan Emil Tsai

Department of Psychiatry, Harbor-UCLA Medical Center, Torrance, CA, USA; Email: etsai@labiomed.org

ABSTRACT

Background: There is a great need to develop new antipsychotic agents. In addition to dopaminergic neurotransmission, glutamatergic neurotransmission has been implicated in the pathophysiology of schizophrenia. The most compelling link between glutamatergic *N*-methyl-D-aspartate (NMDA) neurotransmission and schizophrenia concerns the mechanism of action of the psychotomimetic drug phencyclidine and the dissociative anesthetic, ketamine; both are NMDA antagonists. The psychosis induced by the NMDA antagonists causes not only positive symptoms similar to the action of dopaminergic enhancers but also negative symptoms and cognitive deficits typical of schizophrenia in normal volunteers and worsening of the psychotic symptoms in patients with schizophrenia. Accordingly, enhancing NMDA neurotransmission should benefit the symptoms of schizophrenia. *Methods*: Most clinical trials were done by the addition of the NMDA-enhancing agents, glycine, D-serine, D-alanine, D-cycloserine and sarcosine to the stable regimens of antipsychotics in double-blind, placebo-controlled designs. *Results*: When taken together, the trials of NMDA-enhancing agents in patients with chronic schizophrenia receiving stable dose of antipsychotics, the NMDA-enhancing agents were effective in the domains of negative symptoms, cognition, depression, positive symptoms and general psychopathology. The agents also significantly improved extrapyramidal symptoms. No significant side-effects or safety concerns emerged. *Interpretation*: In addition to testing more lead compounds, dose-finding and long-term trials are required to determine the optimal dose and functional improvement capacity of NMDA receptor agonist. The agents may also be applied to prevention and the treatment for prodromal phases of the illness.

Key words: D-serine, glutamate, glycine transporter, NMDA, sarcosine, schizophrenia.

Correspondence should be addressed to: Guochuan E. Tsai, MD, PhD, Department of Psychiatry, Harbor-UCLA Medical Center, F9, 1000 W, Carson Street, Torrance, CA 90509, USA; Ph: +1 310 222 2890; Email: etsai@labiomed.org

Introduction

There is a great need to develop new antipsychotic agents, providing benefits for the substantial portion of patients with schizophrenia who are only partially responsive or resistant to the treatment of available antipsychotics. Also, given that both conventional and new generation atypical antipsychotics cause significant side-effects, it would be critically important that the new antipsychotic treatment is devoid of debilitating side-effects like extrapyramidal symptoms, tardive dyskinesia or metabolic syndrome (Henderson, 2005). The objective of this paper is to review the clinical trials of new treatments of schizophrenia based upon the hypofunction hypothesis of N-methyl-D-aspartate (NMDA) neurotransmission of schizophrenia.

Until the neurobiology of schizophrenia is elucidated, new therapies will be based upon pharmacological models of schizophrenia. Current antipsychotics are related to the dopaminergic and serotoninergic models of schizophrenia. In addition to dopaminergic and serotoninergic neurotransmission, glutamatergic neurotransmission has been implicated in the pathophysiology of schizophrenia (Tsai & Coyle, 2001; Olney et al., 1999). NMDA receptors, a subtype of ionotropic glutamate receptors, play an important role in neurodevelopment and cognition (Robbins & Murphy, 2006). The most compelling link between the NMDA system and schizophrenia concerns the mechanism of action of the psychotomimetic drug phencyclidine and the dissociative anesthetic, ketamine; both are NMDA antagonists (for reviews, see Tsai & Coyle, 2001; Halberstadt, 1995). The psychosis induced by the NMDA antagonists causes not only positive symptoms similar to the effects of dopaminergic agonists but also negative symptoms and cognitive deficits typically associated with schizophrenia in normal volunteers and worsening of the psychotic symptoms in patients with schizophrenia (Malhotra et al., 1997; Lahti et al., 1995; Krystal et al., 1994). These findings are in agreement with hypofunction of NMDA neurotransmission in schizophrenia, and it is postulated that the psychotomimetic effects may not be limited to the non-competitive antagonists but could result from any dysfunctional attenuation of NMDA neurotransmission (Olney & Farber, 1995).

The pharmacological model of NMDA hypofunction has been strengthened recently by two lines of studies. First, glutamate and glycine (or D-serine, D-alanine) serve as co-agonists at the NMDA receptor with activation of both the glutamate and "glycine" binding sites required for channel opening (Thomson et al., 1989). Inasmuch as agonists on the NMDA recognition site are excitotoxic, molecules acting on the obligatory glycine co-agonist site of the NMDA receptor (NMDA-glycine site) are more promising therapeutic candidates. Several agents, directly or indirectly enhancing NMDA function via the NMDA-glycine site (NMDA-enhancing agents) have been tested to determine their efficacy for the treatment of schizophrenia within the past 10–15 years. These include the agonists of the

NMDA-glycine site, glycine (Diaz *et al.*, 2005; Heresco-Levy *et al.*, 2004; 1999; 1996; Javitt *et al.*, 2001; 1994; Evins *et al.*, 2000; Potkin *et al.*, 1999; 1992; Leiderman *et al.*, 1996; Costa *et al.*, 1990; Rosse *et al.*, 1989; Waziri, 1988), D-serine (Heresco-Levy *et al.*, 2005; Tsai *et al.*, 1999; 1998), D-alanine (Tsai *et al.*, 2006) and a partial agonist D-cycloserine (Goff *et al.*, 2005; 1999a, b; 1996; 1995; Duncan *et al.*, 2004; Evins *et al.*, 2002; Heresco-Levy *et al.*, 2002; 1998; van Berckel *et al.*, 1999; 1996; Rosse *et al.*, 1996; Cascella *et al.*, 1994). Of these agents, D-cycloserine is marketed (use in schizophrenia is off-label), the rest are simple amino acid natural compounds. Most of the studies of the NMDA-enhancing agents showed significant improvement in multiple symptom domains of schizophrenia including positive, negative, cognitive and depressive symptoms. However, the effect of D-cycloserine is limited to negative symptoms (Goff *et al.*, 2005; 1999a, b; 1996; 1995; Duncan *et al.*, 2004; Evins *et al.*, 2002; Heresco-Levy *et al.*, 2002; 1998; van Berckel *et al.*, 1999; 1996; Rosse *et al.*, 1996; Cascella *et al.*, 1994).

Another approach to enhance NMDA neurotransmission is to block the reuptake of glycine through the glycine transporter-1 (GlyT-1). GlyT-1 plays a pivotal role in maintaining the concentration of glycine within synapses at a sub-saturating level. The anatomical distribution of GlyT-1 is parallel to that of the NMDA receptor (Smith *et al.*, 1992). Supporting the critical role GlyT-1 plays in NMDA neurotransmission, the GlyT-1 inhibitor, a sarcosine analog – *N*[3-(4'-fluorophenyl)-3-(4'-phenylphenoxy)propyl]sarcosine – and the GlyT-1 knockdown mutation have been shown to enhance NMDA neurotransmission (Tsai *et al.*, 2004b; Chen *et al.*, 2003; Kinney *et al.*, 2003; Bergeron *et al.*, 1998). Sarcosine is an endogenous inhibitor of GlyT-1. Supporting its NMDA-enhancing and antipsychotic function, sarcosine had shown clinical efficacy when added to conventional and atypical antipsychotics (Tsai *et al.*, 2004a).

The second line of studies supporting hypofunction of NMDA neurotransmission in schizophrenia exploits a common defect involving the glutamatergic synapses in families and established by a series of genetic linkage studies (Harrison & Owen, 2003). NMDA neurotransmission is influenced in one way or another by most if not all of the putative susceptibility genes including proline dehydrogenase, dysbindin, neuregulin 1, disrupted-in-schizophrenia 1, V-akt murine thymoma viral oncogene homolog 1, regulator of G-protein signaling-4 (Robbins & Murphy, 2006) and metabotropic glutamate receptor-3 (Harrison & Weinberger, 2005). Of these risk genes identified, D-amino acid oxidase (DAAO) and G72, a primate specific activator of DAAO, are directly involved in NMDA neurotransmission. G72, a primate specific gene, encodes a protein that activates DAAO, the enzyme that catabolizes D-serine and D-alanine (Chumakov *et al.*, 2002). DAAO appears to be the critical determinant of D-serine levels as its activity correlates inversely with D-serine levels both regionally and developmentally

(Hashimoto, 2002). If G72 function is facilitated, it upregulates DAAO activity and consequently, metabolism of D-serine and D-alanine are enhanced to contribute to hypofunction of NMDA neurotransmission. Over the last 3 years, seven studies have demonstrated an association of G72 with the risk for schizophrenia and two with the risk for bipolar disorder (Korostishevsky et al., 2006; 2004; Addington et al., 2004; Chen et al., 2004; Schumacher et al., 2004a, b; Wang et al., 2004; Hattori et al., 2003; Chumakov et al., 2002). The replication of the association of G72 with the risk for schizophrenia is intriguing, given recent findings that serum and cerebrospinal fluid (CSF) levels of D-serine are reduced in schizophrenic subjects (Hashimoto et al., 2005; 2003). Consistent with the NMDA hypofunction hypothesis of schizophrenia, one study reported increased expression of G72 in prefrontal cortex (Hattori et al., 2003).

Trials of NMDA-Enhancing Treatment

Overall, 22 randomized, double-blind trials of the NMDA-enhancing agents involving about 500 schizophrenic patients are published. Most are small proof of concept trials; with few exceptions, most trials enrolled 10–40 subjects. Also, most studies are of short-term duration of 4–8 weeks. Of these studies, nine studied the efficacy of glycine (Diaz et al., 2005; Heresco-Levy et al., 2004; 1999; 1996; Javitt et al., 2001; 1994; Evins et al., 2000; Potkin et al., 1999; 1992), seven studied D-cycloserine (Goff et al., 2005; 1999; Duncan et al., 2004; Heresco-Levy et al., 2002a; 1998; van Berckel et al., 1999; Rosse et al., 1996), three studied D-serine (Heresco-Levy et al., 2005; Tsai et al., 1999; 1998) and two with sarcosine (Lane et al., 2006a; Tsai et al., 2004a). There was a single study examining the effect of D-alanine (Tsai et al., 2006). In addition, there is one study comparing D-serine and sarcosine in patients with acute exacerbations of schizophrenia (Lane et al., 2005).

Standard symptom rating scales, including the Brief Psychiatric Rating Scale, Positive and Negative Syndrome Rating Scale (PANSS) and Scale for the Assessment of Negative Symptoms were applied in all trials. Although most of the trials of NMDA-enhancing agents reveal positive findings, there are many questions regarding NMDA-enhancing treatment that remain unaddressed. The effects of the NMDA-enhancing agents on different symptom domains are inconsistent, with earlier reports suggesting that the actions are mainly on the negative symptoms and later reports extending to the positive, cognitive and depressive symptoms. Furthermore, it is unclear which of the NMDA-enhancing agents – full agonists or partial agonists of the NMDA-glycine site or GlyT-1 inhibitor – are superior to the others; or whether they are similar in their efficacy possibly due to their final common action of enhancing the NMDA neurotransmission. In addition, most studies applied an add-on strategy and the concomitant antipsychotics were variable with no clear evidence that NMDA-enhancing agent is better for patients receiving conventional antipsychotics or the atypical antipsychotics, including clozapine. Moreover, it remains unclear whether NMDA enhancers alone can serve as antipsychotics for schizophrenia.

Overall Effects of NMDA-Enhancing Agents on Key Symptom Domains

Collectively, compared with placebo, NMDA-enhancing agents added on to antipsychotics were effective in improving the critical symptom domains of negative, positive, cognitive and depressive symptom of schizophrenia. In contrast to early studies which suggested that the therapeutic effects were mainly on negative symptoms (Javitt *et al.*, 2001; 1994; Goff *et al.*, 1999), we found that the effects extend to positive, cognitive and depressive symptoms. Overall, the effect sizes (ES) are in the small to medium range similar to those of the atypical antipsychotics (Davis *et al.*, 2003). When considering all the studies, the pooled ES of clinical efficacy of NMDA-enhancing agents is 0.26 for total psychopathology. The efficacy of the symptom domains is in decreasing order for negative symptoms (ES = 0.29), cognitive symptoms (0.25), depressive symptoms (0.23), positive symptoms (0.14) and general psychopathology (0.10).

The wide spectrum of the therapeutic effects of the NMDA-enhancing agents suggests that these agents can be useful not only for schizophrenia but potentially also for other mental disorders that have psychotic, cognitive or mood manifestations. For the same reason, there is a strong argument for the MDA-enhancing agents to be tested as a sole pharmacotherapeutic agent in addition to add-on treatment for schizophrenia.

Effect of NMDA Receptor Agonists and Concomitant Antipsychotics on Different Symptom Domains

Negative symptoms are often refractory to antipsychotic treatment with the exception of clozapine and, to a lesser degree, the other atypical antipsychotics (Gasquet *et al.*, 2005). NMDA-enhancing agents have a therapeutic effect on the negative symptoms in patients with chronic schizophrenia who were receiving stable doses of antipsychotics before the initiation of the NMDA-enhancing treatments. Most of the patients were resistant to antipsychotic treatment or fulfilled deficit syndrome criteria and were chronically ill (Heresco-Levy *et al.*, 1999; Tsai *et al.*, 1998). The improvement in negative symptoms by NMDA-enhancing agents can have critical implications in the long-term functional outcome of patients with schizophrenia since negative symptoms are one of the main causes of disability and poor outcome (Milev *et al.*, 2005).

Similarly, neurocognitive impairment also is associated with the outcome and adaptive function of patients with schizophrenia. It is suggested that cognitive impairment may have a stronger relationship with poor outcome than other symptoms domains (Green, 1996). Although there is a significant effect of the NMDA-enhancing agents on the scores of the PANSS-cognitive subscale, most studies are short-term trials evaluating symptom reduction and lack an assessment of cognitive domains by neurocognitive testing. One study indicated an improvement in performance on the Wisconsin Card Sorting Test (Tsai et al., 1998) and another demonstrated a significant increase in temporal lobe activation during a word fluency task for the patients receiving D-cycloserine (Yurgelun-Todd et al., 2005). However, 66% of the variance in cognitive functioning cannot be explained by the PANSS-cognitive measurement (Good et al., 2004). In addition, long-term functional assessment has not been a focus of these studies except for a negative study of D-cycloserine over 24 weeks (Goff et al., 2005). Taken together, it is premature to draw any conclusion regarding the cognition-improving effect of the NMDA-enhancing agents. At the same time it is critically important to conduct long-term trials and neurocognitive studies to determine whether the symptom reduction, particularly the reductions in negative and cognitive symptoms can improve and sustain the cognition and long-term functional outcome of the patients with schizophrenia.

Effect of Different NMDA-Enhancing Agents

The NMDA-enhancing agents are not a homogenous group. D-serine and glycine treatment have a more comprehensive symptom improvement profile than does D-cycloserine. The ES of D-serine and glycine are larger than that of D-cycloserine in negative symptoms. This may be due to the fact that D-serine and glycine are full agonists and D-cycloserine is a partial agonist which can not fully activate the NMDA receptor; in fact, this agent behaves like an antagonist when there is a substantial agonist on the NMDA synapse (Watson et al., 1990) with significant worsening of the psychosis (van Berckel et al., 1999; Simeon et al., 1970). Consistent with its role as a full agonist and its low brain bioavailability by peripheral administration, higher doses of glycine are more effective for negative symptoms than the earlier studies using lower doses (Heresco-Levy et al., 2004; 1999; Javitt et al., 2001).

Although one of the three studies is a negative trial in patients receiving clozapine (Tsai et al., 1999), D-serine significantly improved negative, positive, cognitive, depressive and total psychopathology when the three studies were pooled together. The ES of D-serine was similar to that of glycine in negative, cognitive, depressive and total psychopathology. In addition, D-serine, but not glycine, improved the positive symptoms (Heresco-Levy et al., 2005; Tsai et al., 1998). This may be due to the better central bioavailability of serine (Oldendorf, 1971) or the existence of scattered inhibitory glycine receptors, GlyT-2, in the forebrain regions

(Zafra *et al.*, 1995) that may render the activation of glycine on NMDA-circuitry involved in positive symptoms insufficient. Since all the D-serine trials applied the same dosing strategy, it is not clear whether there is a dose–response relationship similar to the glycine trials with higher doses inducing better symptom improvement.

D-alanine is another full agonist of the NMDA-glycine site. D-alanine has been tested only by the author's group and it showed a comprehensive efficacy profile as D-serine (Tsai *et al.*, 2006). More studies of D-alanine will have to be conducted to have a meaningful comparison of its efficacy with other NMDA-enhancing agents.

Although there are several GlyT-1 inhibitors in preclinical development (Lechner, 2006), only sarcosine had been tested in three studies; two in chronic stable patients (Lane *et al.*, 2006a; Tsai *et al.*, 2004a) and the other in patients with acute exacerbations (Lane *et al.*, 2005). In the single sarcosine trial in chronic patients receiving stable dose of non-clozapine antipsychotics, the efficacy was similar to D-serine and D-alanine (Tsai *et al.*, 2004a). Subanalysis of the risperidone-treated patients also indicated a therapeutic effect of sarcosine. A recent study suggested that sarcosine can benefit acutely ill patients with schizophrenia on concurrent risperidone therapy (Lane *et al.*, 2005); no improvement in positive symptoms was seen, but the other symptom domains improved significantly. This finding indicates that a GlyT-1 inhibitor may be more efficacious than NMDA-glycine site agonists. Nevertheless, further confirmation and parallel comparison is required to determine the effective dosing ranges and whether the full agonist of the NMDA-glycine site or the GlyT-1 inhibitor is more efficacious in treating schizophrenia.

D-cycloserine has a very narrow therapeutic window, with doses higher than 100 mg worsening the symptoms of schizophrenia (van Berckel *et al.*, 1999; Goff *et al.*, 1995). D-cycloserine also worsens the symptoms of patients receiving clozapine, which raises an intriguing possibility that part of clozapine's effects may involve the NMDA-glycine site. This hypothesis is consistent with the negative finding of glycine, D-serine and sarcosine in patients receiving clozapine (Lane *et al.*, 2006a; Evins *et al.*, 2000; Potkin *et al.*, 1999; Tsai *et al.*, 1999) and the preclinical study which showed that clozapine can inhibit the system A amino acid transporter (Javitt *et al.*, 2005). This is not consistent with the report of Heresco-Levy *et al.* that four treatment-resistant patients taking clozapine responded favorable to glycine treatment (Heresco-Levy *et al.*, 1996). Most patients treated with clozapine are treatment resistant to other antipsychotic and represent a subpopulation of severe pathology. However, clozapine's efficacy has extended to a wide range of partial responders including stable outpatients with moderate symptoms (Breier *et al.*, 1994). It is possible that an augmenting effect of the NMDA-enhancing agents might be observed in less severely ill clozapine-treated subjects if the treatment effects depend on the disease severity, not the effect of clozapine on NMDA neurotransmission.

Almost all the studies of the NMDA-enhancing agents were performed with patients on stable doses of concomitant antipsychotics. The type of concomitant antipsychotics may affect the efficacy of the NMDA-enhancing agents. NMDA-enhancing agents as a whole are highly efficacious for patients on non-clozapine antipsychotics, including both typical and atypical antipsychotics. Agents added on atypical antipsychotics (risperidone and olanzapine), resulted in significant improvement in total psychopathology (ES = 0.47), negative symptoms (0.49), cognitive symptoms (0.30) and depressive symptoms (0.38), and there was a trend toward improvement in positive symptoms. These findings underscore the significance of NMDA enhancement as a new therapeutic approach in an era when the atypical antipsychotics are becoming the primary agents for the majority of the patients with schizophrenia. In addition, the ES for patients receiving concomitant non-clozapine atypical antipsychotics are larger than those receiving typical antipsychotics in negative and total psychopathology, which suggests there may exist synergistic therapeutic effects of the atypical antipsychotics and NMDA-enhancing agents. If this is confirmed, it provides an intriguing augmentation strategy for the patients who are partially responsive or resistant to the atypical antipsychotics. However, only two studies enrolled subjects receiving solely risperidone or olanzapine (Heresco-Levy et al., 2005; 2004); most studies include a small percentage of patients receiving typical antipsychotics. Therefore, the synergistic effects of the NMDA-enhancing agent in patients receiving atypical antipsychotics, not typical antipsychotics, should be considered preliminary.

Tolerability, Side-Effects and Safety

NMDA-enhancing agents were well tolerated and have been found to significantly improve extrapyramidal symptoms, in both Simpson Angus Scale (ES = 0.11) and Abnormal Involuntary Movement Scale measurements (0.20). These effects are largely driven by a D-serine study (Heresco-Levy et al., 2005) and the observation require confirmation. NMDA-enhancing agents may reduce the dosage of antipsychotic required to improve schizophrenic symptoms and the add-on strategies may lead to reduction of dose-related side-effects from the conventional and atypical antipsychotics.

No systemic side-effects were attributed to the NMDA-enhancing agents except for gastro-intestinal upset and nausea in some glycine trials (Heresco-Levy et al., 2004; 1999). Other side-effects were not different between those receiving treatment with placebo and those on NMDA-enhancing agents. Adding NMDA-enhancing agents to other antipsychotics also produced few side-effects; they did not worsen the side-effects of concomitant antipsychotics, which are mediated by D2, 5-HT2, histamine, muscarinic or other receptors (Lane et al., 2006a; 2005; Tsai et al., 2006; 2004a; 1999; 1998; Diaz et al., 2005;

Goff *et al.*, 2005; 1999a, b; 1996; 1995; Heresco-Levy *et al.*, 2005; 2004; 2002; 1999; 1998; 1996; Duncan *et al.*, 2004; Evins *et al.*, 2002; 2000; Javitt *et al.*, 2001; 1994; Potkin *et al.*, 1999; 1992; van Berckel *et al.*, 1999; 1996; Leiderman *et al.*, 1996; Rosse *et al.*, 1996; 1989; Cascella *et al.*, 1994; Costa *et al.*, 1990; Waziri, 1988). Nevertheless, long-term study is required to thoroughly evaluate their safety. If confirmed by more studies, NMDA-enhancing agents would be safe antipsychotic agents devoid of the side-effects of extrapyramidal symptoms, tardive dyskinesia and metabolic syndrome. These advantages will help a substantial portion of patients who develop serious side-effect while taking conventional or atypical antipsychotics.

Perspective

NMDA-enhancing agents have been tested as add-on treatments for patients who are on stable antipsychotic regimens. The only exception was a study using D-cycloserine as the sole agent and it failed to improve positive symptoms (van Berckel *et al.*, 1996). This may be due to the limited efficacy of D-cycloserine on positive symptoms or to issues of study design. NMDA-enhancing agents should be tested as monotherapy for psychosis.

The application of NMDA-enhancing agents is not limited to schizophrenia. These agents have been shown to be beneficial in Alzheimer's disease (Tsai *et al.*, 1999), post-traumatic stress disorder (Heresco-Levy *et al.*, 2002b), autism (Posey *et al.*, 2004) and phobias (Ressler *et al.*, 2004). In theory, any neuropsychiatric disorder which has a component of attenuated NMDA function can benefit from the strategy of enhancing NMDA activity. The potential conditions range from learning disorders in childhood to dementia in the elderly.

Early in the disease process of schizophrenia, NMDA hypofunction may be more prominent and consequently, the disease may be more amendable to NMDA-enhancing agents (Olney *et al.*, 1999). Correction of NMDA hypofunction early on may not only benefit the symptoms but also may improve the disease course given that hypo-NMDA neurotransmission plays a role in neurotoxicity and the developmental risks of schizophrenia (Tsai & Coyle, 2001; Olney *et al.*, 1999). This concept is supported by our recent pilot finding that antipsychotic-naïve patients benefit more from sarcosine therapy than patients who had been previously treated with antipsychotics (Lane *et al.*, 2007). It will be important to explore the role of NMDA enhancement treatment not only in symptom treatment but also in illness prevention and long-term functional outcome. Further larger placebo-controlled studies are warranted to compare NMDA-enhancing agents versus antipsychotics to determine their respective strengths and weaknesses. Treatment may be individually tailored in the future when adding NMDA-enhancing agents is an option.

Conclusion

In summary, although the results of the studies of NMDA-enhancing agents are encouraging, there are some negative or equivocal findings (Goff *et al.*, 2005; 1999; Evins *et al.*, 2000; Tsai *et al.*, 1999; van Berckel *et al.*, 1999; Potkin *et al.*, 1992). Add-on treatments with NMDA-enhancing agents usually improve symptoms of chronically stable schizophrenia. However, most studies are small series and the optimal dose for each individual agent is unknown, except possibly for D-cycloserine. Not all studies are positive; several recent reports did not demonstrate clinical efficacy including those by Carpenter *et al.* (2004), Duncan *et al.* (2004) and Goff *et al.* (2005). This suggests that the approach of enhancing NMDA neurotransmission is still developing. However, NMDA-enhancing agents as a group, when added to stable antipsychotic treatment, improve a wide spectrum of the symptoms of schizophrenia. The side-effects and safety profile are satisfactory. Among the three agents analyzed, the full agonists, D-serine and glycine, and the GlyT-1 inhibitor, sarcosine, are associated with better outcomes than the partial agonist, D-cycloserine, with their efficacy extending to the positive symptom domain. Large trials exploring the optimal doses are required to determine efficacy and limitations for the treatment of schizophrenia. Enhance NMDA neurotransmission may bring benefits not only to schizophrenia but also to other neuropsychiatric conditions as well.

Acknowledgement

D-cycloserine, D-serine, D-alanine and sarcosine are protected by US patents 6228875, 6667297, 6420351, for which Dr. Tsai is an inventor. Dr. Tsai is supported in part by Los Angeles Biomedical Institute and a NARSAD Independent Research Award.

References

Addington, A.M., Gornick, M., Sporn, A.L., Gogtay, N., Greenstein, D., Lenane, M., Gochman, P., Baker, N., Balkissoon, R., Vakkalanka, R.K., Weinberger, D.R., Straub, R.E., & Rapoport, J.L. (2004). Polymorphisms in the 13q33.2 gene G72/G30 are associated with childhood-onset schizophrenia and psychosis not otherwise specified. *Biological Psychiatry*, 55, 976–980.

Bergeron, R., Meyer, T., Coyle, J., & Greene, R. (1998). Modulation of *N*-methyl-D-aspartate receptor function by glycine transport. *Proceedings of the National Academy of Sciences of the United States of America*, 95, 15730–15734.

Breier, A., Buchanan, R.W., Kirkpatrick, B., Davis, O.R., Irish, D., Summerfelt, A., & Carpenter Jr., W.T. (1994). Effects of clozapine on positive and negative symptoms in outpatients with schizophrenia. *American Journal of Psychiatry*, 151, 20–26.

Carpenter Jr., W.T., Buchanan, R.W., Javitt, D.C., Marder, S.R., Schooler, N.R., Heresco-Levy, U., & Gold, J.M. (2004). Is glutamatergic therapy efficacious in schizophrenia? *Neuropsychopharmacology*, 29, S110.

Cascella, N.G., Macciardi, F., Cavallini, C., & Smeraldi, E. (1994). D-cycloserine adjuvant therapy to conventional neuroleptic treatment in schizophrenia: an open-label study. *Journal of Neural Transmission General Section*, 95, 105–111.

Chen, L., Muhlhauser, M., & Yang, C.R. (2003). Glycine transporter-1 blockade potentiates NMDA-mediated responses in rat prefrontal cortical neurons *in vitro* and *in vivo*. *Journal of Neurophysiology*, 89, 691–703.

Chen, Y.S., Akula, N., Detera-Wadleigh, S.D., Schulze, T.G., Thomas, J., Potash, J.B., DePaulo, J.R., McInnis, M.G., Cox, N.J., & McMahon, L.F.J. (2004). Findings in an independent sample support an association between bipolar affective disorder and the G72/G30 locus on chromosome 13q33. *Molecular Psychiatry*, 9, 87–92.

Chumakov, I., Blumenfeld, M., Guerassimenko, O., Cavarec, L., Palicio, M., Abderrahim, H., Bougueleret, L., Barry, C., Tanaka, H., La Rosa, P., Puech, A.,Tahri, N., Cohen-Akenine, A., Delabrosse, S., Lissarrague, S., Picard, F.P., Maurice, K., Essioux, L., Millasseau, P., Grel, P., Debailleul, V., Simon, A.M., Caterina, D., Dufaure, I., Malekzadeh, K., Belova, M., Luan, J.J., Bouillot, M., Sambucy, J.L., Primas, G., Saumier, M., Boubkiri, N., Martin-Saumier, S., Nasroune, M., Peixoto, H., Delaye, A., Pinchot, V., Bastucci, M., Guillou, S., Chevillon, M., Sainz-Fuertes, R., Meguenni, S., Aurich-Costa, J., Cherif, D., Gimalac, A., Van Duijn, C., Gauvreau, D., Ouellette, G., Fortier, I., Raelson, J., Sherbatich, T., Riazanskaia, N., Rogaev, E., Raeymaekers, P., Aerssens, J., Konings, F., Luyten, W., Macciardi, F., Sham, P.C., Straub, R.E., Weinberger, D.R., Cohen, N., & Cohen, D. (2002). Genetic and physiological data implicating the new human gene G72 and the gene for D-amino acid oxidase in schizophrenia. *Proceedings of the National Academy of Sciences of the United States of America*, 99, 13675–13680.

Costa, J., Khaled, E., Sramek, J., Bunney Jr., W., & Potkin, S.G. (1990). An open trial of glycine as an adjunct to neuroleptics in chronic treatment-refractory schizophrenics. *Journal of Clinical Psychopharmacology*, 10, 71–72.

Davis, J.M., Chen, N., & Glick, I.D. (2003). A meta-analysis of the efficacy of second generation antipsychotics. *Archives of General Psychiatry*, 60, 553–564.

Diaz, P., Bhaskara, S., Dursun, S.M., & Deakin, B. (2005). Double-blind, placebo-controlled, crossover trial of clozapine plus glycine in refractory schizophrenia negative results. *Journal of Clinical Psychopharmacology*, 25, 277–278.

Duncan, E.J., Szilagyi, S., Schwartz, M.P., Bugarski-Kirola, D., Kunzova, A., Negi, S., Stephanides, M., Efferen, T.R., Angrist, B., Peselow, E., Corwin, J., Gonzenbach, S., & Rotrosen, J.P. (2004). Effects of D-cycloserine on negative symptoms in schizophrenia. *Schizophrenia Research*, 71, 239–248.

Evins, A.E., Fitzgerald, S.M., Wine, L., Rosselli, R., & Goff, D.C. (2000). Placebo-controlled trial of glycine added to clozapine in schizophrenia. *American Journal of Psychiatry*, 157, 826–828.

Evins, A.E., Amico, E., Posever, T.A., Toker, R., & Goff, D.C. (2002). D-cycloserine added to risperidone in patients with primary negative symptoms of schizophrenia. *Schizophrenia Research*, 56, 19–23.

Gasquet, I., Haro, J.M., Novick, D., Edgell, E.T., Kennedy, L., & Lepine, J.P. (2005). Pharmacological treatment and other predictors of treatment outcomes in previously untreated patients with schizophrenia: results from the European Schizophrenia Outpatient Health Outcomes (SOHO) study. *International Clinical Psychopharmacology*, 20, 199–205.

Goff, D.C., Tsai, G., Manoach, D.S., & Coyle, J.T. (1995). Dose-finding trial of D-cycloserine added to neuroleptics for negative symptoms in schizophrenia. *American Journal of Psychiatry*, 152, 1213–1215.

Goff, D.C., Tsai, G., Manoach, D.S., Flood, J., Darby, D.G., & Coyle, J.T. (1996). D-cycloserine added to clozapine for patients with schizophrenia. *American Journal of Psychiatry*, 153, 1628–1630.

Goff, D.C., Henderson, D.C., Evins, A.E., & Amico, E. (1999a). A placebo-controlled crossover trial of D-cycloserine added to clozapine in patients with schizophrenia. *Biological Psychiatry*, 45, 512–514.

Goff, D.C., Tsai, G., Levitt, J., Amico, E., Manoach, D., Schoenfeld, D.A., Hayden, D.L., McCarley, R., & Coyle, J.T. (1999b). A placebo-controlled trial of D-cycloserine added to conventional neuroleptics in patients with schizophrenia. *Archives of General Psychiatry*, 56, 21–27.

Goff, D.C., Herz, L., Posever, T., Shih, V., Tsai, G., Henderson, D.C., Freudenreich, O., Evins, A.E., Yovel, I., Zhang, H., & Schoenfeld, D. (2005). A six-month, placebo-controlled trial of D-cycloserine co-administered with conventional antipsychotics in schizophrenia patients. *Psychopharmacology (Berlin)*, 179, 144–150.

Good, K.P., Rabinowitz, J., Whitehorn, D., Harvey, P.D., & DeSmedt, G., & Kopala, L.C. (2004). The relationship of neuropsychological test performance with the PANSS in antipsychotic naive, first-episode psychosis patients. *Schizophrenia Research*, 68, 11–19.

Green, M.F. (1996). What are the functional consequences of neurocognitive deficits in schizophrenia? *American Journal of Psychiatry*, 153, 321–330.

Halberstadt, A.L. (1995). The phencyclidine-glutamate model of schizophrenia. *Clinical Neuropharmacology*, 18, 237–249.

Harrison, P.J., & Owen, M.J. (2003). Genes for schizophrenia? Recent findings and their pathophysiological implications. *Lancet*, 361(Suppl. 9355), 417–419.

Harrison, P.J., & Weinberger, D.R. (2005). Schizophrenia genes, gene expression, and neuropathology: on the matter of their convergence. *Molecular Psychiatry*, 10(Suppl. 1), 40–68.

Hashimoto, A. (2002). Effect of the intracerebroventricular and systemic administration of L-serine on the concentrations of D- and L-serine in several brain areas and periphery of rat. *Brain Research*, 955, 214–220.

Hashimoto, K., Fukushima, T., Shimizu, E., Komatsu, N., Watanabe, H., Shinoda, N., Nakazato, M., Kumakiri, C., Okada, S., Hasegawa, H., Imai, K., & Iyo, M. (2003). Decreased serum levels of D-serine in patients with schizophrenia: evidence in support of the *N*-methyl-D-aspartate receptor hypofunction hypothesis of schizophrenia. *Archives of General Psychiatry*, 60, 572–576.

Hashimoto, K., Engberg, G., Shimizu, E., Nordin, C., Lindstrom, L.H., & Iyo, M. (2005). Reduced D-serine to total serine ratio in the cerebrospinal fluid of drug naive schizophrenic patients. *Progress in Neuropsychopharmacol and Biological Psychiatry*, 29, 767–769.

Hattori, E., Liu, C., Badner, J.A., Bonner, T.I., Christian, S.L., & Maheshwari, M. (2003). Polymorphisms at the G72/G30 gene locus, on 13q33, are associated with bipolar disorder in two independent pedigree series. *American Journal of Human Genetics*, 72, 1131–1140.

Henderson, D.C. (2005). Schizophrenia and comorbid metabolic disorders. *Journal of Clinical Psychiatry*, 66(Suppl. 6), 11–20.

Heresco-Levy, U., Javitt, D.C., Ermilov, M., Mordel, C., Horowitz, A., & Kelly, D. (1996). Double-blind, placebo-controlled, crossover trial of glycine adjuvant therapy for treatment-resistant schizophrenia. *British Journal of Psychiatry*, 169, 610–617.

Heresco-Levy, U., Javitt, D.C., Ermilov, M., Silipo, G., & Shimoni, J. (1998). Double-blind, placebo-controlled, crossover trial of D-cycloserine adjuvant therapy for treatment-resistant schizophrenia. *International Journal of Neuropsychopharmcology*, 1, 131–135.

Heresco-Levy, U., Javitt, D.C., Ermilov, M., Mordel, C., Silipo, G., & Lichtenstein, M. (1999). Efficacy of high-dose glycine in the treatment of enduring negative symptoms of schizophrenia. *Archives of General Psychiatry*, 56, 29–36.

Heresco-Levy, U., Ermilov, M., Shimoni, J., Shapira, B., Silipo, G., & Javitt, D.C. (2002a). Placebo-controlled trial of D-cycloserine added to conventional neuroleptics, olanzapine, or risperidone in schizophrenia. *American Journal of Psychiatry*, 159, 480–482.

Heresco-Levy, U., Kremer, I., Javitt, D.C., Goichman, R., Reshef, A., Blanaru, M., & Cohen, T. (2002b). Pilot-controlled trial of D-cycloserine for the treatment of post-traumatic stress disorder. *International Journal of Neuropsychopharmacology*, 5, 301–307.

Heresco-Levy, U., Ermilov, M., Lichtenberg, P., Bar, G., & Javitt, D.C. (2004). High-dose glycine added to olanzapine and risperidone for the treatment of schizophrenia. *Biological Psychiatry*, 55, 165–171.

Heresco-Levy, U., Javitt, D.C., Ebstein, R., Vass, A., Lichtenberg, P., Bar, G., Catinari, S., & Ermilov, M. (2005). D-serine efficacy as add-on pharmacotherapy to risperidone and olanzapine for treatment-refractory schizophrenia. *Biological Psychiatry*, 57, 577–585.

Javitt, D.C., Zylberman, I., Zukin, S.R., Heresco-Levy, U., & Lindenmayer, J.P. (1994). Amelioration of negative symptoms in schizophrenia by glycine. *American Journal of Psychiatry*, 151, 1234–1236.

Javitt, D.C., Silipo, G., Cienfuegos, A., Shelley, A.M., Bark, N., Park, M., Lindenmayer, J.P., Suckow, R., & Zukin, S.R. (2001). Adjunctive high-dose glycine in the treatment of schizophrenia. *International Journal of Neuropsychopharmacology*, 4, 385–391.

Javitt, D.C., Duncan, L., Balla, A., & Sershen, H. (2005). Inhibition of system A-mediated glycine transport in cortical synaptosomes by therapeutic concentrations of clozapine: implications for mechanisms of action. *Molecular Psychiatry*, 10, 275–287.

Kinney, G.G., Sur, C., Burno, M., Mallorga, P.J., Williams, J.B., Figueroa, D.J., Wittmann, M., Lemaire, W., & Conn, P.J. (2003). The glycine transporter type 1 inhibitor N-[3-(4′-fluorophenyl)-3-(4′-phenylphenoxy)propyl]sarcosine potentiates NMDA receptor-mediated responses *in vivo* and produces an antipsychotic profile in rodent behavior. *Journal of Neuroscience*, 23, 7586–7591.

Korostishevsky, M., Kaganovich, M., Cholostoy, A., Ashkenazi, M., Ratner, Y., & Dahary, D. (2004). Is the G72/G30 locus associated with schizophrenia? Single nucleotide polymorphisms, haplotypes, and gene expression analysis. *Biological Psychiatry*, 56, 169–176.

Korostishevsky, M., Kremer, I., Kaganovich, M., Cholostoy, A., Murad, I., Muhaheed, M., Bannoura, I., Rietschel, M., Dobrusin, M., Bening-Abu-Shach, U., Belmaker, R.H., Maier, W., Ebstein, R.P., & Navon, R. (2006). Transmission disequilibrium and haplotype analyses of the G72/G30 locus: suggestive linkage to schizophrenia in Palestinian Arabs living in the North of Israel. *American Journal of Medical Genetics Part B Neuropsychiatric Genetics*, 141, 91–95.

Krystal, J.H., Karper, L.P., Seibyl, J.P., Freeman, G.K., Delaney, R., Bremner, J.D., Heninger, G.R., Bowers Jr., M.B., & Charney, D.S. (1994). Subanesthetic effects of the noncompetitive NMDA antagonist, ketamine, in humans. Psychotomimetic, perceptual, cognitive, and neuroendocrine responses. *Archives of General Psychiatry*, 51, 199–214.

Lahti, A.C., Koffel, B., LaPorte, D., & Tamminga, C.A. (1995). Subanesthetic doses of ketamine stimulate psychosis in schizophrenia. *Neuropsychopharmacology*, 13, 9–19.

Lane, H.Y., Chang, Y.C., Liu, Y.C., Chiu, C.C., & Tsai, G.E. (2005). Sarcosine or D-serine add-on treatment for acute exacerbation of schizophrenia: a randomized, double-blind, placebo-controlled study. *Archives of General Psychiatry*, 62, 1196–1204.

Lane, H.Y., Huang, C.L., Wu, P.L., Liu, Y.C., Chang, Y.C., Lin, P.Y., Chen, P.W., & Tsai, G. (2006a). Glycine transporter I inhibitor, N-methylglycine (sarcosine), added to clozapine for the treatment of schizophrenia. *Biological Psychiatry*, 60, 645–649.

Lane, H.-Y., Liu, Y.C., Huang, C.-L., Chang, Y.-C., Liau, C.-H., & Tsai, G.E. (2007). Sarcosine (N-methylglycine) treatment for acute schizophrenia. *Biological Psychiatry* (In Press).

Lechner, S.M. (2006). Glutamate-based therapeutic approaches: inhibitors of glycine transport. *Current Opinion in Pharmacology*, 6, 75–81.

Leiderman, E., Zylberman, I., Zukin, S.R., Cooper, T.B., & Javitt, D.C. (1996). Preliminary investigation of high-dose oral glycine on serum levels and negative symptoms in schizophrenia: an open-label trial. *Biological Psychiatry*, 39, 213–215.

Malhotra, A.K., Pinals, D.A., Adler, C.M., Elman, I., Clifton, A., Pickar, D., & Breier, A. (1997). Ketamine-induced exacerbation of psychotic symptoms and cognitive impairment in neuroleptic-free schizophrenics. *Neuropsychopharmacology*, 17, 141–150.

Milev, P., Ho, B.C., Arndt, S., & Andreasen, N.C. (2005). Predictive values of neurocognition and negative symptoms on functional outcome in schizophrenia: a longitudinal first-episode study with 7-year follow-up. *American Journal of Psychiatry*, 162, 495–506.

Oldendorf, W.H. (1971). Brain uptake of radiolabeled amino acids, amines, and hexoses after arterial injection. *American Journal of Physiology*, 221, 1629–1639.

Olney, J.W., & Farber, N.B. (1995). Glutamate receptor dysfunction and schizophrenia. *Archives of General Psychiatry*, 52, 998–1007.

Olney, J.W., Newcomer, J.W., & Farber, N.B. (1999). NMDA receptor hypofunction model of schizophrenia. *Journal of Psychiatric Research*, 33, 523–533.

Posey, D.J., Kem, D.L., Swiezy, N.B., Sweeten, T.L., Wiegand, R.E., & McDougle, C.J. (2004). A pilot study of D-cycloserine in subjects with autistic disorder. *American Journal of Psychiatry*, 161, 2115–2117.

Potkin, S.G., Costa, J., Roy, S., Sramek, J., Jin, Y., & Gulasekaram, B. (1992). Glycine in the treatment of schizophrenia: theory and preliminary results. In: Meltzer, H.Y. (ed.), *Novel Antipsychotic Drugs*. New York: Raven Press, pp. 179–188.

Potkin, S.G., Jin, Y., Bunney, B.G., Costa, J., & Gulasekaram, B. (1999). Effect of clozapine and adjunctive high-dose glycine in treatment-resistant schizophrenia. *American Journal of Psychiatry*, 156, 145–147.

Ressler, K.J., Rothbaum, B.O., Tannenbaum, L., Anderson, P., Graap, K., Zimand, E., Hodges, L., & Davis, M. (2004). Cognitive enhancers as adjuncts to psychotherapy: use of D-cycloserine in phobic individuals to facilitate extinction of fear. *Archives of General Psychiatry*, 61, 1136–1144.

Robbins, T.W., & Murphy, E.R. (2006). Behavioural pharmacology: 40+ years of progress, with a focus on glutamate receptors and cognition. *Trends in Pharmacological Science*, 27, 141–148.

Rosse, R.B., Theut, S.K., Banay-Schwartz, M., Leighton, M., Scarcella, E., Cohen, C.G., & Deutsch, S.I. (1989). Glycine adjuvant therapy to conventional neuroleptic treatment in schizophrenia: an open-label, pilot study. *Clinical Neuropharmacology*, 12, 416–424.

Rosse, R.B., Fay-McCarthy, M., Kendrick, K., Davis, R.E., & Deutsch, S.I. (1996). D-cycloserine adjuvant therapy to molindone in the treatment of schizophrenia. *Clinical Neuropharmacology* 19, 444–450.

Schumacher, J., Jamra, R.A., Freudenberg, J., Becker, T., Ohlraun, S., & Otte, A.C. (2004a). Examination of G72 and D-amino-acid oxidase as genetic risk factors for schizophrenia and bipolar affective disorder. *Molecular Psychiatry*, 9, 203–207.

Schumacher, J., Jamra, R.A., Freudenberg, J., Becker, T., Ohlraun, S., Otte, A.C., Wang, X., He, G., Gu, N., Yang, J., Tang, J., & Chen, Q. (2004b). Association of G72/G30 with schizophrenia in the Chinese population. *Biochemical and Biophysical Research Communication*, 319, 1281–1286.

Simeon, J., Fink, M., Itil, T.M., & Ponce, D. (1970). D-cycloserine therapy of psychosis by symptom provocation. *Comprehensive Psychiatry*, 11, 80–88.

Smith, K.E., Borden, L.A., Hartig, P.R., Branchek, T., & Weinshank, R.L. (1992). Cloning and expression of a glycine transporter reveal colocalization with NMDA receptors. *Neuron*, 8, 927–935.

Thomson, A.M., Walker, V.E., & Flynn, D.M. (1989). Glycine enhances NMDA-receptor mediated synaptic potentials in neocortical slices. *Nature*, 338, 422–424.

Tsai, G., & Coyle, J.T. (2001). Glutamatergic mechanisms in schizophrenia. *Annual Review of Pharmacology and Toxicology*, 42, 165–179.

Tsai, G., Yang, P., Chung, L.C., Lange, N., & Coyle, J.T. (1998). D-serine added to antipsychotics for the treatment of schizophrenia. *Biological Psychiatry*, 44, 1081–1089.

Tsai, G., Falk, W., Gunther, G., & Coyle, J.T. (1999). D-cycloserine improves cognition of Alzheimer's disease. *American Journal of Psychiatry*, 156, 467–469.

Tsai, G.E., Yang, P., Chung, L.C., Tsai, I.C., Tsai, C.W., & Coyle, J.T. (1999). D-serine added to clozapine for the treatment of schizophrenia. *American Journal of Psychiatry*, 156, 1822–1825.

Tsai, G., Lane, H.Y., Yang, P., Chong, M.Y., & Lange, N. (2004a). Glycine transporter I inhibitor, N-methylglycine (sarcosine) added to antipsychotics for the treatment of schizophrenia. *Biological Psychiatry*, 55, 452–456.

Tsai, G., Ralph-Williams, R.J., Martina, M., Bergeron, R., Berger-Sweeney, J., Dunham, K.S., Jiang, Z., Caine, S.B., & Coyle, J.T. (2004b). Gene knockout of glycine transporter 1: characterization of the behavioral phenotype. *Proceedings of the National Academy of Sciences of the United States of America*, 101, 8485–8490.

Tsai, G.E., Yang, P., Chang, Y.C., & Chong, M.Y. (2006). D-alanine added to antipsychotics for the treatment of schizophrenia. *Biological Psychiatry*, 59, 230–234.

van Berckel, B.N., Hijman, R., van der Linden, J.A., Westenberg, H.G., van Ree, J.M., & Kahn, R.S. (1996). Efficacy and tolerance of D-cycloserine in drug-free schizophrenic patients. *Biological Psychiatry*, 40, 1298–1300.

van Berckel, B.N., Evenblij, C.N., van Loon, B.J., Maas, M.F., van der Geld, M.A., Wynne, H.J., van Ree, J.M., & Kahn, R.S. (1999). D-cycloserine increases positive symptoms in chronic schizophrenic patients when administered in addition to antipsychotics: a double-blind, parallel, placebo-controlled study. *Neuropsychopharmacology*, 21, 203–210.

Wang, X., He, G., Gu, N., Yang, J., Tang, J., & Chen, Q. (2004). Association of G72/G30 with schizophrenia in the Chinese population. *Biochemical and Biophysical Research Communication*, 319, 1281–1286.

Watson, G.B., Bolanowski, M.A., Baganoff, M.P., Deppeler, C.L., & Lanthorn, T.H. (1990). D-cycloserine acts as a partial agonist at the glycine modulatory site of the NMDA receptor expressed in Xenopus oocytes. *Brain Research*, 510, 158–160.

Waziri, R. (1988). Glycine therapy of schizophrenia. *Biological Psychiatry*, 23, 210–211.

Yurgelun-Todd, D.A., Coyle, J.T., Gruber, S.A., Renshaw, P.F., Silveri, M.M., Amico, E., Cohen, B., & Goff, D.C. (2005). Functional magnetic resonance imaging studies of schizophrenic patients during word production: effects of D-cycloserine. *Psychiatry Research*, 138, 23–31.

Zafra, F., Aragon, C., Olivares, L., Danbolt, N.C., Gimenez, C., & Storm-Mathisen, J. (1995). Glycine transporters are differentially expressed among CNS cells. *Journal of Neuroscience*, 15, 3952–3969.

Progress in Neurotherapeutics and Neuropsychopharmacology, 3:1, 291–297 © 2008 Cambridge University Press
Printed in the United Kingdom

Subject Index

Progress in Neurotherapeutics and Neuropsychopharmacology, 3:1, 299 © 2008 Cambridge University Press
Printed in the United Kingdom

Author Index